Getting Acquainted With
Wide Complex
Tachycardias

A Workbook for the Electrocardiographically Confused!

Jerry W. Jones, MD FACEP FAAEM

Contents

Foreword

Do you remember your very first ECG class? You were probably taught "wide complex tachycardia = ventricular tachycardia." Ahh, the joy of a high confidence level. Later, you learned about aberrant conduction. "Okay, then..." Sometime later, you probably learned that there is more than one type of ventricular tachycardia – and some forms are much more dangerous than others! "Oh, no! I feel my confidence level slipping."

I could describe myself as the perfect target reader for this workbook. I am an emergency department nurse, paramedic, clinical instructor, cardiac procedures nurse, and ECG instructor. Although I consider myself to be an "intermediate level" practitioner, I know there is so much more to learn.

It feels like Dr. Jones speaks directly to me and at my level. But what is amazing, however, is that he also engages those above and below my level of expertise as well. He takes complex topics that I know something about – but never *fully* understood – and makes them understandable. Better yet, he makes the information practical and usable in a clinical setting. Whether you know only the basics of ECG interpretation or are a practice expert, this workbook will help add to your toolbox and hone your skills. You will become more fluent in the interpretation of wide-complex rhythms. Fluency makes our jobs easier, quicker, and more fun. Dr. Jones understands that the more accurate we are, the more confident we are, and the easier our jobs become.

In this workbook format, Dr. Jones involves the reader by giving practical quizzes and questions along the way – opportunities to apply and practice what has been learned. I recommend that, no matter what your current skill level is, you start at the beginning of this book and progress through it. If you are already an expert, you will find pearls and helpful tips throughout. If you are an ECG instructor, you will find yourself including new insights learned from this book in your classes.

Jerry W. Jones, MD FACEP FAAEM is a sought-after ECG instructor. He teaches his **Masterclass in Advanced Electrocardiography** and **Masterclass in Advanced Dysrhythmias** in person all over the world. He is also very generous in sharing his knowledge on social media and other ECG instructors' websites, including my own.

Dr. Jones has a very unique skill: he can take complex topics and make them understandable without over-simplifying to the point of inaccuracy. He gives us the advantage of his more than forty years of clinical and teaching experience, allowing us to avoid pitfalls he himself experienced. I would go so far as to say he has even made it FUN!

Dawn B. Altman, RN, EMT-Paramedic
Owner, ECGGuru.com

Preface

I began my medical career knowing absolutely nothing about ECGs. No one taught me *anything*. As a first-year resident in internal medicine, I was told to buy a book and read it. The medical school bookstore had only one copy of one book, Dubin's *Rapid Interpretation of EKGs* – first edition. It was very thin back then and I read it in less than an hour.

"Wow... that was easy! Now I can read EKGs!"

The next morning I arrived on the floor and a nurse handed me a 12-lead ECG. I looked at it very carefully. And I looked at it. And then I turned it upside down and looked at it some more. I still had absolutely no idea what I was looking at!

Today there are hundreds of books, all telling you how "easy" it is to read ECGs and that you can be an ECG "expert" in just 3 days, and so on.

What I've learned is that the most *basic* tenets of electrocardiography are indeed not difficult – but neither are they particularly useful in real-life situations. It's like being very proud of yourself for the ability to spell the word C-A-T as someone is about to give you an examination regarding the literary essays and poetic symbolism of the 18th-century English poet, John Donne.

I totally agree that everyone must start as absolute beginners – I *certainly* had to. *But you should strive to move on from there!* Too many books and online courses simply keep you spinning your wheels in the same place – always feeding you the *same introductory material* at the *same introductory level!*

I didn't call this workbook *Wide Complex Tachycardias Made Easy* because there's nothing "easy" about this subject. I just hope that I have made it more understandable and accessible for you.

Do NOT attempt to cover too much at one time. Let the knowledge sink in and give those synapses time to connect. But you CAN accomplish this. As Henry Ford once said:

"Whether you think you can, or think you can't. You're right!"

Acknowledgements

There are two people I am very indebted to for making many of the ECGs and rhythm strips available to me:

Dawn Altman, RN EMT-P (ECGGuru.com)

and

Mike Cadogan, MD (LITFL.com)

Thank you both for your kindness and generosity.

There is also someone very special without whom this book would not be possible.

You know who you are.

Introduction

This is a *training manual* and *workbook*. It is not an academic reference text. Therefore, you will find a lot of repetition in this book – *it's there for a reason!*

It does not contain any original research on my part. It does not contain a thesis with footnotes justifying any new, original claims. It does contain information from academic, reputable sources – including many of the founding fathers of electrocardiography – and also some untested, unvalidated, but for me – very useful tips, tricks, and pearls – I've accumulated over almost forty years of reading and interpreting ECGs.

I present these tachydysrhythmias in the context of what you will experience *in real life*. As in both my Masterclasses, I use *real, original ECGs*. I do not use computer-generated tracings nor do I use tracings that have been "cleaned up" or altered in any way to make interpretation "easier" (other than to conceal patient identification data). You would not have the benefit of such alterations in an ER or a critical care unit at 3 a.m., so why train you on altered ECGs?

I found that in studying the algorithms and methods for distinguishing supraventricular tachycardias from ventricular tachycardias, what may seem very simple in a textbook example can often turn to frustration and increased stress when confronted with a real patient, or a real-life ECG, *and things aren't as easy as the algorithm implied they would be!*

We will not immediately jump into looking at wide complex tachycardias in this book. Had you had a *proper* introduction to the knowledge and skills needed to be an effective ECG interpreter *before* taking on wide complex tachycardias, you wouldn't be here today reading this book!

For almost forty years I stood where you stand every day and every night. I had no one to teach me and there weren't any easily accessible books on ECG interpretation – much less wide complex tachycardias. Internet? *We didn't even have computers!* I learned the hard way – by self-study and by making a lot of mistakes! But I learned and I strived for improvement and increased skill. Now, I teach classes in advanced electrocardiography and I have written this book so you can get started faster and easier – and hopefully without as many mistakes.

I have labeled all ECGs that I obtained – *with permission* – from other sources. If an ECG is not labeled, then it is from my private collection.

One of my strongest admonitions to all my students is "**NEVER DIAGNOSE A DYSRHYTHMIA – ESPECIALLY A TACHYCARDIA – FROM A RHYTHM STRIP! YOU MUST SEE A 12-LEAD ECG!**" And then what do I do? I give you a bunch of rhythm strips to look at! Let me assure you: all these rhythm strips were either taken from a 12-lead ECG or else they were from patients who had already had 12-lead ECGs recorded.

In addition to some background anatomy and physiology in Chapter 1, I am going to train you to recognize the subtlety inherent in so many tracings. DO THE EXERCISES in this workbook! You have my permission to make photocopies of the exercises for your personal use so you can review them several times without marking in the book. Your most efficient practice will consist of studying the same exercises and rhythm strips again and again until you feel very comfortable recognizing everything that I have put before you. *Then* get on the internet and start looking at different ECGs. You aren't going to learn all this in a day or a week. You have to keep at it. Just know that – aside from all the algorithms and methods – there *is* an approach to interpreting and diagnosing a wide complex tachycardia that will enable you to confidently take control of the situation.

That's what you should learn from this workbook.

Chapter 1

Things You MUST Know Before We Begin...

I know you want to jump right in and start looking at wide complex tachycardias and ventricular tachycardias. But following that path is exactly what brought you HERE! You tried analyzing WCTs by approaching them directly before acquiring the tools you needed to be successful! Complete or perform the exercises as I have suggested. I have been teaching this subject for almost forty years, and before that, *I had to learn all this myself*. I *know* which skills I had to develop, and I am going to pass on those skills to you. If you wish to become proficient in the diagnosis and management of wide complex tachycardias, *you are going to need these skills!* This isn't "Wide Complex Tachycardias Made Easy!" *This isn't easy!*

OK... let's get started!

Aberrancy

Aberrancy – as a *medical* term **– is a bundle branch block due to the arrival of a supraventricular impulse at a bundle branch during its relative or absolute refractory period**. That's all! It does NOT refer to an *abnormal-appearing* QRS complex due to just *any* reason! (It's a **term of art** – its meaning in electrocardiography is very *specific* and *different* from its use in general conversation.) Aberrancy presents usually as a RIGHT bundle branch block. Right bundle branch block aberrancy can occur in a *normal* ventricle or a *diseased* ventricle. Left bundle branch block aberrancy occurs far less frequently and is typically associated with a *diseased* left ventricle. Why is this?

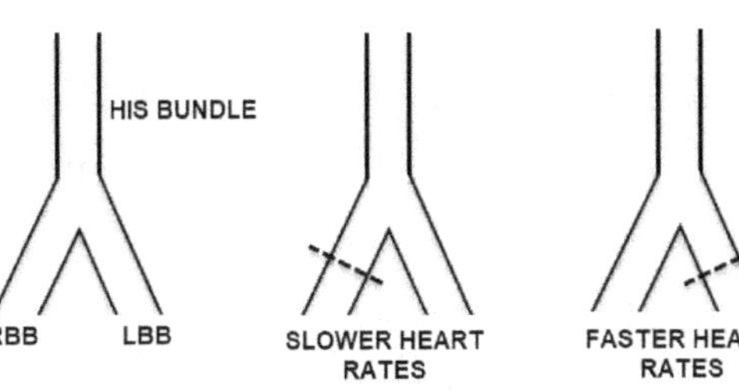

Figure 1-1

With slower tachycardias (up to around 120 – 130/minute), even under *normal circumstances*, the right bundle branch has a longer refractory period than the left bundle branch. At faster rates, the left bundle branch develops a longer refractory period. *This is seen very infrequently.* If an impulse arrives at the right bundle branch a little too early under most normal circumstances, it will find it refractory. If the right bundle is in its *absolute refractory period*, there will be a complete right bundle branch block (cRBBB). This longer refractory period of the right bundle branch is *physiologic* – it does *not* imply any conduction system defect or disease.

An atrial ectopic beat (P′) occurring too soon after the QRS (short R-P′ interval) is a very common cause of right bundle branch block aberrancy. An aberrantly conducted beat can *look exactly* like a classic bundle branch block or it may simply *resemble* a bundle branch block. Here is an example of a **classic right bundle branch block** (Figure 1-2):

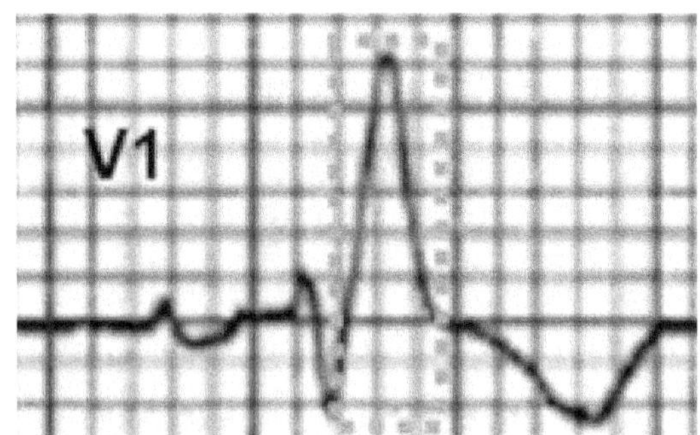

Figure 1-2

This is a sinus-conducted beat. It begins normally and then the aberrant portion appears (dotted rectangle). All bundle branch blocks fit the definition of *aberrant conduction* because *that's exactly what aberrant conduction is*: **a bundle branch block!**

Here is an example of an ectopic beat (Figure 1-3):

This (Figure 1-3) is a **premature ventricular complex** – a **PVC**. It likely arose spontaneously in the left ventricular conduction system although PVCs can originate in working myocardium under specific conditions.

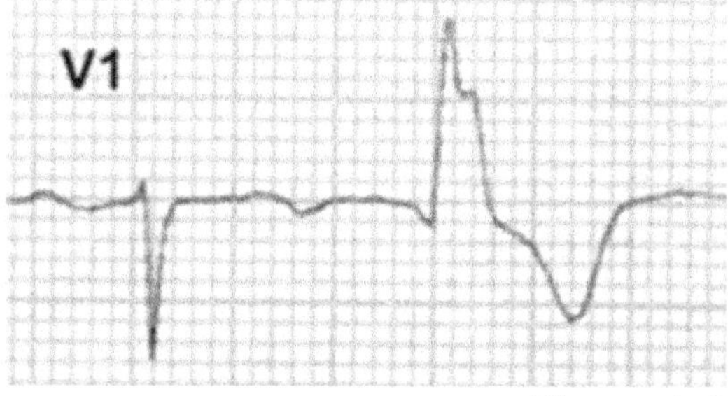

Figure 1-3

PEARL | Beats with a RIGHT bundle branch morphology in Lead V1 originate in the LEFT ventricle! Beats with a LEFT bundle branch block morphology in Lead V1 originate in the RIGHT ventricle!

Let's compare aberrancy with ectopy:

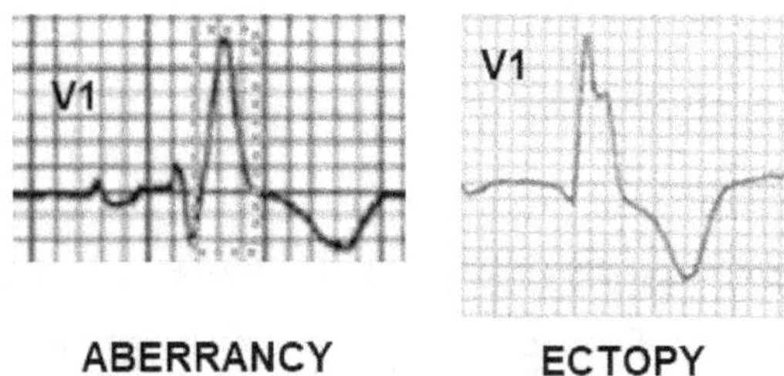

Figure 1-4

As you can see, the only thing this PVC representing **ECTOPY** has in common with the classic bundle branch block representing **ABERRANCY** is the fact that both are positive, upright complexes in Lead V1. Look at them for a moment. Both have the same type of repolarization abnormality. Why is that? It's because both **DEPOLARIZATION** (QRS complex) and **REPOLARIZATION** (ST-T) originated in the **SUBENDOCARDIUM**. As a rule, when the QRS and the T wave are on the same side of the baseline, *depolarization* began in the *endocardium* and *repolarization* began from the *epicardium*, their vectors traveling in opposite directions. That is *normal!* When they are on *opposite* sides of the baseline, depolarization and repolarization both began from the *endocardium* – and that is *abnormal!*

Now let's take a look at a snippet of an *aberrantly conducted* beat that appeared too soon after the previous beat, finding the right bundle branch still in its absolute refractory period (the arrow lengths depicting the refractory period of the right bundle branch are *estimates*):

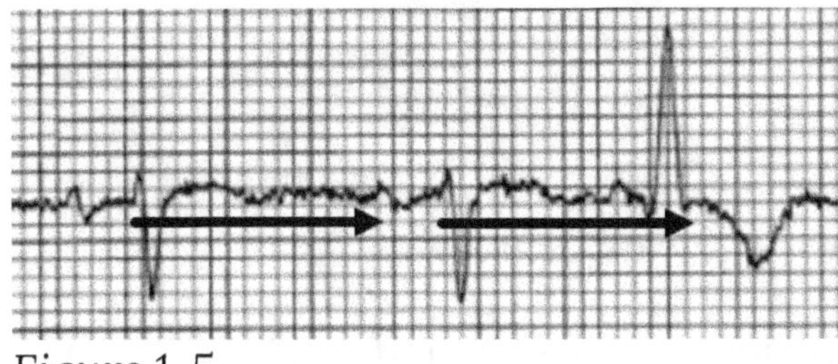

Figure 1-5

This (Figure 1-5) is an example of the **Ashman phenomenon** during sinus rhythm. A long R-R interval is followed immediately by a shorter R-R interval that is terminated by a premature atrial complex (PAC) with an aberrantly conducted QRS. Why is that?

PEARL | What is the one absolute requirement for aberrant conduction that we often forget? The aberrantly conducted impulse must originate *above the division of the His bundle* into the right and left bundle branches. And, since the division into the two bundle branches actually occurs *within* the His bundle, the impulse is more likely to be generated by an atrial ectopic focus or in the very proximal portion of the His bundle. To get the typical bundle branch block morphology, the impulse must descend through the His-Purkinje system. An ectopic impulse does not do that, so the *only thing it has in common with an aberrantly conducted beat is that it activates one ventricle before the other.* As always in medicine, there are a few, rare exceptions you will learn about later.

Each R-R interval determines the length of the refractory period for the *next* R-R interval. When an R-R interval is *long*, the refractory period of the *next* R-R interval will also be *long* (*bundle branches and Purkinje fibers only*); when the R-R interval is *short*, the refractory period of the *next* R-R interval will be *short*. The Ashman phenomenon occurs when a *premature* beat appears soon after a QRS, creating a *short* R-R interval following a *longer* R-R interval. *The premature beat falls within the lengthened refractory period caused by the previous long R-R interval and finds the right bundle branch in its refractory state; therefore, it is conducted aberrantly* (Figure 1-5). A QRS that follows the aberrantly conducted QRS would most likely be normal, but it would have benefited from a *shortened* refractory period because of the short R-R interval between the aberrantly conducted beat and the preceding sinus beat.

The aberrantly-conducted QRS in Figure 1-5 has a qR morphology with a classic repolarization abnormality. The ST segment should begin *at the baseline or no more than 1 mm (one small square) below the baseline* (in the case of RBBB morphology). If more than 1 mm below the baseline, then you should consider the presence of ischemia. The J-point of the aberrantly-conducted QRS in Figure 1-5 is no more than 1 mm below the baseline, so it's OK.

The aberrantly conducted beat will usually look like a *classic* right bundle branch block, but the morphology *can* vary a bit – depending on other factors, such as the presence of ischemia or scarring, electrolyte status, or medication effects, to name a few.

Ectopy

Ectopic impulses are impulses that develop outside the SA node and can arise in *conducting fibers* or in the *working myocardium* (in this case, *ventricular* myocardium).

Since all supraventricular impulses that enter the ventricles via the AV node will have a normal initial deflection, this is how we will base our comparison. *Ventricular ectopic impulses* that arise in the working myocardium will be *wide from the very first inscription of the QRS complex* while the first portion of *aberrantly conducted beats* will be conducted normally.

In Figure 1-6 you can see the initial wide r wave followed by a wide S wave and then a tall, upright T wave. This is typical of the ectopic beat that originates in the working myocardium. It will be **wide from the beginning**. An ectopic impulse originating in, or immediately adjacent to, conducting tissue may be narrower, however.

Figure 1-6

OK... let's practice!

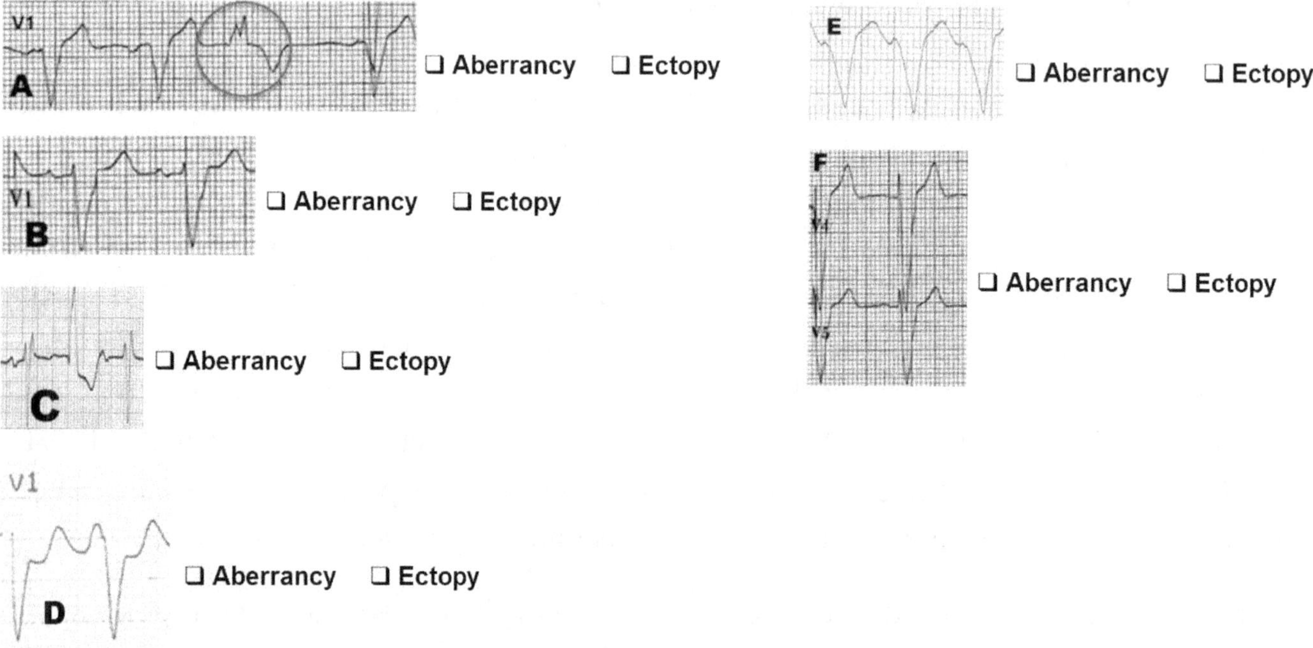

Figure 1-7

Discussion (Figure 1-7).

A – The deflection in question represents *ectopy*. It is a left-sided PVC since it is primarily positive (upright) in Lead V1. While it grossly resembles a QRS with RBBB (somewhat), it is not a classic aberrantly conducted beat. Besides, an aberrantly conducted beat would likely have a P wave in front of it (apart from a junctional ectopic beat which is relatively infrequent). All the other beats represent actual LBBB and each is preceded by a P wave. As you will notice, some real LBBBs (aberrancy) can look ectopic because the downslope of the S wave is not always as sleek, smooth, and pristine as you would expect. It's usually much easier to distinguish true RBBB (aberrancy) from left-sided PVCs (ectopy). The morphology of the aberrantly conducted LBBB beats is likely the result of disease in the right ventricle or septum (remember: the first part of an LBBB represents conduction in the RIGHT ventricle – not the LEFT!

B – This is an example of real LBBB that is (fortunately) more characteristic with a small and very narrow r wave followed by a smooth downslope of the S wave. Also, each is preceded by a P wave. Remember: except for junctional ectopic beats – which are infrequent – there should always be a P wave in front of an aberrantly conducted beat. Look for them; sometimes they are hidden in T waves!

C – This is a left-sided PVC. It is ectopic! Remember: if the PVC is upright in Lead V1, it came from the LEFT ventricle; if it is negative (inverted) in Lead V1, it originated in the RIGHT ventricle. ***But only Lead V1 can distinguish reliably between right and left.***

D – This is an *ectopic* rhythm, i.e. *ventricular tachycardia*. Notice how incredibly wide the r waves are in Lead V1. Compare them to the r waves in **B**. Whenever you start seeing "daylight" between the ascending and descending limbs of the r waves in Lead V1, you should seriously consider that you are viewing an ectopic rhythm (though *hyperkalemia* and *Class I anti-arrhythmic toxicity* are two other possibilities). Often the small r waves in V1 will have a rounded top when ectopic.

E – Look at the r waves in this snippet! They also have a lot of daylight between the ascending and descending limbs. And look at the downslope of the S wave. It has a very decreased slope which indicates slow conduction through the myocardium.

> **PEARL** | Here are two things to remember: as a slope *increases*, it becomes *more vertical*, whether the deflection is positive or negative. And as the slope *decreases*, it becomes less vertical and *more horizontal*. The ECG is just a graph of *voltage* against *time*, and time is on the *horizontal* axis. So... *the more vertical a line, the less time it takes and therefore, the faster the conduction! The more "slanted" the line (i.e., less slope), the more time it takes and the slower the conduction.*

TRICK | I used to have trouble remembering which axis was "X" and which was "Y." I knew that TIME was on the horizontal axis but I could never remember if that was the "X" or "Y" axis. One day a colleague said, "Are you familiar with TIMEX watches?" "Of course!" "Then just remember TIME-X. "TIME" is on the "X" axis!"

Don't confuse the wide r waves with P waves! Remember: if P waves are producing those wide QRS complexes, they still must cross through the AV node and the PR interval will remain relatively constant. A P wave that directly touches the onset of a QRS complex *did not produce that* QRS complex (or that *portion* of the QRS if pre-excited)! A dissociated rhythm can present with P waves encroaching on QRS complexes and will occasionally appear during slower wide complex tachycardias.

F – This is *aberrant* conduction. Look at the r waves – they are very narrow and there's no daylight between the limbs. And look at the downslope of the S waves – *smooth, sleek,* and *almost vertical.* The only thing that will conduct that fast in the heart is the His-Purkinje system.

> **PEARL |** The first half of an aberrantly conducted beat is conducted normally – *it's the second half that is aberrant!*

Look at the beginnings of the QRS complexes. Are the lines straight and nearly vertical or are they angled, irregular, or notched? Straight, nearly vertical upward or downward lines without notches or slurs indicate *rapid conduction* which is more likely to occur in the conducting Purkinje fibers. This would suggest aberrancy because initial activation during aberrant conduction always indicates ventricular entry via the AV node and His-Purkinje system. If the onset of the QRS includes lines with less slope, more slanted lines, and lines that have some curves or irregularities or even notches, then you are likely seeing depolarizations that originated in the ventricles and likely outside the conducting system.

> **TIP |** RBBB aberrancy is usually much easier to recognize because the initial part of the deflection (often referred to as the "first 0.04 seconds) follows the characteristic morphology more closely than LBBB aberrancy. LBBB aberrancy can often look like right ventricular ectopy (and vice versa), so sometimes it isn't as easy to distinguish them.

Vector Direction and the QRS Complex

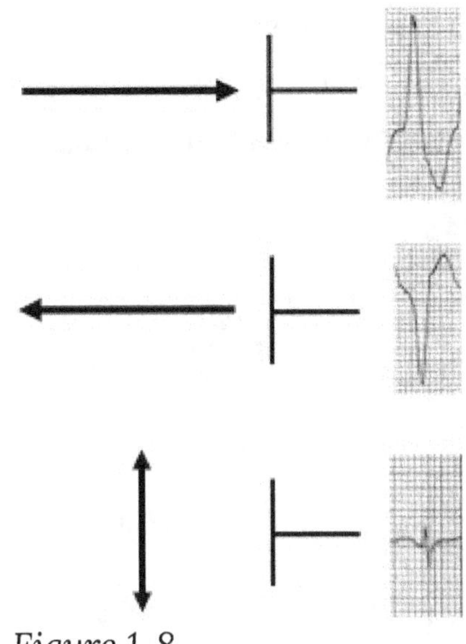

Figure 1-8

You probably know this already, but just to refresh your memory: when a vector travels TOWARD the POSITIVE pole of a lead (i.e., the recording electrode on the skin surface), that lead will inscribe a deflection. If that impulse represents *depolarization*, then the vector will have a POSITIVE HEAD and a NEGATIVE TAIL and there will be a *positive* QRS in that lead. And, since the only positive deflection in a QRS is the R wave, that lead will manifest a dominant R wave. However, on the contrary, if a depolarization impulse travels AWAY FROM the POSITIVE pole of a lead, that lead will see the NEGATIVE TAIL and will inscribe a *negative* deflection. There are two possibilities here for a negative deflection – Q wave and S wave – it will *usually* concern an S wave (or QS). A depolarization vector traveling in a path that is *perpendicular* to the recording electrode will inscribe either an *isoelectric* deflection (one that is less than 1 mm in amplitude, essentially *flat*) or a deflection that is *equiphasic* (R wave and S wave have equal magnitude).

A repolarization vector, on the other hand, has a NEGATIVE HEAD and a POSITIVE TAIL, and under normal circumstances, it travels from the epicardium to the endocardium. That means that during repolarization, the recording electrode will see the positive tail and inscribe a positive deflection – an *upright* T wave.

It is very important to remember that an ectopic impulse ("X" in Figure 1-9) doesn't travel in only *one* direction. It creates vectors in many different directions, though most of them never appear on the ECG because of *the cancellation of forces* (their opposite directions cancel each other). It has been estimated that the vast majority of electrical activity in the heart is never recorded on the ECG tracing due to the cancellation of forces! Just remember that when an ectopic pacemaker focus sends out a vector traveling to the left, there is usually a vector traveling to the right. These opposite vectors are not necessarily equal in magnitude because one may travel through a larger amount of myocardium, thus increasing its voltage, while the other may quickly extinguish due to a lack of conducting myocardium to support it. What we see on the ECG is the *mean* (average) *value* for all these vectors. **This is a very important point to remember when we get to "Precordial Transition" later.**

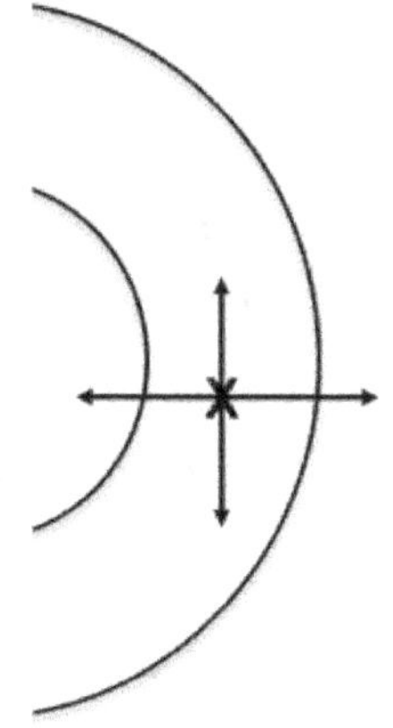

Figure 1-9

Thus, you can very easily know the direction of a depolarization impulse just by noting the net voltage of the QRS complex in a particular lead. And we are only concerned with the POSITIVE poles of a lead; don't worry about the negative poles. An R wave means the vector (impulse) is traveling TOWARD the *positive* pole of a lead and a Q or S wave (or QS wave) means the vector is traveling AWAY FROM the *positive* pole of a lead. Again, you needn't worry about negative poles.

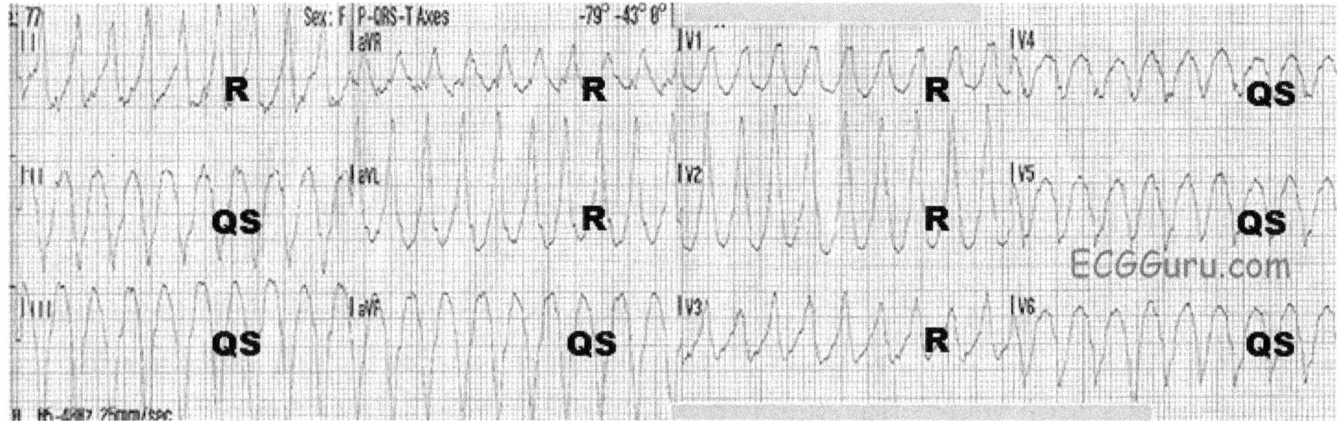

Figure 1-10

Look at each of the 12 leads on this ECG (Figure 1-10) and decide whether the depolarization impulse is traveling toward the positive pole of the lead or away from it. Since you haven't completed Chapter 4 and may have difficulty with some of the QRS morphologies, I have given you a little "hint" in each lead. But you're NOT finished yet! If you would like to enhance your skill even further, then I want you to decide where each impulse *originated*. Feel free to refer to the hexaxial reference grids in the next section. For example, there is a QS in Lead III. That indicates an impulse traveling AWAY FROM the left foot electrode; therefore, it must be originating in the *lower (apical) area* of the left ventricle.

  TIP | We are more interested in where the impulse is *coming from* (its origin) than *where it is going*. You will be reminded of this again and again in this workbook.

The ECG machine (electrocardiograph) does not detect, record, or inscribe EVERY vector created by the depolarizing and repolarizing currents traveling around the heart. It records *mean* or averaged vectors. It records the mean QRS axis (ÂQRS) in the frontal plane – not EVERY QRS axis.

As you will see in a moment, Lead I is a left-sided lead. If it has a tall R wave then you already know two very important pieces of information: the impulse is traveling TOWARD Lead I and, in that case, it must be originating further to the RIGHT of Lead I. A *depolarization impulse can't travel to the left unless it is coming (at least somewhat) from the right!*

The Hexaxial Reference Grid

This is an absolute requirement! *You cannot become proficient in the interpretation of ECGs without a thorough knowledge of the Hexaxial Reference Grid (HRG).*

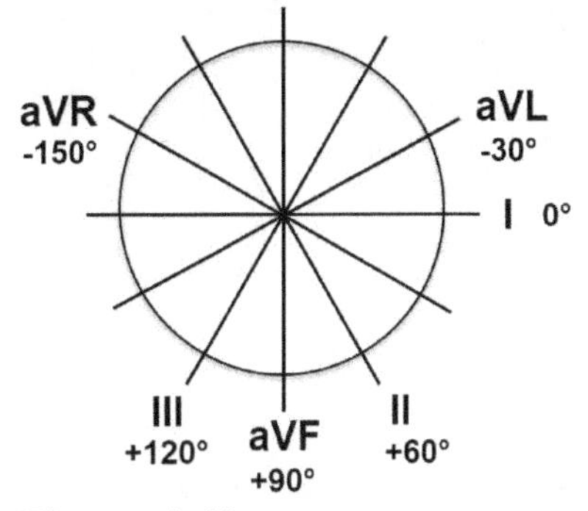

Figure 1-11

There's a lot to understand about the HRG (Figure 1-11), but for now, we only need to concentrate on the location of the frontal plane leads (NOTE: there are *only frontal plane leads* on an HRG).

There are six leads represented on the hexaxial reference grid and they are labeled at their *positive* poles. Again, you needn't concern yourself with the negative poles at this time.

The HRG is also divided into SUPERIOR and INFERIOR sections by the Lead I AXIS (*horizontal* line). Leads aVR and aVL are *superior* leads. Leads II, aVF, and III are *inferior* leads. Lead I is neither superior nor inferior. To designate that a vector is *above* the Lead I axis, we place a minus sign (–) in front of the number of degrees. That's all that it means – there is no mathematical, algebraic, or geometric significance. Likewise, for all vectors *below* the Lead I axis, we place a plus sign (+) in front of the number of degrees. Again, there is no mathematical, algebraic, or geometric significance. If we were to add +30° to –30°, the answer would be 60°, *not* 0°.

The Lead aVF axis (vertical line) divides the HRG into RIGHT and LEFT. Leads aVL, I, and II are all LEFT-SIDED leads. Leads aVR and III are RIGHT-SIDED leads. Lead aVF is neither right- nor left-sided.

Welcome back to the sixth paragraph! A lead may have two orientations: Lead aVR is not only a superior lead, but also a right-sided lead. Lead aVL is also not just a superior lead, but also a left-sided lead.

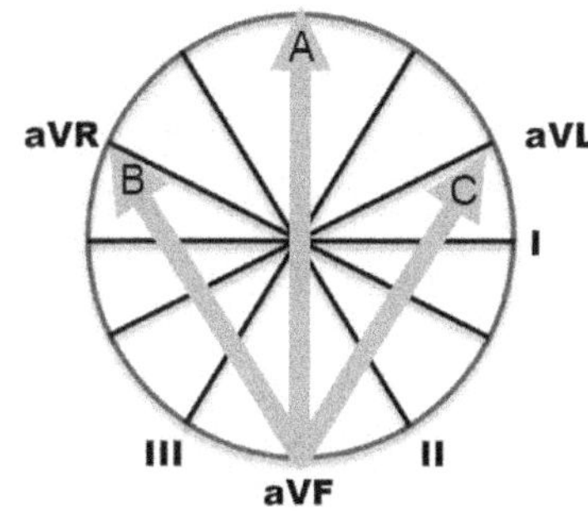

Figure 1-12

The same applies to Leads II and III.

Here's what you need to learn from the HRG...

Impulses originating in the apical region travel upward (Figure 1-12, **Vector A**). Because the positive poles of Leads aVR and aVL are located in the superior portion of the HRG, they will both record *positive* deflections (R waves) in their leads. But what if the vector – though traveling upward – is directed *more* toward Lead aVR than Lead aVL (Figure 1-12, **Vector B**)? Both Leads aVR and aVL will record R waves, but the R wave in Lead aVR will be taller – it will have a greater amplitude – than the R wave in Lead aVL. If the vector is directed more toward Lead aVL, the R wave in aVL will be greater than the R wave in Lead aVR (Figure

1-12, **Vector C**). But you aren't going to be looking at hexaxial reference grids when confronted with a patient having palpitations. You will be given a 12-lead ECG (hopefully it's *all 12-leads* and not just a rhythm strip!). What does all this look like on an ECG?

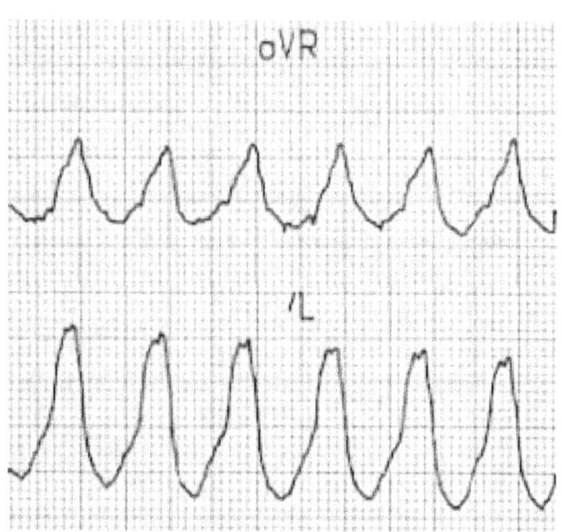

Figure 1-13 Courtesy of LITFL.com

In this snippet (Figure 1-13), in which direction is the depolarization impulse traveling? (*Depolarization impulse* means QRS complex). Here we are looking at Leads aVR and aVL. Both have positive, upright depolarizations (*QRS complexes* which manifest as *monophasic R waves*). We know, from just a few paragraphs ago, that Leads aVR and aVL are *superior* leads. Both are located 30° *above* the horizontal Lead I axis. Is the depolarization impulse traveling UP... or DOWN? *A depolarization impulse traveling in the general direction of a lead's positive pole will create a positive, upright QRS in that lead.* On the other hand, *when a depolarization impulse travels AWAY FROM the positive pole of a lead, that lead will record a negative QRS complex. The more it travels directly toward the recording electrode, the greater the amplitude of the QRS.* Since both Leads aVR and aVL are located superiorly and both have positive QRS complexes, then the impulse must be traveling UPWARDS and *generally* toward both of them. When we are thinking in terms of the HRG and also in terms of mean vectors or mean axes – we are only considering straight lines. Of course, impulses within the heart cannot travel in perfectly straight lines – they wander about, avoiding random, non-conducting obstacles and opting for the path of least resistance.

> **TIP |** Here is a very important piece of information (*one more time!*): we don't care in which direction the impulse is going – we are interested only in *where it is coming from!* The *origin* of the impulse is what matters here.

Looking at the snippet in Figure 1-13, can you add any information about the depolarization impulse other than the fact that it originated low in the ventricle – *presumably in the apical area* – and is traveling upward? Does one of the leads have an R wave that is greater in amplitude? Lead aVL has a larger R wave, so that means that, although the impulse is traveling upward, it's traveling *more in the direction of the recording electrode for Lead aVL, i.e. toward its positive pole.*

Let's consider another:

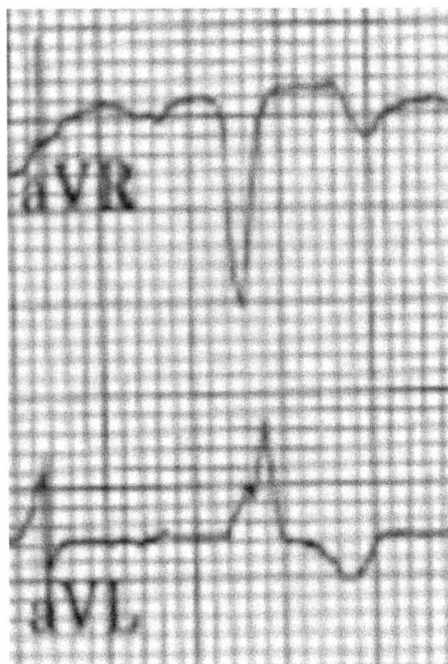

Figure 1-14

Here (Figure 1-14) we have a very different situation. Leads aVR and aVL have *opposite* polarities. How can we decide if the impulse is directed more toward one lead as opposed to the other – or is the impulse even traveling vertically UP or DOWN?

OK… we are going to have to use our knowledge of the HRG here. First, is the impulse traveling vertically at all – either UP or DOWN? The answer is "likely not," since the two leads have opposite polarities. However, the HRG can help us find the resolution to this confusing situation. The answer to this is in the *sixth paragraph* of this section. Read it again and see if *you* can resolve this issue (*now you know what that sentence meant!*).

The answer lies in the fact that both Lead aVR and Lead aVL have TWO orientations. Both are superior leads because they are located above the horizontal Lead I axis, but… Lead aVR is also a RIGHT-sided lead and Lead aVL is also a LEFT-sided lead.

TIP | When a depolarization impulse travels AWAY FROM the positive pole of a lead, that lead will record a negative QRS complex (hence the negative QRS in Lead aVR). If that same depolarization impulse is traveling TOWARD the positive pole of another lead, that lead will record an upright QRS complex (hence the positive QRS in Lead aVL). Now look at those two leads again on the HRG. This impulse is traveling from RIGHT to LEFT, from Lead aVR to Lead aVL – not bottom to top! (Having trouble? Refer back to Figure 1-8.)

What to remember of all this:

1. Know where the positive poles of the leads are located on the HRG. Their position corresponds approximately to their actual physical location with respect to the heart.

2. The positive deflections tell you where the impulse is going – it is going TOWARD those leads with positive QRS complexes and AWAY FROM those leads with negative QRS complexes. We are interested only in where it is coming FROM – its ORIGIN… its SOURCE!

PEARL | An ECG can't speak up and *tell* you where the problem is… *but it can certainly point to it!*

Inferior and Superior Axes

We frequently speak of the *mean* QRS axis in the frontal plane (ÂQRS) and it is used quite often in diagnosing wide complex tachycardias. But you will very often hear or read about a SUPERIOR axis or INFERIOR axis. We use those terms to denote the direction (up or down) an impulse is traveling.

> **PEARL |** We are usually a lot more interested in where an impulse is coming FROM – its ORIGIN – than where it is going (its destination). The important information within a wide complex tachycardia lies in the ORIGIN of the impulse – NOT its DESTINATION!

So, why are we concerned with the direction the impulse is traveling when what we really want to know is its *origin*?

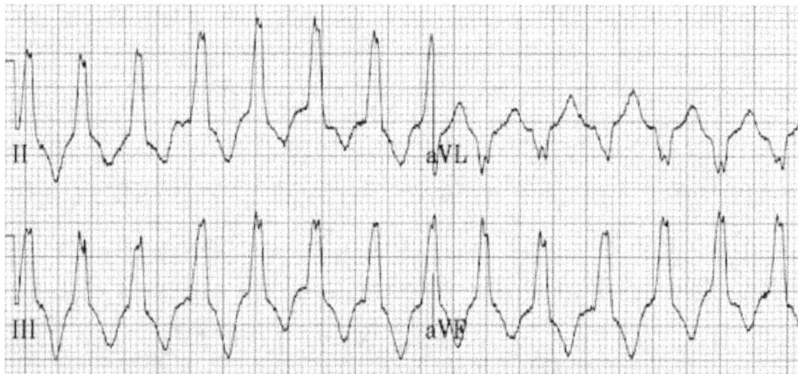

Figure 1-15 *Origin in the outflow tract*

I don't have a good answer to that question. I find it ludicrous that we are using misleading terms (i.e., an *inferior axis* for the *superior origin* of an ectopic impulse). I just look at the QRS complexes in the inferior leads and I immediately know in which part of the ventricle – upper or lower – the origin is located.

Here's an easy way to keep from getting confused:

> **TRICK |** When you are trying to decide whether a superior axis or an inferior axis is present, just think of the QRS complexes in the inferior leads as *pointing to the ORIGIN of the impulse.* Remember: the ECG can't talk but it can sure *point!*

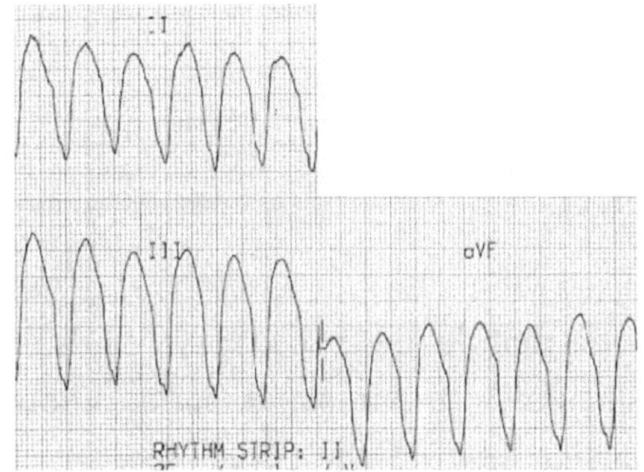

Figure 1-16 Origin in the apex

If all the inferior leads have tall R waves (Figure 1-15), they are pointing up to the ORIGIN of the impulse. An impulse that develops in the superior right ventricle can only travel downward with an inferior axis (an *axis* represents the direction of an impulse). If all the inferior leads have rS or QS complexes – *pointing downward* – then the origin of the impulse is in the lower ventricle, or apex (Figure 1-16). Since the impulse arises in the apex, it can only travel up – therefore, it represents a *superior axis*. If there is any disagreement or inconsistency among the three inferior leads, *follow the direction that Lead aVF is pointing.*

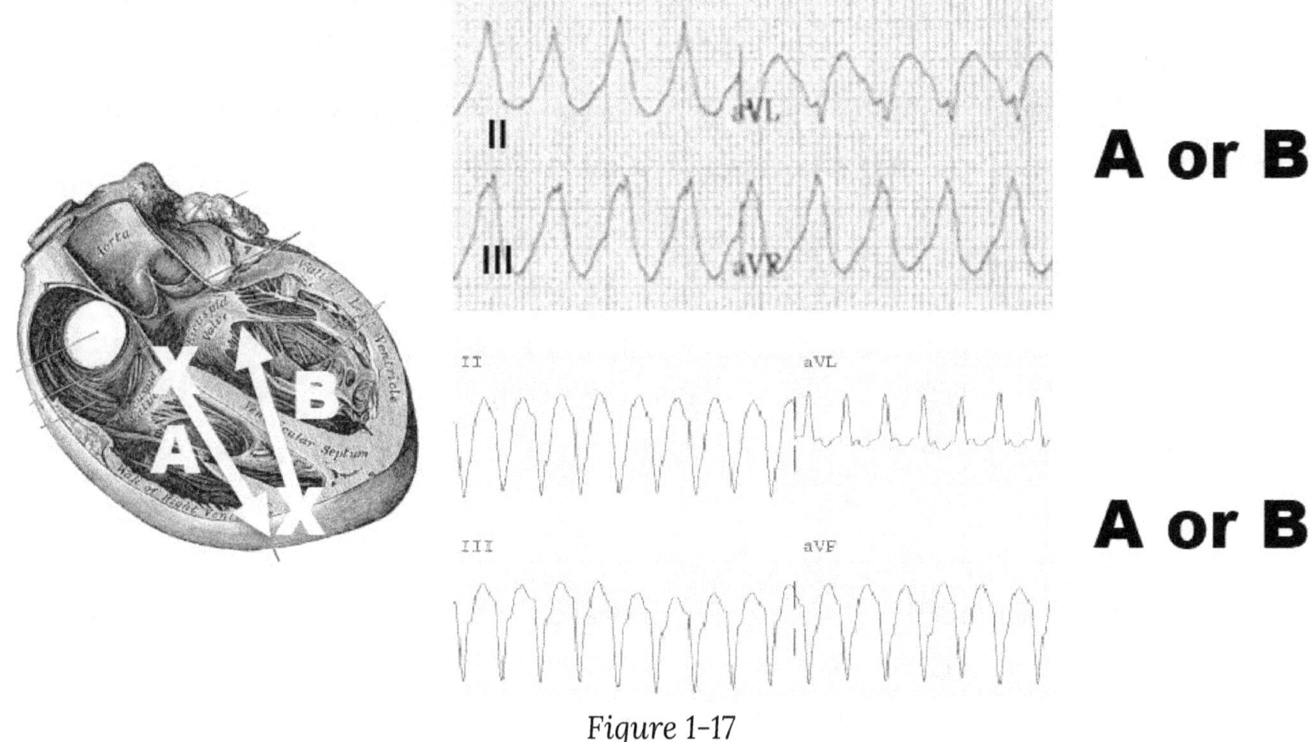

Figure 1-17

Determining whether there is a superior or inferior axis for a ventricular tachycardia originating in the right ventricle can mean the distinction between a very benign dysrhythmia (right ventricular outflow tract) or a very dangerous and lethal one (apex). It is a very important characteristic and one with which you should be very familiar. Now match the white arrows (A and B) to the correct snippet of leads II, III, and aVF (Figure 1-17). And remember: it's the *origin* of the tachycardia that tells us what we want to know.

Answer | The top snippet is (A) and the bottom snippet is (B).

Essential Coronary Anatomy

Let's begin with some terms you may have heard but were never sure exactly what they meant.

BASE and APEX

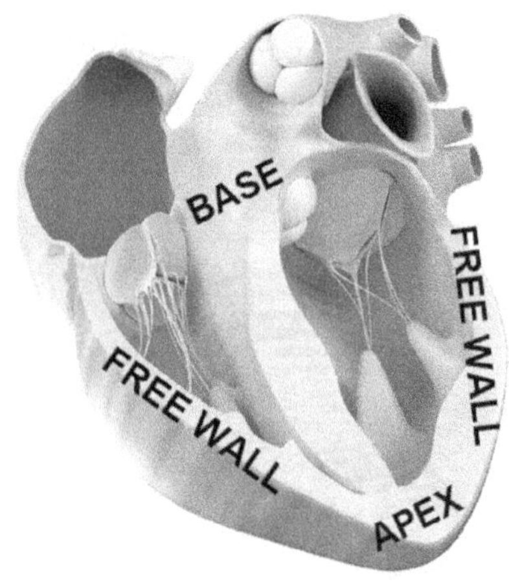

Figure 1-18

The *base* of the heart is the area that divides the atria from the ventricles. All four valves are basically in that same plane. When you hear a reference to the *basilar septum*, then you know that person is referring to the part of the septum that is located at the entrance into the ventricles near the base. How about *the basolateral wall*? That's the area of the left ventricular wall that is near the mitral valve annulus – formerly the "high lateral" wall. And you can see where the *apex* is located.

We often speak of the right free wall or the left free wall. Now you see where they are located.

The Septum and the Outflow Tracts

The *right ventricular outflow tract* is the area just below the pulmonary valve and the *left ventricular outflow tract* is the area just below the aortic valve (and even around the valve itself).

There is a quirky bit of anatomical trivia here. If you look at Figure 1-19, you will see that if we start at the apex and follow the septum upwards, it begins to become thinner as we reach the base and it also *curves around to the left*. Essentially, the right ventricular outflow tract wraps itself around the aorta and the left ventricular outflow tract. The septum changes from a thick muscular wall to a much thinner membranous structure. The interventricular septum (the "septum") is not thick for its full length.

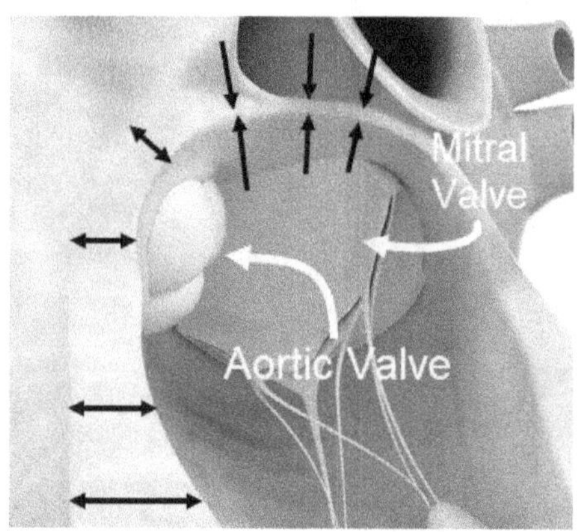

Figure 1-19

> **PEARL |** A wide complex tachycardia with an LBBB pattern in Lead V1 – but an *early* precordial transition – is likely originating in the upper part of the right ventricular outflow tract (RVOT) that is slightly to the left of the LVOT.

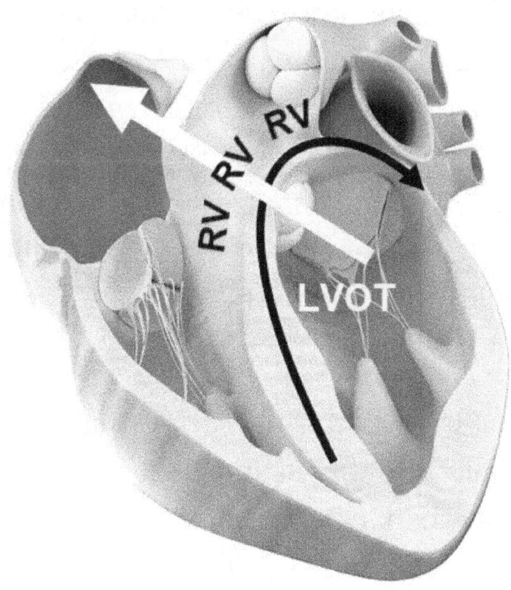

In Figure 1-20, you will also notice that the "RVs" indicating the right ventricular outflow tract curve around to the left until the *right* ventricular outflow tract is to the left of the *left* ventricular outflow tract, indicated by the white arrow. This results in some incongruities regarding precordial transition. We normally think of left-sided impulse origins as having *early* precordial transitions and right-sided impulse origins as having *late* precordial transitions. However, in that leftward portion of the *upper* right ventricular outflow tract, a right-sided PVC or rhythm could have a precordial transition very similar to a left-sided origin.

Figure 1-20

Also, an impulse originating on the left side of the septum in that area may actually discharge into the right ventricle creating an LBBB pattern *caused by a left-sided impulse!*

Let's take a look at precordial transitions. We will be using them a lot in diagnosing WCTs.

Precordial Transition

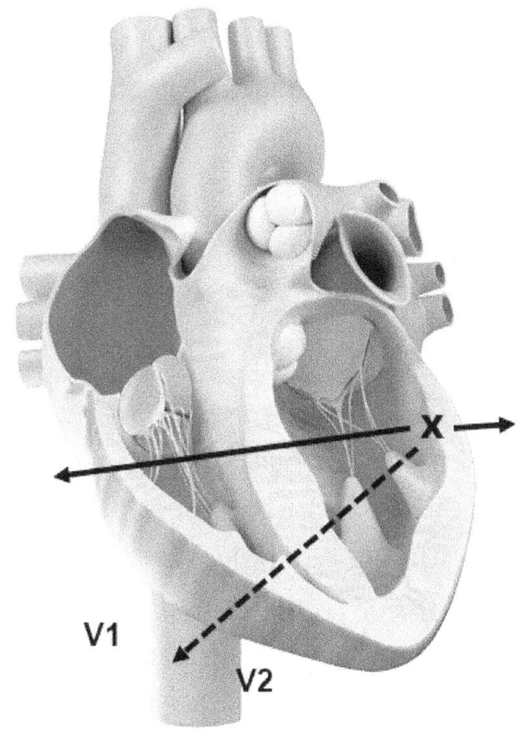

You have learned how to determine within which ventricle the ectopic impulse is originating by looking at the QRS morphology in Lead V1. You have learned to use the inferior leads in the frontal plane (II, III, aVF) to determine the vertical location of an impulse's origin within a ventricle: if the inferior leads have tall R waves *pointing up*, the origin of the impulse is in the *outflow tract* located in the upper ventricle (right or left). If the inferior leads manifest deep S waves pointing down, the impulse is originating in the apical region.

But what if we want to localize the impulse origin even more specifically along a horizontal (lateral-medial-lateral) axis that runs right-to-left and left-to-right? Then we must look at the *precordial transition*. Finally... after all these years you are just now learning how to use the precordial transition. It's been pretty useless information until now, hasn't it?

Figure 1-21

Precordial transition is a concept used very frequently in the discussion of ventricular tachy-cardias – especially the idiopathic VTs. When an impulse originates in the far-left ventricular wall (which we now know to be located posteriorly) it will have an *early precordial transition,* usually *before* Lead V3 (Figure 1-21). As you recall, an ectopic impulse sends out vectors in all directions, though most of them cancel each other. In Figure 1-21 the impulse ("X") is located on the endocardial surface of the lateral wall of the left ventricle. It sends vectors transmurally to the LEFT (toward the epicardial surface) creating a small r wave and to the RIGHT – most notably toward the right ventricle, creating a deeper S wave.

Just as the QRS axis in the frontal plane is a mean vector, *so is the vector that determines the precordial transition.* The precordial transition is equivalent to the mean QRS axis in the horizontal plane. It measures rotation a bit more specifically than "clockwise" or "counter-clockwise." A *mean vector* (Figure 1-21) is pointing between Leads V1 and V2. It is derived from the left and right vectors mentioned above. That is where the QRS will appear with an R wave equal to an S wave; in other words, where the R/S ratio = 1.0. That is the *transition point* – but there's just one problem: *the ECG didn't record it.* It only records what is beneath the individual electrodes. What you would see on the ECG would be an rS complex in Lead V1 and an Rs complex in Lead V2, indicating that the transition occurred AFTER Lead V1 but BEFORE Lead V2. You may also encounter definitions of precordial transition as the lead with *the first R/S complex in which the R > S.* Although this definition is *technically* not correct (transition occurs at the point that R = S), *it is reasonable for practical purposes* because most criteria that require use of precordial transition require the designation of a *specific lead* in which the transition takes place. Unfortunately, that is not always possible since true precordial transitions (R = S) frequently occur *between* leads.

> **TIP |** When an impulse originates in the far-left ventricular wall it will have an *early precordial transition, usually before Lead V3.*

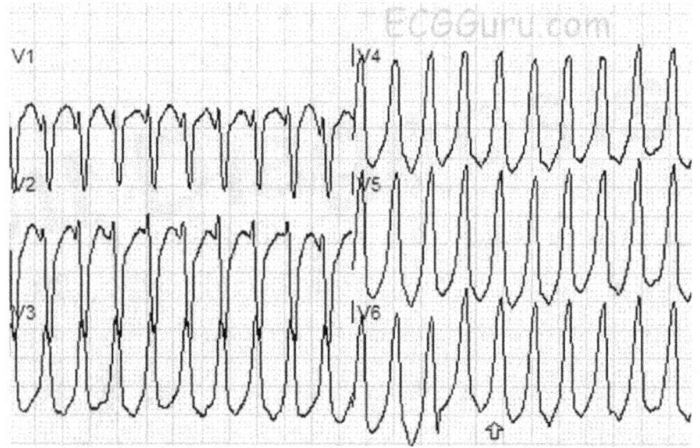

Figure 1-22

Here is an ECG with an *early precordial transition* (Figure 1-22). The transition has occurred between Leads V2 and V3. This sometimes creates confusion for some people. Where exactly is the precordial transition? How do I know that it occurred *between* those leads? I know because true precordial transition occurs when the R wave amplitude EQUALS the S wave amplitude – an R/S ratio = 1.0. Because the QRS in Lead V2 is an rS complex and the

QRS in Lead V3 is a monophasic dominant R wave, the transition could only occur *between* those two leads – which is not recordable. Therefore, for practical reasons, we usually say that the transition lead is the first lead with a dominant R wave or a QRS having an obvious R/S ratio = 1.0.

PEARL | Just remember that **the transition *lead* is not necessarily the transition *point*!**

PEARL | Precordial transition is NOT just a change in polarity of the QRS complex – it must change FROM a QRS with a dominant S wave (rS) TO a QRS with a dominant R wave (Rs). When the transition occurs at or before Lead V1, it is not unusual for the QRS complexes to revert to an rS morphology before Lead V6 – but that is not a precordial transition!

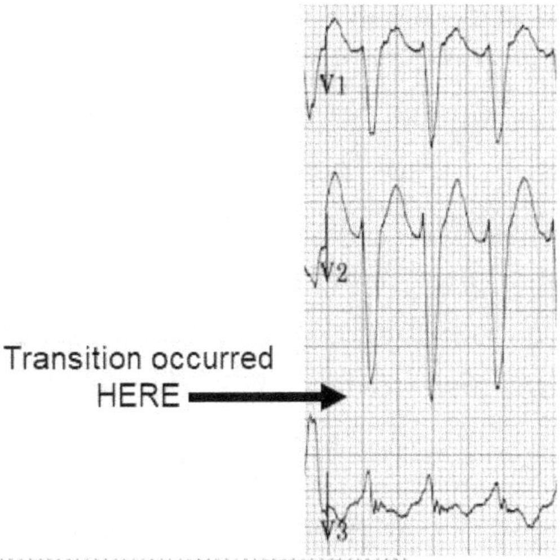

Transition occurred HERE

igure 1-23

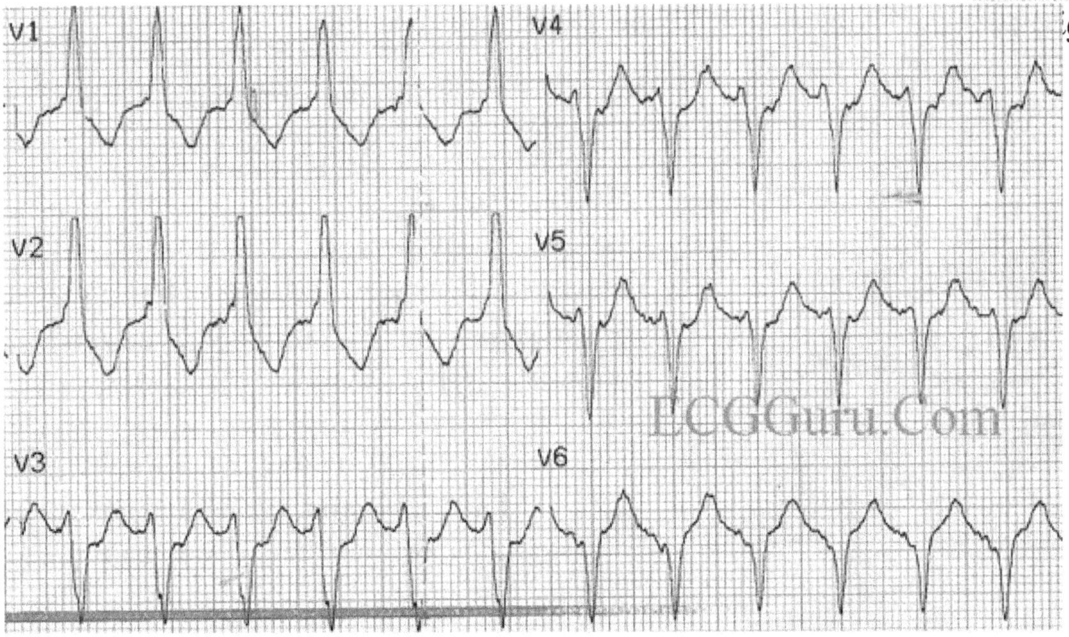

Figure 1-24

The precordial transition in *this* ECG (Figure 1-24) occurred BEFORE Lead V1. It is not unusual for the precordial leads to begin with a dominant R wave in Lead V1 and then revert to rS waves before V6. **The transition in this ECG does NOT occur at V3 with the change to an rS morphology.** The precordial transition occurs *only* when the morphology changes from an rS complex *to* a QRS complex with an R/S ratio ≥ 1.0. The leads with the dominant R waves are

NOT obligated to extend to Lead V6 and beyond. They certainly CAN – *but it is not required that they do so.*

Now let's move the ectopic pacemaker focus more to the right, but still on the *left* side of the interventricular septum (Figure 1-25). How does that affect the precordial transition? The ectopic focus is almost midway in the heart. Therefore, its mean vector is pointing toward Lead V3 *in this instance.* The greater thickness of the left ventricular walls could add some voltage and draw the mean vector more towards Lead V4 (remember: as an impulse travels through more and more myocardium, it increases in voltage). Does something look familiar to you here? *This is exactly what happens during a <u>normal</u> precordial transition!* Look again where the ectopic focus is located – **it's exactly where a normal sinus impulse initiates ventricular activation!**

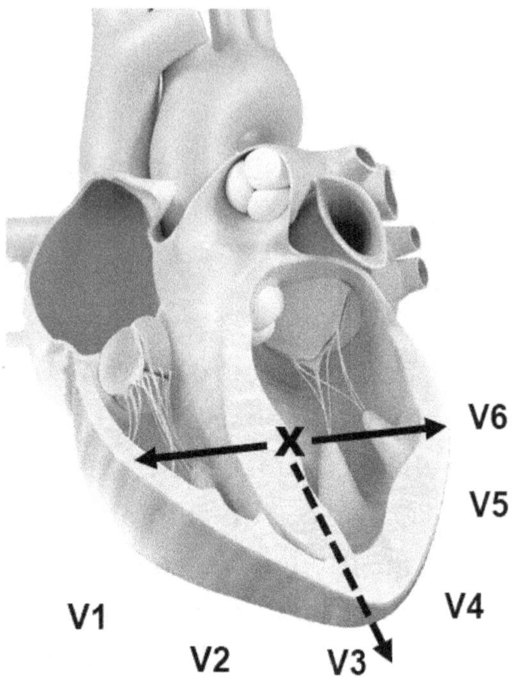

Figure 1-25

Let's continue to move further to the right – to the right side of the interventricular septum (Figure 1-26). Now observe the opposing vectors created by the ectopic focus:

There is much less myocardial mass on the right, so the mean vector is going to be more heavily skewed to the left. In this example, it is pointing slightly past Lead V4 – definitely a *late* precordial transition. If, however, there were just a bit more myocardial mass in the right ventricle, the mean vector could point more toward Lead V3.

Do you see the problem developing here? Both RIGHT ventricular *and* LEFT ventricular ectopic foci can manifest as a precordial transition in Lead V3. Just be aware of that!

In this ECG (Figure 1-27, precordial leads only), the precordial transition occurs between Leads V4 and V5. That is a LATE PRECORDIAL TRANSITION.

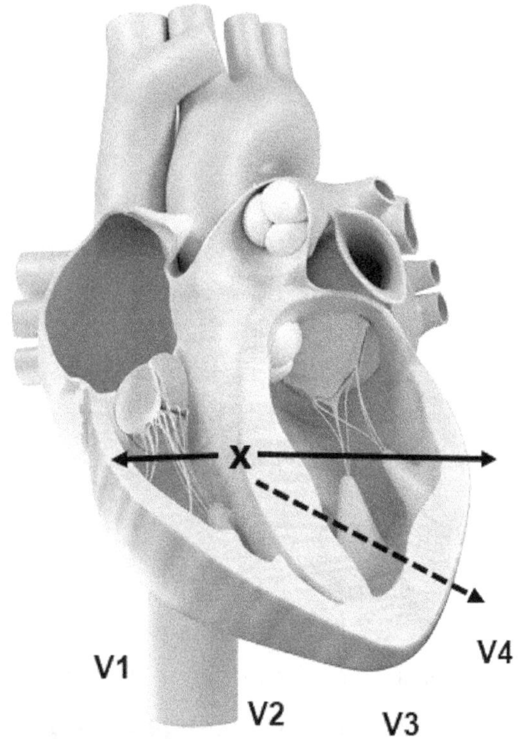

Figure 1-26

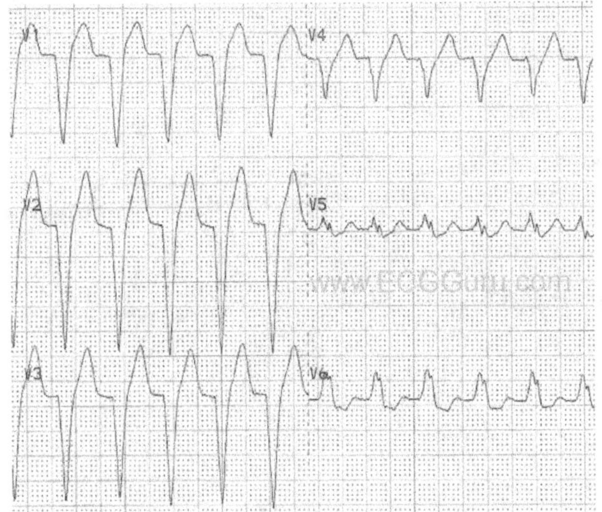

Figure 1-27

The precordial transition doesn't manifest on this ECG until Lead V5, the first lead with a dominant R wave (yes, it's small, but it's still *dominant!*). What does that suggest to you?

First, it should suggest that the origin of the tachycardia is in the RIGHT ventricle.

Second, it should suggest that the ectopic focus may be on the right side of the interventricular septum, which typically results in a precordial transition in Lead V4 or even Lead V3.

TRICK | During a ventricular tachycardia we can use the precordial transition to better localize the impulse origin along a horizontal (right-left) plane. The inferior leads give us a vertical orientation; the precordial transition can give us a more specific horizontal orientation rather than just the right ventricle or left ventricle.

An impulse originating in the free wall of the right ventricle (Figure 1-28) will have a *late precordial transition* – probably around V5 or V6. We use precordial transitions to help validate whether an impulse originated in the right ventricle or the left. "Doesn't the QRS complex in Lead V1 tell us that?" you ask. It does, but the precordial transition can sometimes add clarification and greater specificity.

It can be used to distinguish locations *within a single ventricle.* For example, an impulse arising in the *free wall of the right ventricle* may have a precordial transition at Lead V6 while an impulse arising on the *right side of the septum* may have a precordial transition at Lead V4.

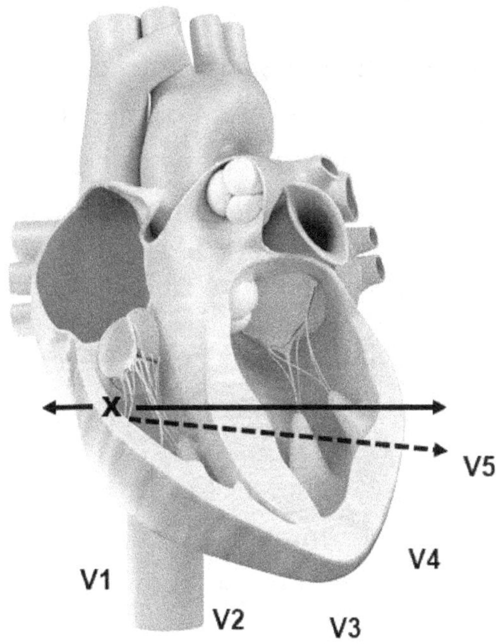

Figure 1-28

PEARL | The *precordial transition* in the transverse plane serves the same purpose as the *mean QRS axis* in the frontal plane. Just remember that the transition occurs *only* when the QRS complex changes from an **rS** to an **Rs** – *not* vice versa.

An impulse that arises in the upper part of the right ventricular outflow tract (RVOT) is physically located much further
left than the rest of the right ventricle (Figure 1-29). Thus,
an impulse originating in that area will paradoxically present
with a precordial transition that is much more leftward than
most impulses of right ventricular origin. When you see a wide
complex tachycardia with a LBBB-like morphology in Lead V1
(indicating a *right* ventricular origin) yet the precordial transition occurs before Lead V3 (as one would expect with a *left*
ventricular origin), then suspect that the impulse is arising
in the upper part of the RVOT located to the left of the left
ventricular outflow tract (LVOT)!

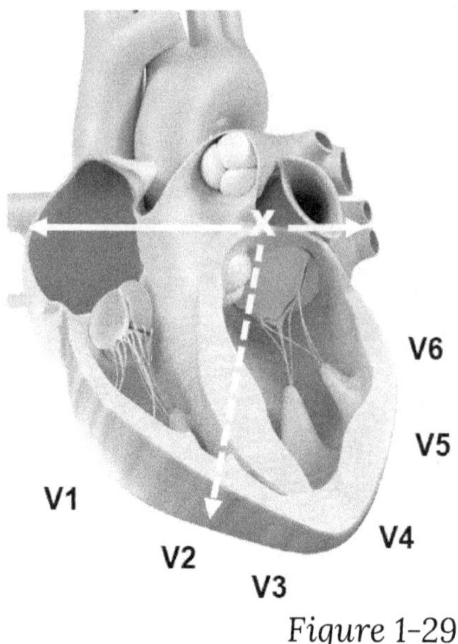

Figure 1-29

Pearl | Foci in the superior portion of the RVOT can have precordial transitions at
or even slightly before Lead V3.

Precordial Transitions and the Impulse Origins

By knowing in which ventricle the impulse origin is located (based on the QRS morphology
in Lead V1), the status of the QRS complexes in the inferior frontal plane leads (II, III, aVF)
and the precordial transition based on the 12-lead ECG... we can determine with reasonable
accuracy the location of the site of origin (SoO) of an ectopic impulse. Let's try it...

Here's the procedure to follow...

1. Look at Lead V1 and determine in *which
   ventricle* the impulse originated.

2. Next, look at Leads II, III, and aVF and
   determine if the impulse originated in
   the *outflow tract* or *apex*.

3. Finally, look at the six precordial leads
   and determine *where the precordial
   transition occurred.*

Let's see how well and quickly we can assess
this 12-lead ECG... you go first (Figure 1-31):

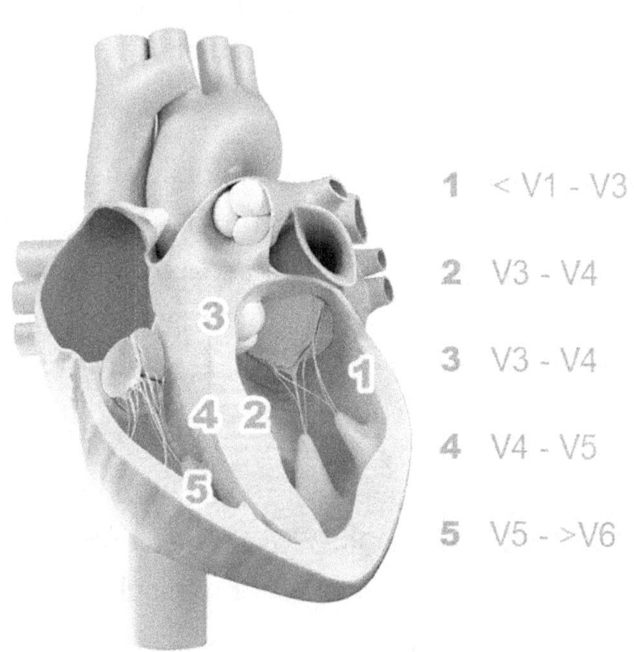

Figure 1-30

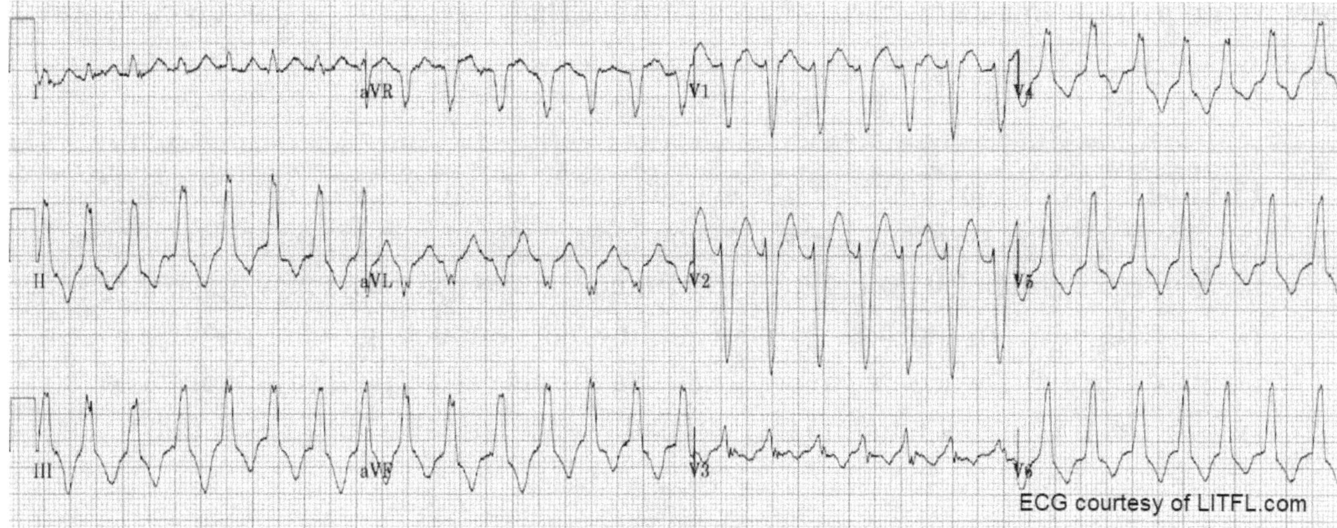

Figure 1-31

OK… it took me about 5 seconds to determine that the impulse originated in the *upper septal region of the right ventricular outflow tract* (and it took me *that* long only because I need new glasses!).

The negative QRS (LBBB-like morphology) in Lead V1 told me that the impulse was coming from the RIGHT ventricle. The QRS complexes in the inferior leads were all tall R waves pointing upward toward the origin of the impulse, so I knew it was coming from the right ventricular outflow tract. The precordial transition occurred *before* Lead V3 which is *very, very early* for an impulse originating in the right ventricle, so it *had* to be coming from the upper septal region of the outflow tract, which you will recall, is actually to the left of the left ventricular outflow tract.

PEARL | The more specifically you can localize the origin of a wide complex tachycardia or VT, the more specifically you can assess prognosis.

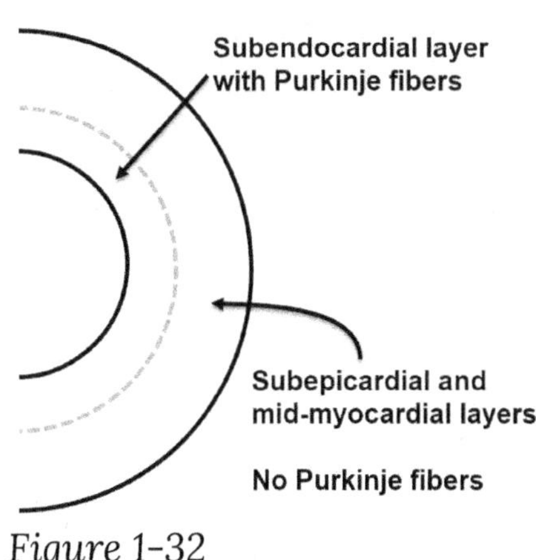

Figure 1-32

If you wish to do more reading about ventricular tachycardias, you will need to thoroughly understand precordial transition because it is mentioned *a lot!*

Epicardial to Endocardial Transmission

Most ectopic rhythms, including ventricular tachycardias, originate in the subendocardial layer. However, some can originate in the epicardium (Figure 1-32). Epicardial ectopic foci will conduct very slowly because the transmission will be cell-to-cell. Rapidly conducting Purkinje fibers generally do not extend past the inner 1/3 of the ventricular wall. That, essentially, is the subendocardial layer.

> **PEARL |** Many ectopic impulses are a combination of cell-to-cell conduction and conducting fibers. Whereas aberrantly conducted beats begin in normal conducting pathways and finish via cell-to-cell conduction, ectopic beats may begin in the working myocardium (cell-to-cell) but finish in conducting fibers. (Example: an antidromic SVT will enter the ventricle via the accessory pathway followed by cell-to-cell transmission but it must ultimately enter the His-Purkinje system to get through the AV node and into the right atrium.)

Difference Between rS and QS During an Ectopic Rhythm

During a regular sinus rhythm, rS and QS complexes have a very different meaning than when those morphologies appear during an ectopic rhythm. During sinus rhythm, an rS complex may represent a conduction delay or block and a QS complex may indicate an area of previous infarction. However, conduction during an ectopic tachycardia doesn't occur in the same way as during sinus rhythm. These morphologies represent the *origin of an ectopic focus* and not a conduction delay or diversion or necessarily an area of infarction.

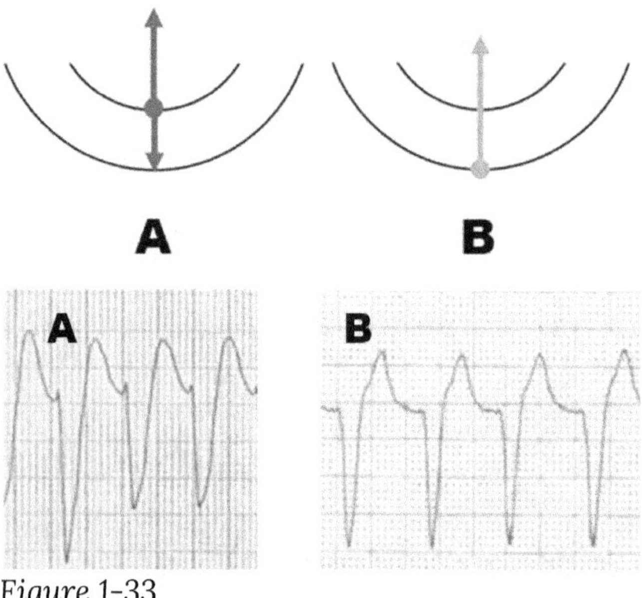

Figure 1-33

These two diagrams (Figure 1-33) represent the wall of the *left* ventricle (but the *right* ventricle acts the same way). If an ectopic focus is located on or very near the endocardial surface (A), it can transmit in two directions: toward the epicardium – a relatively short distance and toward the interior of the heart – a much longer distance. A positive electrode overlying that area will record an rS complex: small r because of the short distance the impulse traveled toward it and an upper case S because of the longer distance the impulse traveled in the opposite direction. If an ectopic focus is located on the epicardial layer (B), it can travel in only one direction – toward the interior of the heart and away from the recording electrode, resulting in a QS complex.

PEARL | As an impulse travels through more and more functional myocardium, its voltage will increase in proportion to the distance traveled and will produce a proportionally larger R wave (or S wave, depending on the recording electrode and direction of travel).

TIP | Many authors on this subject feel strongly that for a Q wave to indicate a previous myocardial infarction during an ectopic tachycardia, it must be followed by an R wave. During ventricular tachycardia, *a QS complex simply represents an impulse traveling directly away from the epicardium beneath the positive pole of a lead and not a previous infarction.*

A Few Exercises to Use What You Have Learned

For each snippet, state:

1. Whether the origin of the tachycardia is in the apex or the outflow tract (don't worry about which ventricle)

2. Whether there is an inferior axis or a superior axis

Snippet #1

___Apex

___Outflow tract

___Superior axis

___Inferior axis

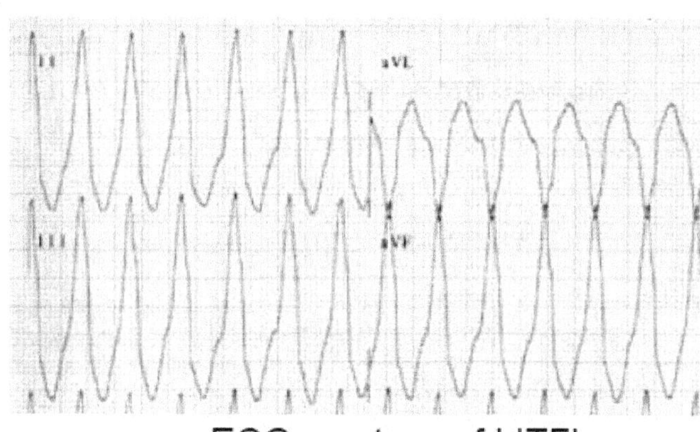

ECG courtesy of LITFL.com

Figure 1-34

Snippet #2

___Apex

___Outflow tract

___Superior axis

___Inferior axis

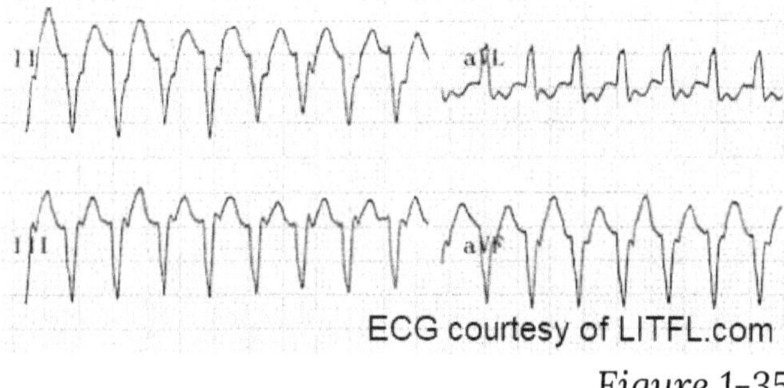

ECG courtesy of LITFL.com

Figure 1-35

Snippet #3

___Apex

___Outflow tract

___Superior axis

___Inferior axis

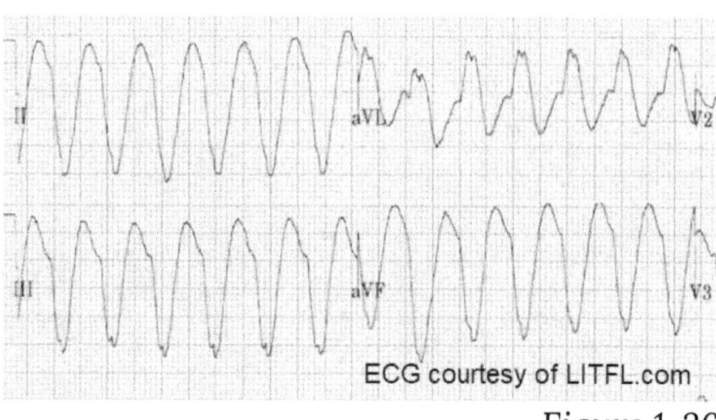

ECG courtesy of LITFL.com

Figure 1-36

Snippet #4

___Apex

___Outflow tract

___Superior axis

___Inferior axis

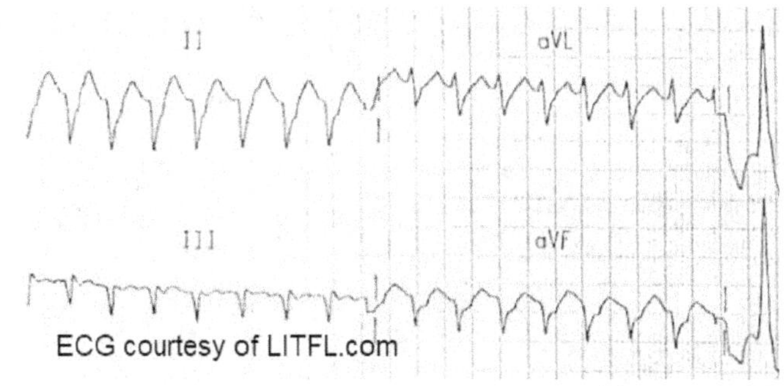

Figure 1-37

Select which location(s) in the heart could produce the precordial transition shown in each snippet.

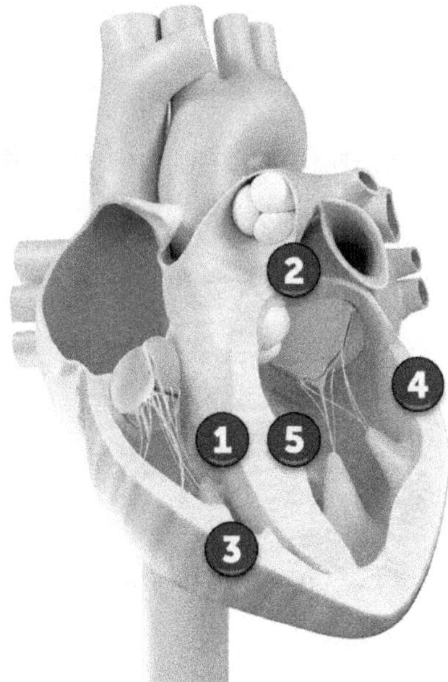

Figure 1-38

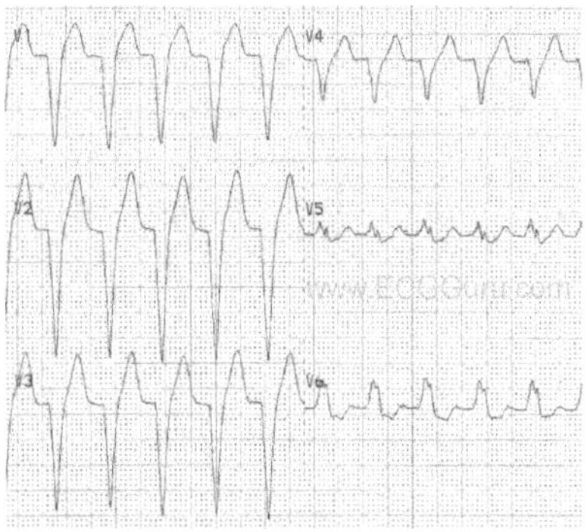

Circle the site(s) that could result in this precordial transition

1   2   3   4   5

Figure 1-39

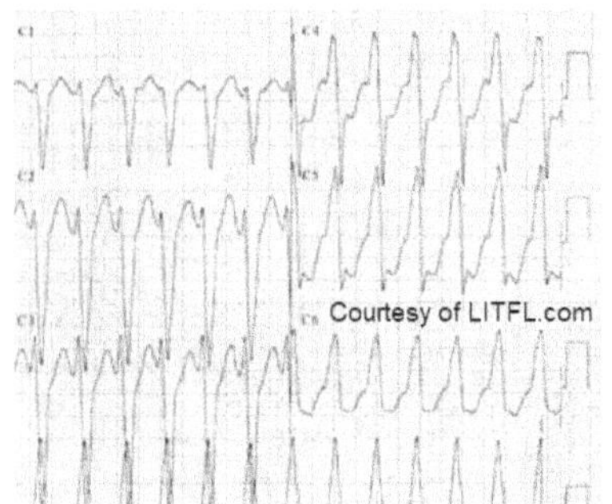

Figure 1-40

Circle the site(s) that could result in this precordial transition

1   2   3   4   5

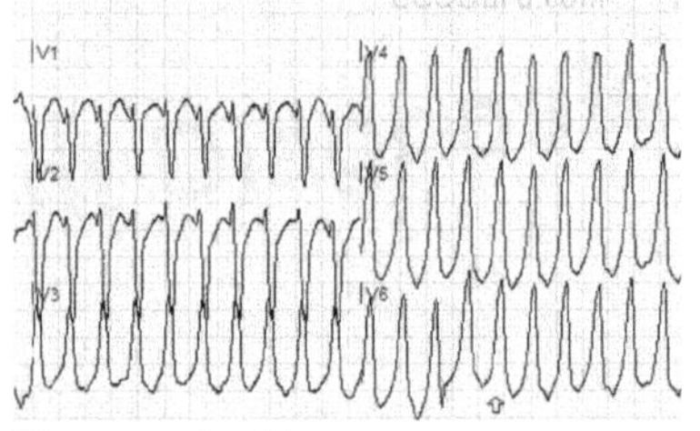

Figure 1-41

Circle the site(s) that could result in this precordial transition

1   2   3   4   5

Circle the site(s) that could result in this precordial transition

1   2   3   4   5

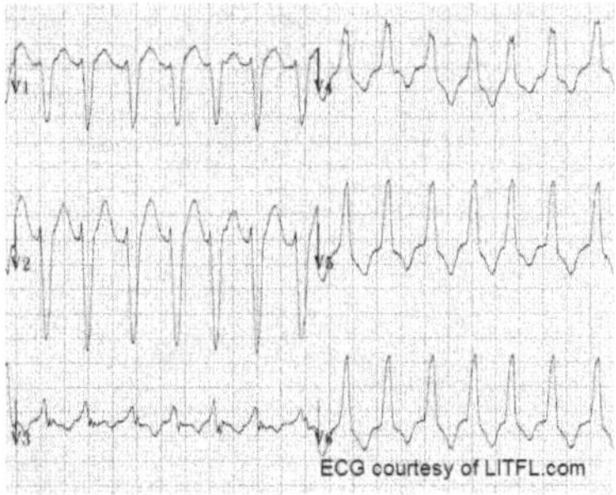

Figure 1-42

Circle the site(s) that could result in this precordial transition

1   2   3   4   5

Figure 1-43

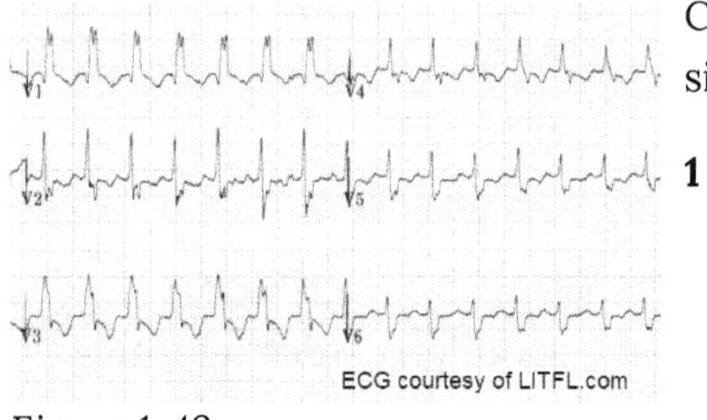

Circle the site(s) that could result in this precordial transition

1   2   3   4   5

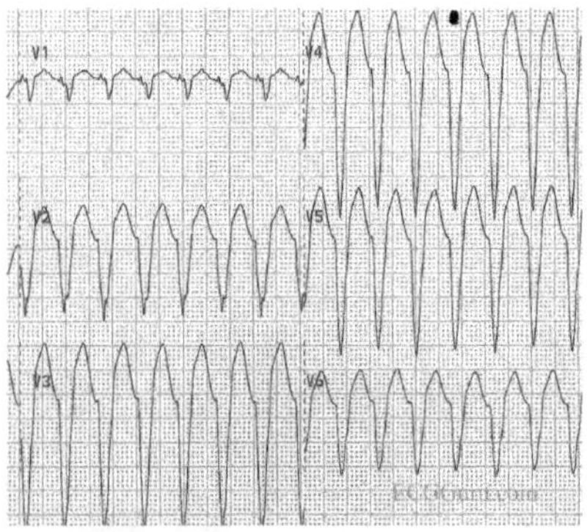

Figure 1-44

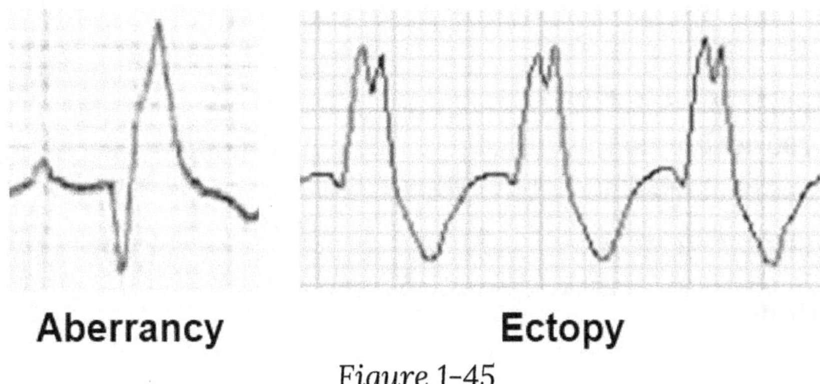

Figure 1-45

Here's a final question for you to ponder (you should be able to answer it by now):

Both snippets in Figure 1-45 are from Lead V1. On the left is a ventricular depolarization with a **QR** morphology that has occurred during a supraventricular rhythm, likely sinus. It represents aberrant conduction – a complete right bundle branch block (cRBBB). On the right is a ventricular depolarization with a **qR** morphology that is an ectopic rhythm with a right bundle branch block-like morphology. The difference in amplitude between the "Q" and "q" waves is not a factor here.

QUESTION | Why is it that a qR complex in Lead V1 during sinus rhythm represents *aberrant conduction* while the *same* morphology in Lead V1 during a wide complex tachycardia is much more likely to represent *ectopy*?

Answer on the next page.

Answers:

Snippet #1 | Outflow tract, inferior axis
Snippet #2 | Apex, superior axis
Snippet #3 | Apex, superior axis
Snippet #4 | Apex, superior axis

Precordial Transitions
Figure 1-39 | 1
Figure 1-40 | 1
Figure 1-41 | 2, 4
Figure 1-42 | 2, 4
Figure 1-43 | 3
Figure 1-44 | 3

ANSWER (Figure 1-45) | The QR of the aberrant conduction (left) is a result of the refractory states of the bundle branches at the time of activation – which occurred through the His-Purkinje system. The deeper Q wave *may or may not* be due to an old anteroapical infarction. The qR of the ventricular tachycardia (ectopy, right) simply reflects the site of origin of the ectopic ventricular impulse since it did not involve the His-Purkinje system.

Recommended Reading:

Cohen SI, MD, Lau SH, MD, Stein E, MD, Young MW, MD, Damato AN, MD. Variations of Aberrant Ventricular Conduction in Man: Evidence of Isolated and Combined Block Within the Specialized Conduction System. *Circulation.* Volume 38, November, 1968; pp. 899-916.

Fisch C, Zipes DP, McHenry PL. Rate Dependent Aberrancy. *Circulation.* 1973;48:714-724.

You can find the online version of this article at: http://circ.ahajournals.org/content/48/4/714.This is one of the *classics* of electrocardiographic literature. Dr. Fisch was a true pioneer in dysrhythmias. He wrote several books – now out of print – that are still available at online booksellers.

Marriott HJL, Schwartz NL, Bix HH. Ventricular Fusion Beats. *Circulation.* 1962;26:880-884.

Another *classic* paper. I think you should focus on being able to recognize *fusion beats.* Capture beats are much easier to see because they always create an interruption in the rhythm and the difference in their morphology is usually very apparent. Many people fail to recognize AV dissociation because there may be only a few fusion beats and no capture beats.

Mazur, A, MD, Kusniec J, MD, Strasberg B, MD. Bundle Branch Reentrant Tachycardia. *Indian Pacing and Electrophysiology Journal.* 5(2); 86-95; (2005).

Nelson W, MD. Abnormalities of Impulse Formation and Conduction. *Card Electrophysiol Clin.* 4 (2012) 469–478.

You can find the online version of this article at: http://dx.doi.org/10.1016/j.ccep.2012.08.035.

Pollack ML, MD, Chan TC, MD, Brady WJ, MD. Electrocardiographic Manifestations: Aberrant Ventricular Conduction. *The Journal of Emergency Medicine.* Vol. 19, No. 4, pp. 363–367, 2000.

Here are some online medical journals from which you can download all but their latest articles at no cost:

Arrhythmia and Electrophysiology Review (Requires that you register with Radcliffe Cardiology *for free*)
Circulation
Circulation Research
Circulation: Arrhythmia and Electrophysiology
Europace
Indian Pacing and Electrophysiology Journal

Clinical Electrophysiology
Journal of Arrhythmia
Journal of the American College of Cardiology (JACC)
Journal of the American Heart Association
Portuguese Review of Cardiology (in English)
Revista Española de Cardiología (in English)
Texas Heart Institute Journal

There are many other excellent journals, but I suggest you begin with these.

Chapter 2

The Action Potential

Repolarization and Dysrhythmias

Many dysrhythmias relate to problems in the action potential – but what *is* the action potential? The action potential is basically an ECG of just ONE cell! It uses the same graph as a regular ECG (voltage in mV on the vertical (Y) axis and time in msec on the horizontal (X) axis). Just as a 12-lead ECG measures the depolarization and repolarization of the atria and ventricles (millions of cells), the action potential measures the depolarization and repolarization of a *single* cell.

Depolarization and repolarization are controlled by the opening and closing of ion channels in the cell membrane (sarcolemma). These "pores" in the cell membrane allow positively charged ions to move in and out... *or not!*

> **PEARL |** The only ions that concern us are Na^+, K^+, and Ca^{++}. Other ions (Cl^-, Mg^{++}) are involved at different points, but you don't need to consider them.

The *resting* working myocyte – in between depolarizations and repolarizations – has an interior charge of approximately -90 mV *relative* to the exterior. This is all *relative*: we say the interior is -90 mV because we *arbitrarily set the exterior to 0 mV.*

Most of the tachydysrhythmias we will be dealing with in this workbook have their origins in abnormalities of the action potential – *during repolarization*, in particular. The repolarization of the myocyte is a struggle between incoming Ca^{++} ions and outgoing K^+ ions. (See? You have only TWO ions to think about!)

(Figure 2-1) The Ca^{++} ions entering the cell through the L-type Ca^{++} channels (the main entry of calcium into the cell) tend to make the interior more POSITIVE because each calcium ion carries a charge of +2. Maintaining the cellular interior positive near or just above 0 mV acts to *prolong* Phase 2. In other words, Ca^{++} influx keeps the cell *depolarized.*

K$^+$, on the other hand, is exiting the cell in an attempt to bring the resting membrane potential back to -90 mV and is THE major force in the *repolarization* of the myocyte. The K$^+$ channels are trying to *shorten* Phases 2 and 3 and repolarize the myocyte.

PEARL | *Depolarizing* (incoming) currents work to *lengthen* the action potential. *Repolarizing* (outgoing) currents work to *shorten* the action potential.

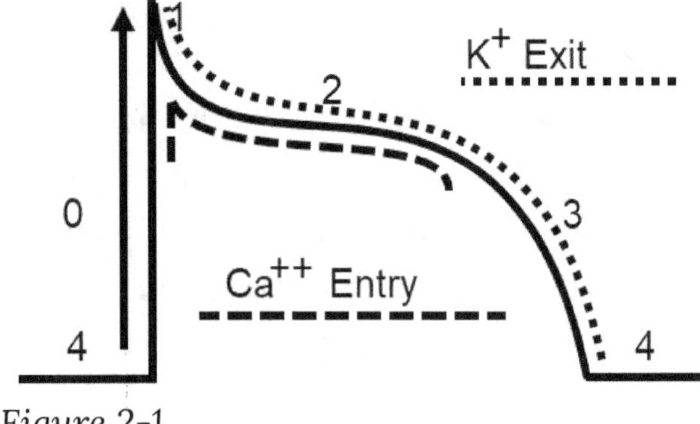

Figure 2-1

TIP | There are three types of action potentials: nodal, Purkinje, and working myocyte. We will deal only with the *working myocyte* action potential.

Figure 2-1 is a normal working myocyte action potential. Ca^{++} entry via the L-type Ca^{++} channels begins during Phase 0 at around -30 to -40 mV and it ends at the end of Phase 2. It is also evident that the K$^+$ exit begins with Phase 1 and continues throughout Phases 2 and 3 and stops at the beginning of Phase 4. At that point – under normal circumstances – the resting membrane potential (RMP) is back to -90 mV.

Let's play with this a little bit by altering the effectiveness of the Ca^{++} and K$^+$ ion channels and see what happens to the QT interval and the shape of the T wave. So many tachycardias have their origin in abnormalities of repolarization, so it's very important that you understand well what is happening during that time. Let's review a few facts before we start to make this a lot easier and more understandable...

1. K$^+$ channels are open and conducting K$^+$ *out of the cell* throughout Phases 1 – 3. So a change in the effectiveness of K$^+$ exit will affect the **ST segment** AND the **T wave**. The K$^+$ channels we are most concerned with during late repolarization are the *delayed rectifying K$^+$ channels* (in case anyone asks).

2. The L-type Ca^{++} channels are open and conducting Ca^{++} *into the cell* throughout Phases 1 and 2, but we are concerned mostly with Phase 2. The Ca^{++} channels are just beginning to open as the Na$^+$ channels are closing, so Ca^{++} will not affect Phase 0 (the QRS complex). And there is no Ca^{++} being conducted during Phase 3 (the T wave) – so the T wave should show no effect from any changes in the Ca^{++} current Figure 2-1).

OK... let's work with a few examples to get a feel for this...

Exercise:

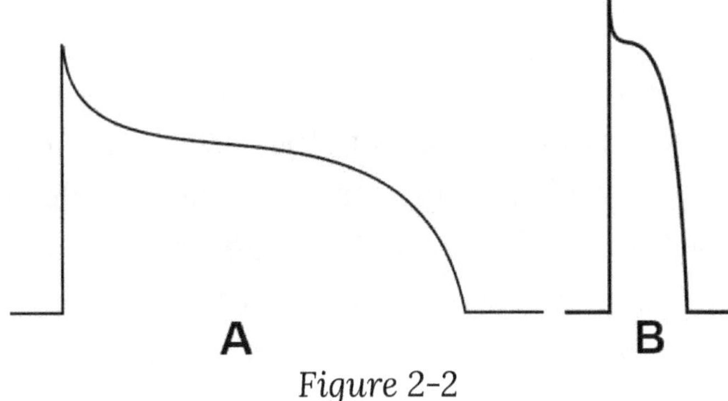

Figure 2-2

Each condition (1-3) describes one of the two action potentials. Match the correct action potential (**A** or **B**) to conditions 1, 2, and 3.

1. Ca^{++} entry is increased
   K^+ exit is decreased

2. Ca^{++} entry is normal
   K^+ exit is increased

3. Ca^{++} entry is normal
   K^+ exit is decreased

ANSWERS | 1: A, 2: B, 3: A

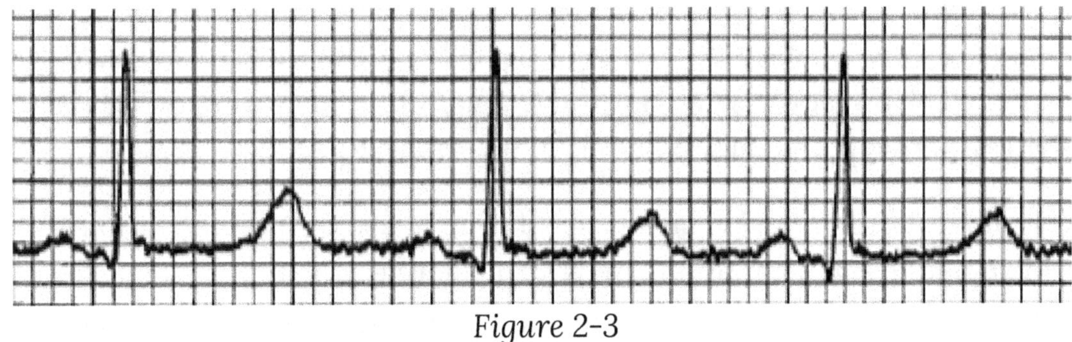

Figure 2-3

Figure 2-3 is a snippet from Lead II of an ECG. The QTc is 471. What are your thoughts about why the QT interval is prolonged? Let's assume there is no medication effect and there are no electrolyte abnormalities. There is either an issue with the Ca^{++} channels or an issue with the K^+ channels.

1. An increase in Ca^{++} conductance (more Ca^{++} entering the cell) or a decrease in K^+ conductance (less K^+ exiting the cell) could do this. Or a combination of both.

2. Only one of the ion channels will have an effect on the T wave. Which one? Has it indeed had any effect?

Discussion:

Only one of the ion channels (K⁺) would affect *both* the *ST segment* AND the *T wave*. A decrease in the exit of K⁺ from the cells would prolong the ST segment by delaying repolarization and also widen the T wave. The T waves, however, don't appear especially widened. It would be unusual for a decrease in K⁺ conductance to have such an effect on the ST segment but not the T wave.

A prolongation of Ca^{++} entry could extend the ST segment without any effect on the T wave – other than to delay it and move it further away from the QRS complex. This likely represents an increase in the Ca^{++} conductance with little or no alteration in K⁺ conductance.

> **TIP |** The K⁺ ions cannot compete with the Ca^{++} ions on a 1:1 basis because the charge on the Ca^{++} is twice the charge on the K⁺ ions. K⁺ ions would have to exit by at least twice the number of Ca^{++} ions just to neutralize the Ca^{++} entry.

This is fun! Let's do one more (I promise just ONE! But it's going to be *very* interesting!): let's say there is a *loss-of-function* mutation in the gene encoding the L-type Ca^{++} channels and entry of Ca^{++} ions into the cell is dramatically *reduced*. Think about that for a second. At the same time, there is a *gain-of-function* mutation in the genes encoding the various components of the K⁺ channels causing K⁺ to *exit the myocyte very rapidly and in very large amounts*. Knowing that the exit of K⁺ from the cell begins during Phase 1 and continues through the end of Phase 3, what do you think the ECG will look like? Just visualize very little Ca^{++} entering the cell but at the same time huge amounts of K⁺ exiting the cell – *and exiting very rapidly!* The action potential should resemble Figure 2-2B.

Since there is no exit of K⁺ (in such quantities) during Phase 0 – *depolarization* – the QRS complex should not be significantly affected by the increased K⁺ exit, if at all. But K⁺ exits the cell throughout *repolarization* – from the beginning of Phase 1 through the end of Phase 3 – so both the ST segment (Phase 2) and the T wave (Phase 3) will be markedly affected. I want you to think about these questions:

1. What effect will this have on Phase 2 and the ST segment on the ECG?

2. What effect will this have on Phase 3 and the T wave on the ECG?

3. Do you think this actually happens and could there be a name for this condition?

Here is the action potential from this exact situation (Figure 2-4)...

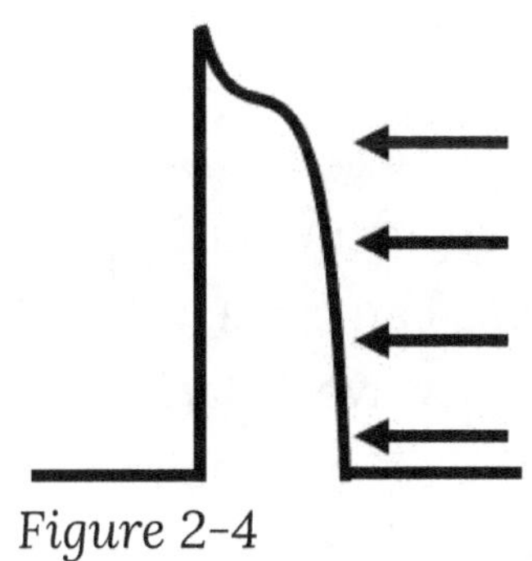

Figure 2-4

Phase 0 looks normal but there are dramatic changes in Phases 1 – 3, especially Phases 2 and 3! Phase 2 is shortened quite a lot. What would this do to the ST segment on the ECG? It would also shorten the ST segment – *quite a lot!* It could virtually disappear from the tracing! What effect did this have on Phase 3? Phase 3 has developed a dramatically *increased downward slope*, with *all of Phase 3 occurring during a much, much shorter length of time.* How would this appear on an ECG?

Let's take a look (Figure 2-5)...

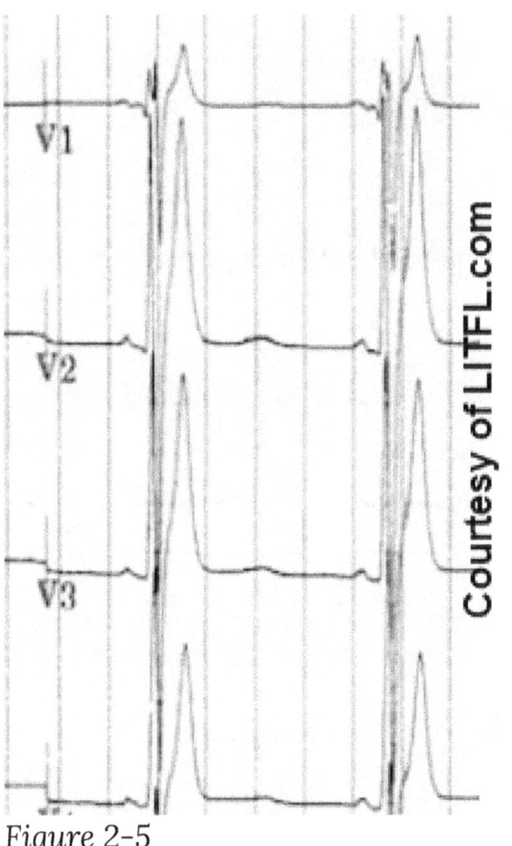

Figure 2-5

PEARL | *Narrowing* on an ECG means *rapid conduction*: a narrow complex was conducted rapidly. *Widening* indicates a *slowing of conduction*. Example: the first half of an RBBB in Lead V1 is narrow because conduction is occurring in rapidly conducting Purkinje fibers in the left ventricle while the second half of the QRS is wide because of slower cell-to-cell conduction in the right ventricle.

This (Figure 2-5) is what happens during a **short QT syndrome** which can lead to a non-torsade polymorphic VT. What other condition can result in T waves like these? **Hyperkalemia!** "But," you protest, "these T waves are narrow because K^+ is *exiting* the cell at such a rapid rate and in increased quantities. That wouldn't happen when the extracellular K^+ level is already increased!" Actually... yes, it would!

TIP | Contrary to intuitive thinking, K^+ exits the cell in *greater* quantities during HYPERkalemia – not during HYPOkalemia. I know... it is completely contrary to common sense – but that's exactly what happens – and there IS a good reason for it (but a little too advanced for this workbook). The increased departure of K^+ from the cell during hyperkalemia can shorten the ST segment (though NOT to this extent!) and it *also* results in an action potential with a *much greater vertical downslope in Phase 3*. **Anything that creates more verticality during Phase 3 of the**

action potential (Figure 2-4) will result in a tall, narrow, and peaked T wave on the ECG.

PEARL | *Hypocalcemia can also cause a significantly prolonged ST segment, but the T wave at the end of that segment will be* normal. *Hypercalcemia can cause a dramatic shortening of the ST segment, but again, no effect on the T wave. Why? Because Ca^{++} has no real effect on Phase 3.* The closing of the L-type Ca^{++} channels marks the *end of Phase 2.* **The K$^+$ channels are the only active channels during Phase 3 (the T wave) during normal conditions.** If you want to know what happens under *abnormal* conditions, that is discussed in Chapter 3, "Afterdepolarizations and Triggered Activity."

When you see an ECG with a **prolonged ST segment**, you should think...

1. Are the K$^+$ channels defective and not working properly to move K$^+$ out of the cells, or

2. Are the Ca^{++} channels extra-active and contributing more than they normally do to moving Ca^{++} into the cells?

When you see an ECG with a **tall, narrow symmetrical, and peaked T wave**, you should think...

1. K$^+$ is exiting the cell faster and in greater quantity than usual!

    a. Is hyperkalemia present?

    b. Is there a *gain-of-function mutation* present and could this be a short QT syndrome?

Exercises in Action Potentials and Abnormalities of Repolarization

Review Figure 2-1 and specifically note:

1. During which phases the Ca++ channels are active. Remember that it is only during those phases that any change in Ca++ entry will have any effect on the ECG. Ca++ exit is not normally noted on the ECG tracing.

2. During which phases the K$^+$ channels are active. Since BOTH Ca^{++} and K$^+$ are active during Phase 2, changes in the ST segment can be caused by either ion. Since there is no activity of the Ca^{++} channels during Phase 3, any changes in the T waves are due to changes in K$^+$ exit. K$^+$ entry is not normally visible on the ECG.

3. Ca^{++} entry serves to LENGTHEN the phase in which it is active – Phase 2 (the ST

segment).

4. K^+ exit serves to SHORTEN the phases in which it is active – Phases 1, 2, and 3 (the ST segment and the T wave).

Select the possible electrolyte processes for each action potential...

Action Potential #1

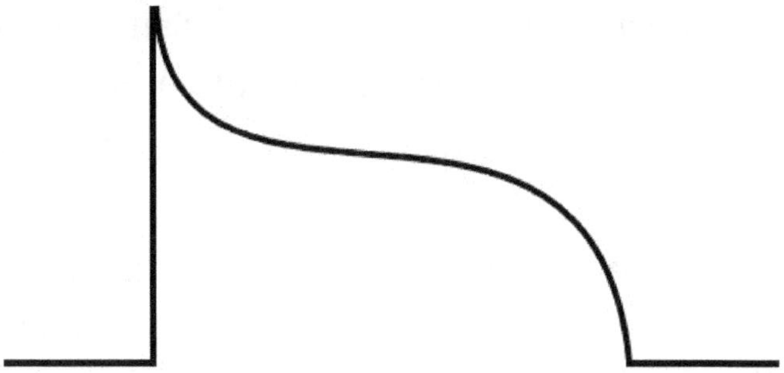

1. Increased activity of Ca^{++} channels

2. Increased activity of K^+ channels

3. Decreased activity of Ca^{++} channels

4. Decreased activity of K^+ channels

5. Normal activity of Ca^{++} channels

6. Normal activity of K^+ channels

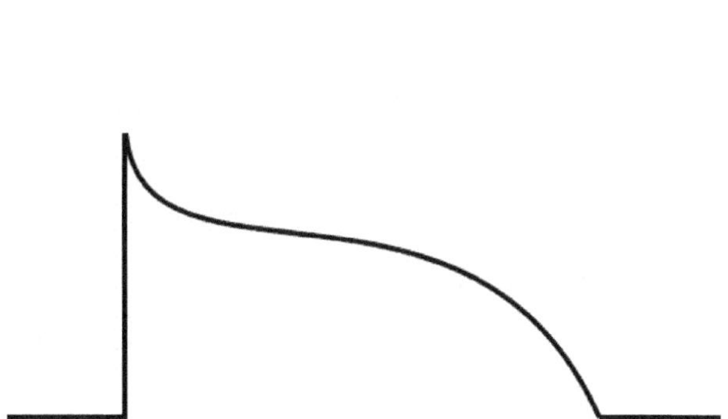

Figure 2-6

Discussion | The total action potential duration appears prolonged, due mainly to the mild prolongation of Phase 2. Phase 3 appears to have its usual slope so it is essentially normal. Both Ca^{++} and K^+ are active during Phase 2 and K^+ remains active during Phase 3. Based on a normal Phase 3, I would say that there is normal activity of the K^+ channels and that the prolongation of Phase 2 must be due to increased Ca^{++} channel activity.

Action Potential #2

1. Increased activity of Ca^{++} channels

2. Increased activity of K^+ channels

3. Decreased activity of Ca^{++} channels

4. Decreased activity of K^+ channels

5. Normal activity of Ca^{++} channels

6. Normal activity of K^+ channels

Figure 2-7

Discussion | On this action potential we see prolongation of both Phase 2 and Phase 3. We know that – since the Ca^{++} channels are not active during Phase 3 – *any change in Phase 3 (the T wave) will be due to K^+ channel activity*, whether increased or decreased. Since a change in K^+ channel activity will have the same effect in Phases 1, 2, and 3 – and Phase 3 is obviously prolonged – there must be decreased activity of the K^+ channels. Are the Ca^{++} channels manifesting increased activity? Maybe, maybe not. In this case, the decreased activity of the K^+ channels would be enough to explain the prolongation of Phases 2 and 3.

Look at this snippet (Figure 2-8) and describe to yourself what the action potential should look like. First, just think about what you observe; then consider the possible ion channel disturbances that may be producing the snippet. I will include a discussion below – but please give it a try before looking at my response.

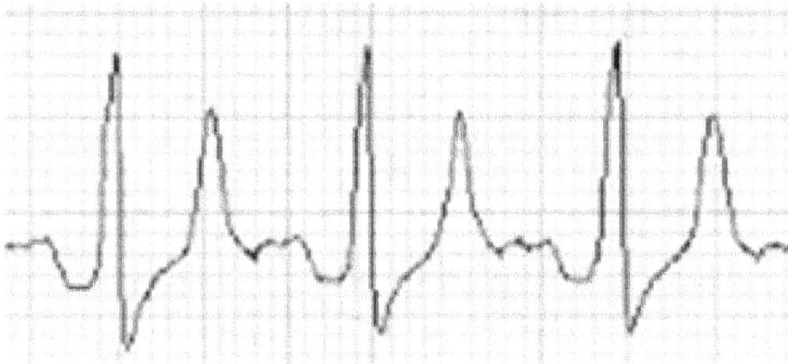

Figure 2-8

Discussion | The ST segment is very short, but it is still present. The T waves are very pointed with narrow bases. This appears to be a situation with very active K^+ channels. The Ca^{++} channels must be depressed because it should not be difficult for Ca^{++} with a charge of 2+ per ion to offset increased K^+ channel activity. The Ca^{++} channels are not very active but the K^+ channels are – which explains this QRS-T pattern. There are two main causes for increased K^+ channel activity: *gain-of-function mutations* in the channel gene and *hyperkalemia*. Yes... contrary to common sense, hyperkalemia causes an increased efflux of K^+ from the myocyte. So this was a case of hyperkalemia.

Chapter 3

Afterdepolarizations and Triggered Activity

The Action Potential and Afterdepolarizations

There is a lot to be said about the action potential, but its role in wide complex tachycardias – more specifically, in *ventricular tachycardia* – can be condensed a bit. I am going to concentrate on the role of Ca^{++} in the production of something called *afterdepolarizations* and *triggered activity*. Let's begin with known facts:

The resting membrane potential of the myocyte is -90 mV – but we don't want it *resting*, we want it *doing* things, like *contracting* and *transmitting impulses*. For that to happen, it must get out of its resting polarized state: it must DEpolarize.

> **PEARL** | Afterdepolarizations and triggered activity are responsible for outflow tract tachycardias, torsade de pointes, and most polymorphic VTs. If you want to feel more comfortable managing wide complex tachycardias – *you need to know this!*

Now let's take a look at a working myocyte action potential (Figure 3-1):

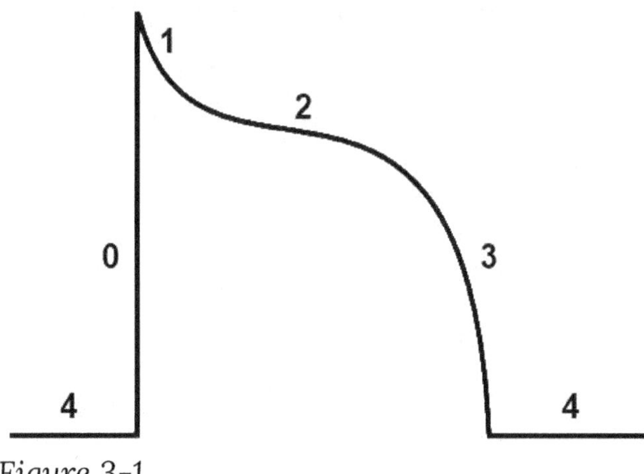

Figure 3-1

On the **action potential**, we have Phases 0, 1, 2, 3, and 4.

On the **ECG**, we have the **QRS** (Phase **0**), the first **onset of repolarization** at the "J" point (Phase **1**), the **ST segment** (Phase 2), the **T wave** (Phase **3**), and the **T-P segment**, or **diastole** (Phase **4**).

Each phase of the action potential has a corresponding event on the ECG (Figure 3-2).

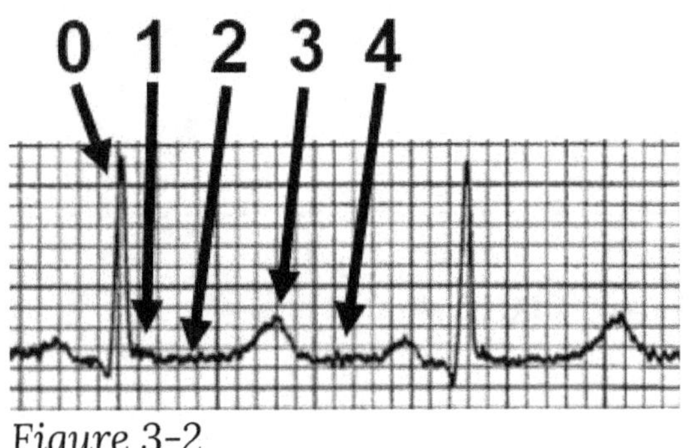

Figure 3-2

And, for a grand finish, the *action potential* on the ECG is called the **QT interval!**

One of the methods of dysrhythmia formation is afterdepolarizations leading to triggered activity. It's a complicated topic, but you needn't bother with all the complicated stuff to properly and effectively manage a patient – let's start with a simple overview of the subject...

1. There are times when there is too much accumulation of intracellular Ca^{++}.

    a. You needn't be concerned about *how* that Ca^{++} got there... yet.

    b. Your only concern right now is at *what point* the cell starts dumping all that extra Ca^{++} and what happens *then!*

2. The cell can start getting rid of the Ca^{++} *during* the action potential – either during Phase 2 or Phase 3 (that's during the ST segment or T wave on the ECG, Figure 3-2), or

3. the cell can start getting rid of the extra Ca^{++} during Phase 4 – after repolarization has occurred (after the end of the T wave).

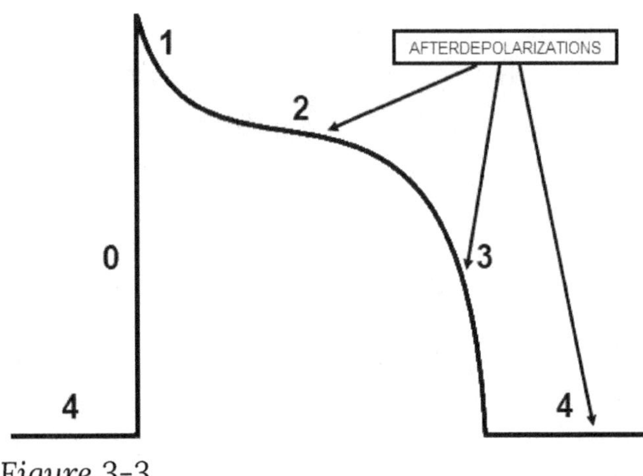

Figure 3-3

Look at Figure 3-3 and see where the cell can start unloading the extra intracellular Ca^{++} – Phases 2, 3 and 4.

Early Afterdepolarizations

Afterdepolarizations that occur during Phase 2 or Phase 3 are called *early afterdepolarizations* **(EADs)**. Afterdepolarizations that occur during Phase 4 are called *delayed afterdepolarizations* **(DADs)**.

TIP | Afterdepolarizations are *not* separate action potentials – they are all part of a *single action potential.* The action potential will last until an afterdepolarization fails to reach the threshold potential and the cells can finally return to their baseline resting membrane potential. *Now that's a lo-o-ong QT interval!*

Keep in mind that there is a very large amount of Ca^{++} to be discharged and the main exit for it will be via the **sodium-calcium exchanger (NCX)** (Figure 3-4). The NCX is a transport mechanism that exchanges three Na^+ ions for one Ca^{++} ion. The surplus Ca^{++} will be removed by the NCX – but that is going to create a strong *inward, positive depolarizing* current as all that extracellular Na^+ enters the cell in exchange for the intracellular Ca^{++}.

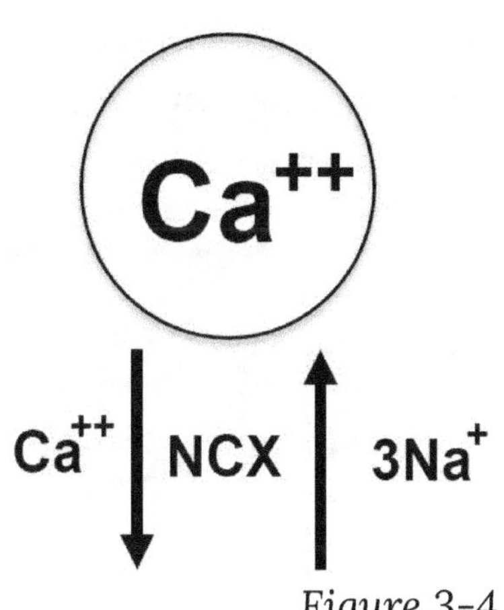

Figure 3-4

> **PEARL |** Na^+ always exchanges in a 3:2 ratio: $3Na^+$ to $2K^+$ or $3Na^+$ to $1Ca^{++}$. Such exchanges are said to be *electrogenic* which means that more ions are being transported in one direction than the other. This will result in a current – sometimes *inward* (depolarizing), sometimes *outward* (repolarizing).

Such a strong, inward current can momentarily counteract the outward repolarizing K^+ current and cause the cell to begin to depolarize once again – even *before* the outward K^+ currents have had a chance to repolarize the cell. These momentary reversals of repolarization (sometimes called "oscillations") caused by the inward Na^+ current resulting from the NCX activity are called **afterdepolarizations**: they occur *after* the *depolarization* of the cell but *before* the cell has had a chance to repolarize. If the afterdepolarization is strong enough, it will reach threshold potential and produce *a single depolarization – a PVC!* The PVC was "triggered" by the initial depolarization, so we call this *triggered activity!*

Look at Phase 2 on the action potential (Figure 3-5). **Afterdepolarizations occurring during Phase 2 typically do not reach threshold; therefore, no triggered activity usually results from afterdepolarizations during Phase 2.**

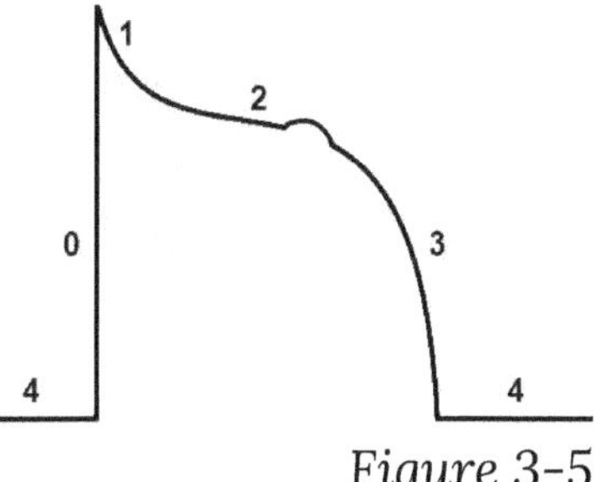

Figure 3-5

Phase 3, however, is a different matter. Afterdepolarizations that occur during Phase 3 can definitely reach threshold potential and produce a PVC.

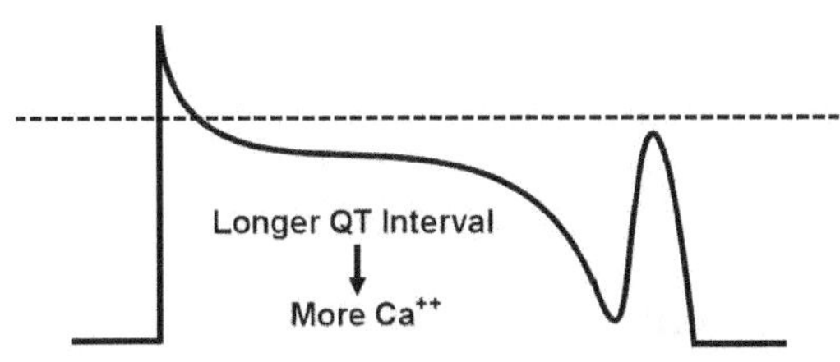

Figure 3-6

A PVC... during Phase 3. Does that mean anything to you? Do you remember which deflection represents Phase 3 on the ECG? The T wave! Triggered activity that occurs during Phase 3 will produce an "R-on-T" phenomenon.

Throughout phases 1, 2, and 3 of the action potential (but especially the latter part of Phase 3) there is a significant variability in the durations of refractoriness of the cells of the ventricular walls. This condition provides an excellent substrate for dangerous reentrant tachycardias. This is why the downslope of the T wave has the nickname "the *vulnerable period.*"

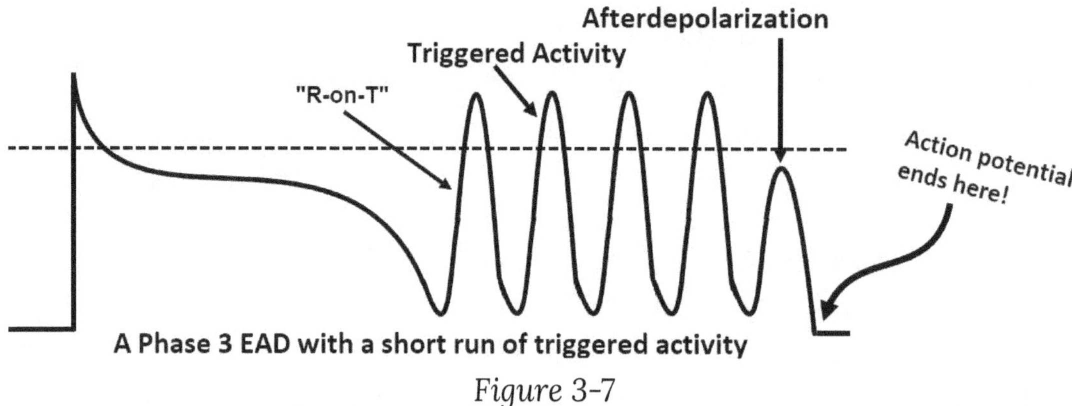

Figure 3-7

In Figure 3-7 we see a Phase 3 afterdepolarization that succeeded in reaching the threshold potential and produced a PVC – an "R-on-T" phenomenon. Each PVC then provoked another afterdepolarization that produced another PVC until one of them failed and the action potential was finally able to return to its baseline resting membrane potential. This entire diagram is just ONE action potential. Triggered activity occurs *before* the action potential has a chance to fully repolarize down to -90 mV. So there can be multiple depolarizations triggered by just one spontaneous depolarization. None of the PVCs in this "train" of depolarizations was spontaneous – each one was "triggered" by the preceding depolarization.

Did you notice something else about the action potential – specifically Phase 2? There is a prolongation of the action potential duration and consequently, a **prolonged QT interval**. Prolongation of the action potential allows much more Ca^{++} to enter the cell. This potentiates early afterdepolarizations and triggered activity. Prolongation of the action potential is the basis for QT prolongation on the ECG. This is the mechanism and origin of **torsade de pointes**. You'll hear more about that later.

We still have delayed afterdepolarizations to discuss, but you already know about 90% of what I am going to say about that topic. Before we move on, let's review what you've just learned...

1. Under some pathological conditions, a marked **excess of Ca^{++}** accumulates within the cytosol (cytoplasm) of the myocyte.

2. In removing the excess Ca^{++}, the **sodium-calcium exchanger (NCX)** goes into action **exchanging three (3) extracellular Na^+ ions for each intracellular Ca^{++} ion.**

3. During the exchange, more Na^+ is entering the cell than the amount of Ca^{++} exiting, so there is an **inward, depolarizing current**.

4. This current – if strong enough – can **reverse the repolarizing activity of the K$^+$ channels** during Phase 3 and attain threshold potential. This results in **another depolarization** before the cell has had a chance to repolarize and reach the normal resting membrane potential of -90 mV.

5. A **prolonged QT interval** is very conducive to the increased intracellular Ca^{++} because it allows **more time for the L-type Ca++ channels** to continue to move Ca++ into the cell.

6. Inward currents – like the resulting Na$^+$ current, also help prolong the action potential duration, i.e., the QT interval... which promotes more triggered activity... which promotes more inward current... which promotes more QT prolongation... which promotes more triggered activity, etc. Now do you see where this is going?

Time to move on to...

Delayed Afterdepolarizations

Delayed afterdepolarizations act very similarly to early afterdepolarizations with THREE major exceptions (hmm... maybe they are not so similar after all!):

1. The cause of the intracellular Ca^{++} overloading is different.

2. There is no inherent prolongation of the action potential (no QT prolongation).

3. And they occur during Phase 4 – diastole. *Nothing is happening in diastole.* Specifically, there is no dispersion of refractory periods creating the substrate for dangerous reentrant tachycardias (Figure 3-8). Although *a few* ventricular tachycardias derived from *delayed* afterdepolarizations are benign – *most are very dangerous and lethal!*

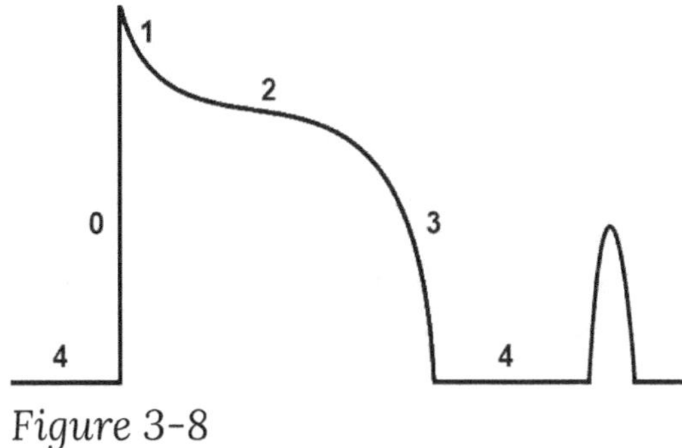

Figure 3-8

There is, however, the same issue with an excess accumulation of cytosolic Ca^{++} and the same mechanism for ridding the cell of the excess Ca^{++}. The same inward Na+ current develops and it does the same thing it did for early afterdepolarizations.

The main factor that contributes to the excess Ca^{++} in the case of delayed afterdepolarizations is an *increase in heart rate.* Because of the increase in heart rate, Ca^{++} begins to accumulate in the cytosol. This shouldn't be a problem because most of us have episodes every day in which our hearts speed up a bit and we don't develop pathological tachycardias. Obviously, there is more going on with a heart in which this can occur. But for managing wide complex tachycardias and ventricular tachycardias, that isn't your concern at this time.

> **PEARL |** An inward, positive current is *depolarizing* and will contribute to the *prolongation* of the action potential. An outward, positive current is *repolarizing* and will contribute to the *shortening* of the action potential.

> **FYI |** All the currents we have discussed (Ca^{++}, Na^+, K^+) are positive currents.

So there... you now have a good, working understanding of early and delayed afterdepolarizations. No, you aren't an expert on the topic yet, but you now know more than 99% of your colleagues (or at least those who haven't read this book yet!) and... you know enough to give you the confidence to handle...

1. Torsade de pointes (early afterdepolarizations)

2. Right ventricular outflow tract tachycardias (delayed afterdepolarizations)

3. Left ventricular outflow tract tachycardias (delayed afterdepolarizations)

4. Polymorphic VT of Brugada syndrome (delayed afterdepolarizations)

5. Short QT syndrome polymorphic VT (delayed afterdepolarizations)

6. Catecholaminergic polymorphic VT (delayed afterdepolarizations)

7. VT due to digitalis toxicity (delayed afterdepolarizations)

Information You Will Need Later On...

Early afterdepolarizations are associated with a *prolonged QT interval*. Most prolonged QT intervals occur in the presence of slow heart rates or rhythm disturbances with lots of pauses. Consequently, when a sinus-conducted beat results in triggered activity, the coupling interval between the last sinus beat and the first "triggered" PVC will be somewhat long – greater than 400 msec (two large squares) and usually much longer than that (500 -700+ msec).

Delayed afterdepolarizations are associated with *increases in heart rate*. The faster rate will result in a shorter coupling interval between the sinus-conducted beat and the triggered PVC that initiates the tachycardia. The coupling interval will almost invariably be shorter than 400 msec (two large squares).

Early Afterdepolarizations – *Torsade de Pointes*

Delayed Afterdepolarizations – *Non-torsade Polymorphic VTs*

This is a very advanced subject and there is a lot more to this than I have mentioned – *a LOT MORE!* But I have exposed you to everything anyone on the front lines of healthcare will need to know to knowledgeably and effectively manage a patient with one of these conditions.

Chapter 4

QRS Morphologies During Wide Complex Tachycardias

Looking at the perfectly formed QRS complexes during sinus rhythm is completely different than looking at the bizarre and almost indecipherable deflections during a wide complex tachycardia. Textbooks teach you the cause of wide complex tachycardias and provide algorithms to help you distinguish between supraventricular rhythms and ventricular ectopic rhythms – but training in the actual *recognition* of the deflections you are trying to analyze was missing until the appearance of my live **Masterclass in Advanced Electrocardiography** and **Masterclass in Advanced Dysrhythmias**. Now I have included much of my teaching in this workbook.

Let's get started!

Confidently Recognizing NORMAL!

There is no possibility of diagnosing or managing a wide complex tachycardia without a thorough and secure knowledge of what a *classic* bundle branch block looks like in Leads V1 and V6. I have found in my classes that while most, if not all, the participants are very familiar with what RBBB and LBBB look like in Lead V1, most have no idea how they should appear in Lead V6. Yet you must thoroughly know their appearance to confidently diagnose wide complex tachycardias. Here are the classic morphologies. Study them and learn them well!

Classic RBBB – Leads V1 and V6

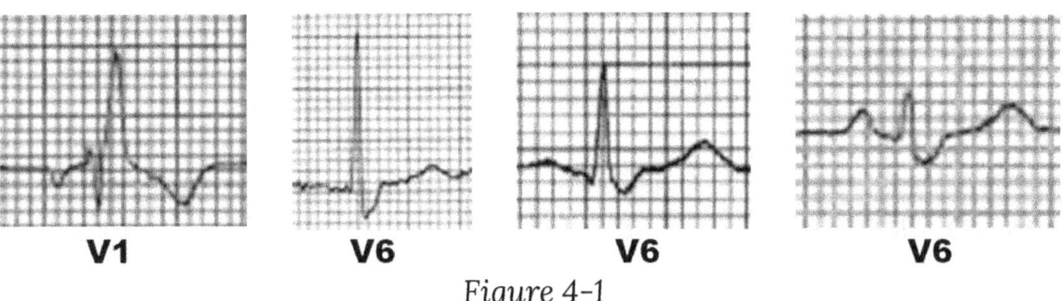

Figure 4-1

I have included three versions of the RBBB morphology in Lead V6 (Figure 4-1). It is often taught as a tall R wave with a wide ("slurred") S wave. My point here is that *it is the S wave that is the most important characteristic* because – like the R′ in Lead V1, it indicates the depolarization of the right ventricle *after* the left ventricle. The R wave may or may not be particularly large, but the R/S ratio should be > 1.0.

Classic LBBB – Leads V1 and V6

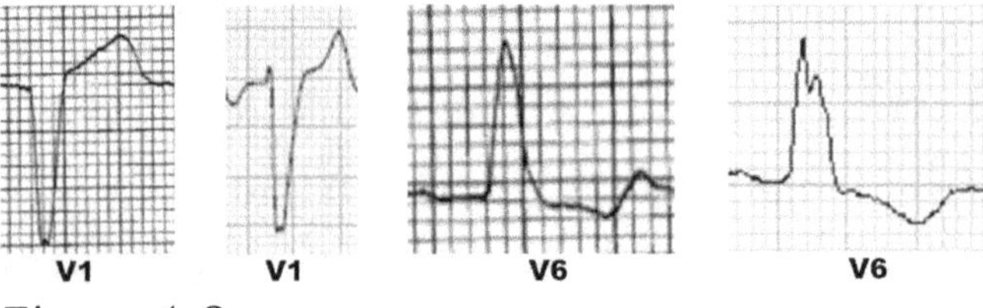

Figure 4-2

I have included two versions each of Leads V1 and V6 (Figure 4-2). For Lead V1, the first is a QS and the second is an rS. Both are accepted as classic LBBB morphology for that lead. There is only ONE version of Lead V6 that is acceptable as classic – a monophasic R with a *slur* or *notch* near the peak (I have included a snippet of each, respectively)!

You must learn these morphologies before going any further. Everything you learn from this point on will be based on a thorough knowledge of these classic bundle branch block morphologies.

QRS morphology in Lead V1

It is very important to know from which ventricle the ectopic or aberrant beat is originating, and **Lead V1 is the <u>only</u> lead that will consistently and reliably distinguish between the RIGHT and LEFT ventricles**.

Some algorithms used in the diagnosis of wide complex tachycardias are based on whether the QRS morphology in V1 is RIGHT bundle branch block-like or LEFT bundle branch block-like.

When we use the term RIGHT bundle branch block-**like**, we do not mean a *classic right bundle branch block*. Far from it! We are simply indicating that the QRS in V1 is more positive than negative, that it has more R wave than S wave. It does *not* have to be triphasic, either. That R wave does NOT have to be an R′ – just more *positive* than *negative*.

A LEFT bundle branch block-**like** QRS would be a QRS that is more *negative* than *positive* in Lead V1 – more S wave than R wave.

Here are a few examples (all are from Lead V1):

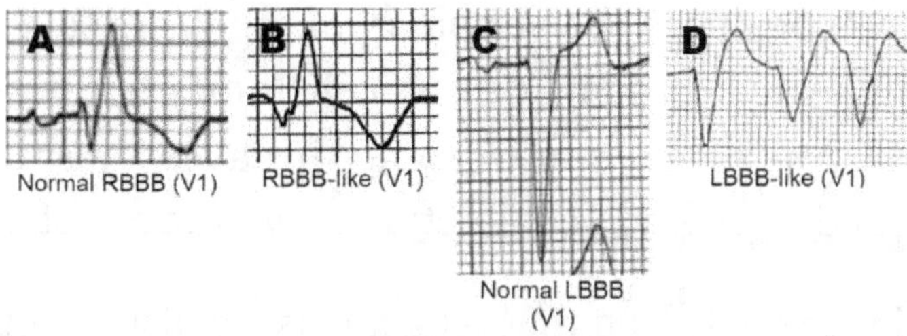

Figure 4-3

The classic RBBB in Lead V1 (Figure 4-3A) has a small r, a deeper S wave, and a tall second R wave called an R′. It should *never* begin with a Q wave and *never* end with an S wave. A terminal S or s wave in Lead V1 *automatically excludes RBBB*. As you can see, the RBBB-like complex (Figure 4-3B) begins with a Q wave. The classic LBBB is a QS wave or occasionally an rS complex. The LBBB-*like* complex looks very similar. If there is an initial r wave, it will be > 40 msec in duration, otherwise, the downslope of the S wave will have a decreased slope. Unfortunately, sometimes the ectopic LBBB-like complex can look very similar to a normal LBBB complex.

Let's practice determining whether the following QRS complexes (Figure 4-4) are RIGHT bundle branch-like or LEFT bundle branch-like (all snippets are from Lead V1):

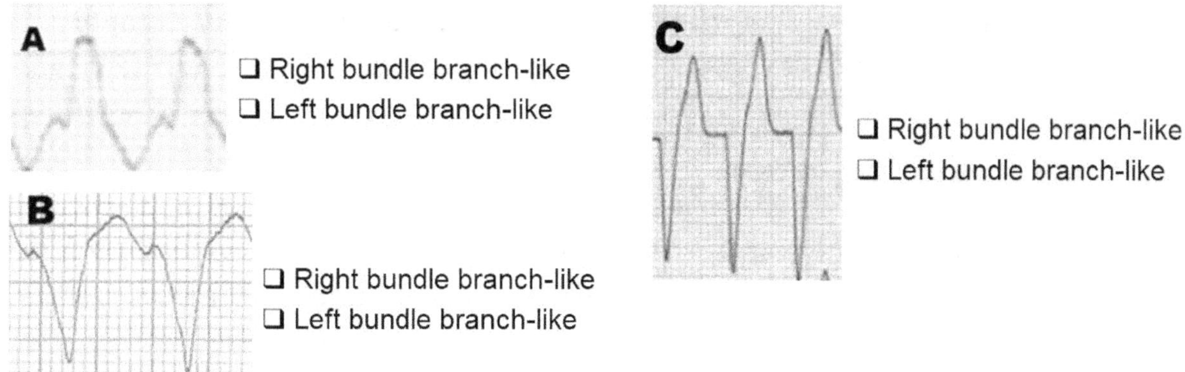

Figure 4-4

Only those impulses originating *above* the division of the His bundle into the right and left bundle branches, or those originating *within the conducting system* of the ventricles (*bundle branch tachycardia* and *fascicular tachycardia*) can produce a *classic* bundle branch block pattern. As you will learn later – *a classic bundle branch block pattern does not automatically rule out ventricular tachycardia*. Fortunately, regarding the two ventricular tachycardias that are not ruled out, both are very infrequent and one is benign. The rule may not be perfect, but, as a rule of thumb, it's OK.

Answers to the quiz in Figure 4-4: **A**-RBBB-like; **B**-LBBB-like; **C**-LBBB-like.

PEARL | Always use Lead V1 to distinguish between RIGHT and LEFT!

If an ectopic depolarization begins in the periphery of the ventricular myocardium, it will typically spread through the myocardium, cell-to-cell. It may occasionally enter a Purkinje fiber, but it often won't be able to conduct *antegrade* because it just depolarized the area where the fiber is going and retrograde conduction may or may not be possible.

As I said before, Lead V1 is the *only* lead that *reliably* distinguishes between right and left. Many people feel that Lead II has the best P waves and is also very good at distinguishing between right and left. Do YOU think so? Let's take a look...

Here (Figure 4-5) we have a left bundle branch block (LBBB), a right bundle branch block (RBBB), a left-sided PVC (ectopic, short run of VT), and a right-sided PVC (ectopic, short run of VT) – all taken from Lead II. They *all* look about the same, don't they? Of the four, only the ectopics manifest a repolarization abnormality. Still think Lead II is good at differentiating between the right and left ventricles?

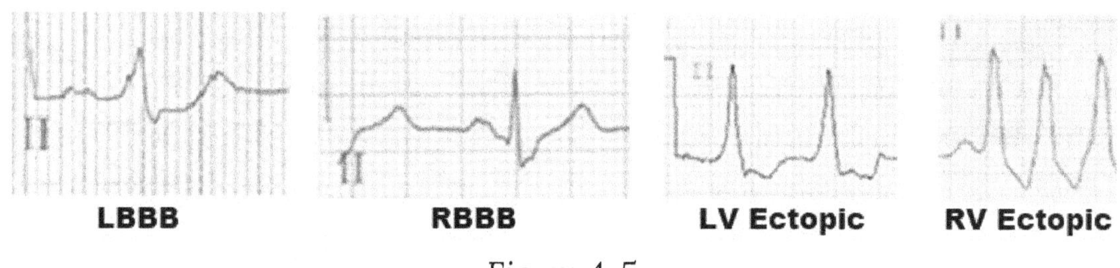

Figure 4-5

The Spread of Depolarization

The further the depolarization wave travels in the myocardium (cell-to-cell), the wider and more bizarre the QRS complex, especially if there is any structural heart disease (scars, fibrosis, etc.) encountered in its path.

> **PEARL |** Purkinje fibers do not extend to the epicardium. They are generally located in the inner one-third of the ventricular wall – in the subendocardium. There are no Purkinje fibers that run transversely through the interventricular septum. Left-to-right septal transmission is cell-to-cell, as is right-to-left conduction.

> **REMINDER |** The *rate* of depolarization (i.e., the heart rate) is based on the firing of an ectopic pacemaker or reentry circuit. It has nothing to do with *conduction velocity*. Conduction velocity is measured by the <u>width</u> of the QRS complex – *not by the <u>frequency</u> of the QRS complexes.*

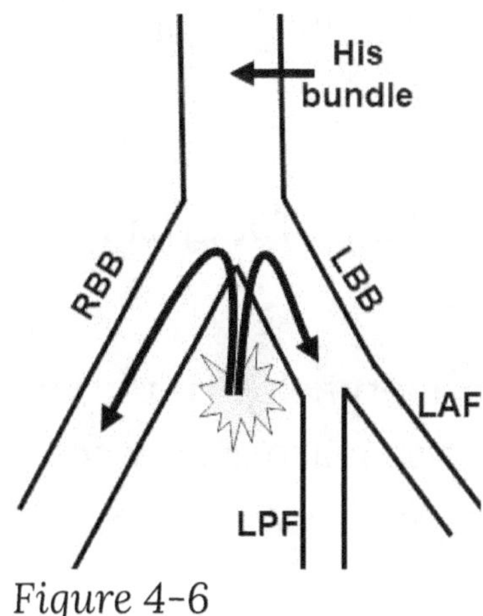

Figure 4-6

If the ectopic focus is located high up in the basilar portion of the ventricular septum and close to the His bundle or the bundle branches, as in Figure 4-6, it can enter those fibers almost simultaneously and then it will conduct throughout both ventricles normally, inscribing a narrow QRS complex *even though it is a ventricular ectopic beat.*

Any impulse that enters the ventricles via the His-Purkinje system will have a QRS complex whose initial forces will resemble the regular QRS complexes.

Aberrant conduction is caused by delay or blockage in the His-Purkinje system – typically one of the bundle branches. Therefore, aberrant conduction should look more like a regular bundle branch block. But it doesn't always and here's why: bundle branch block is not always a *true block* – it is usually simply a *delay due to decreased speed of conduction through an area of the conducting fiber.* The little bit of delay that caused an "incomplete" RBBB may turn into a greater delay due to a longer refractory period or perhaps some problems caused by localized ischemia resulting in a complex that is *wider* and *more bizarre* in appearance. But the bottom line is that *the beginning of the QRS complex should still show evidence of normal conduction.*

The R wave in Figure 4-7A has a duration of about 0.02 seconds; it is from a normal tracing and represents ventricular activation through the His-Purkinje system. The R wave in Figure 4-7B is much broader – about 0.06 seconds – and is from a patient in ventricular tachycardia; therefore, it originated in the myocardium and traveled from cell to cell.

Now we are going to develop your expertise and skill in recognizing different QRS-T morphologies during wide complex tachycardias. Let's look at some examples while I drop a few PEARLS here and there...

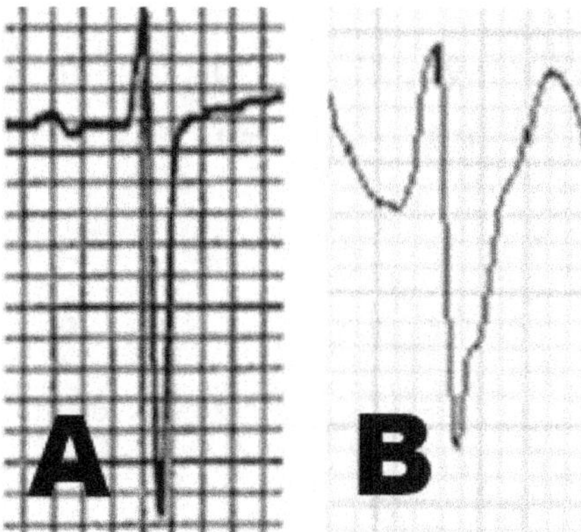

Figure 4-7

Determining the Morphology of the QRS Complex

TIP | Although a BBB-like morphology is NOT a true BBB, it will *help us identify which ventricle is the origin of the tachydysrhythmia.* Its morphology is not based on the presence of a bundle branch delay or block; it's because one ventricle is being activated *before* the other ventricle. Do you recall how to recognize LBBB-like and RBBB-like morphologies? If not, go back and review them.

The bundle branch block-*like* QRS complexes do not have to be monophasic. They just have to be "mostly" positive or negative.

The reason for the similarity between a classic RBBB and an RBBB-*like* morphology is the fact that in both cases the left ventricle is depolarized *first*. Similarly, the resemblance between a true LBBB and an LBBB-*like* morphology is the fact that, in both situations, the right ventricle is activated *first*.

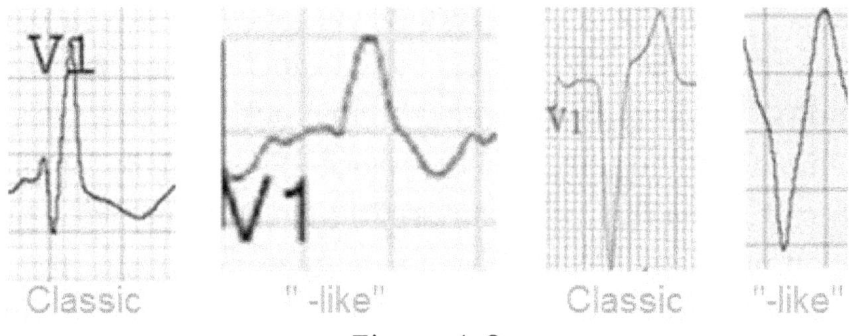

Figure 4-8

Recognizing the Various Deflections in a Wide Complex Tachycardia

When you study ventricular tachycardia in a textbook, you are usually presented with an ECG that appears deceptively simple to interpret.

However, here's what you're apt to face at 3 a.m. in the CCU, ICU, or ER (Figure 4-9):

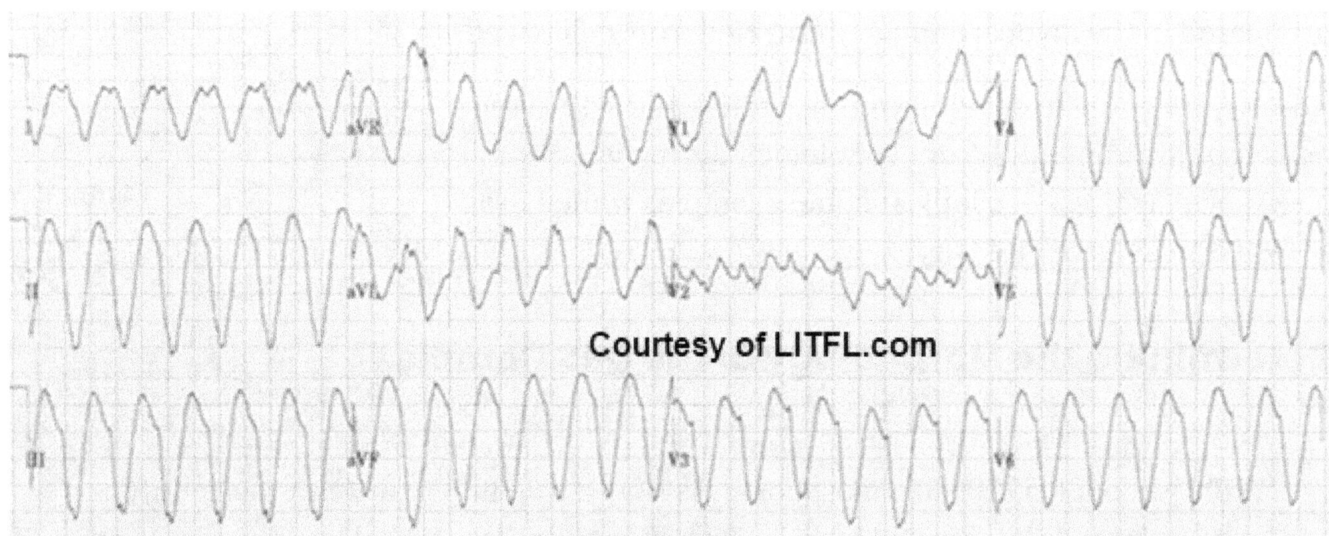

Figure 4-9

Which complexes are positive and which are negative? And what is the QRS morphology in Lead V1 on this tracing? Is this originating in the right or left ventricle? Is the impulse coming from the *outflow tract* or *the apex* of the ventricle? Let's do a little studying and a little practice, and then these questions won't seem so intimidating.

> **PEARL |** During ventricular tachycardia, Leads II, III, and aVF will *tend* to have the same morphology and polarity. They can differ, however, during both normal and ectopic rhythms, but that conduction follows conducting pathways and is subject to an occasional block. An ectopic rhythm usually follows no pathways, so its relationship to the inferior leads reflects its site of origin and direction of propagation.

The following morphologies are real-life examples and not machine-generated.

Morphology #1 – rS complex

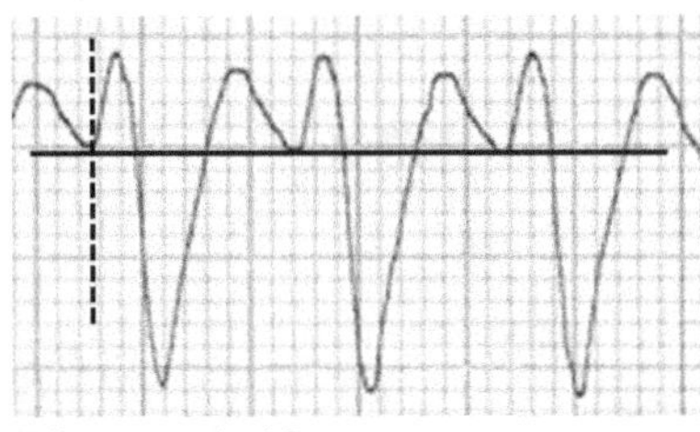

Figure 4-10

This complex represents *a small r wave and a large, wide S wave* (Figure 4-10). The *vertical* dotted line marks the beginning of the r wave and the *horizontal* line represents the otherwise non-existent baseline. Everything above the horizontal "baseline" is either an R wave or a T wave; everything below it is an S wave. Remember that *during a wide complex tachycardia, an rS wave represents an impulse that is in the endocardial layer – it transmits outward* to the surface (r) and inward towards the cavity of the ventricle (S).

Morphology #2 – Monophasic R Complex

This is a monophasic R wave with a very common and very confusing QRS-T morphology (Figure 4-11). Remember that the first part of an S wave is *usually* the continuation of the R wave below the baseline; *it is part of the same line* (Figure 4-12, next page). Back in Figure 4-11, the horizontal thick black line indicates the baseline; everything *above* it is an R wave… but is there an S wave *below* it? Any S wave should be continuous with the downslope of the R wave (represented here by the near-vertical dashed line). The angled dashed line shows very plainly that there is no straight

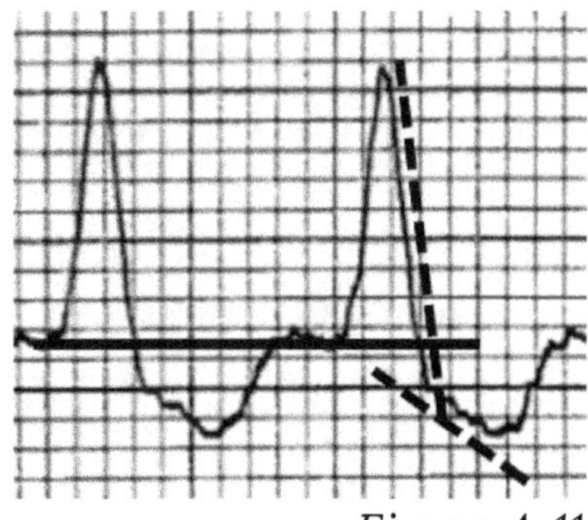

Figure 4-11

continuation with the downslope of the R wave. The lines below the baseline represent *the ST segment* and *inverted T wave*. Remember: **not every QRS complex has to have an S wave, but _every_ QRS complex _must_ have a T wave!** Here are some examples of real RS waves from a normal tracing and two wide complex tachycardias (Figure 4-12):

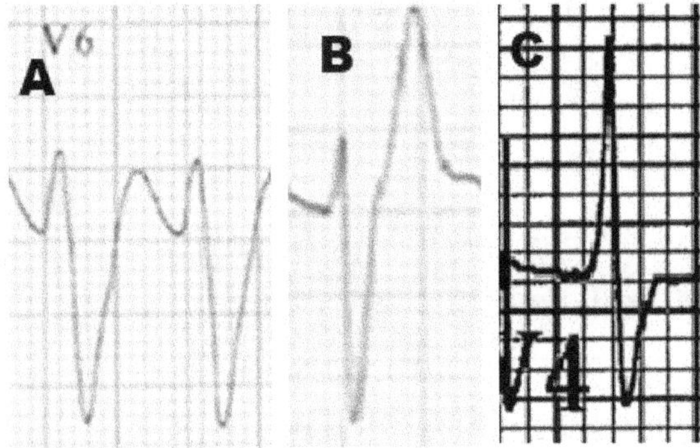

Do you see how the S wave is a continuation of the downslope of the R wave? (Figure 4-12B is normal.) Study the differences between these two sets of complexes (Figures 4-11 and 4-12) so that the distinction is very clear in your mind. These examples of r and S waves are classic and very obvious. In the next section, let's look at some that aren't quite so obvious...

Figure 4-12

PEARL | If you think you see an S wave, then you must <u>*clearly identify the T wave*</u> that follows it! If you can't, then that is *not* an S wave.

Morphology #3 – QS Complex

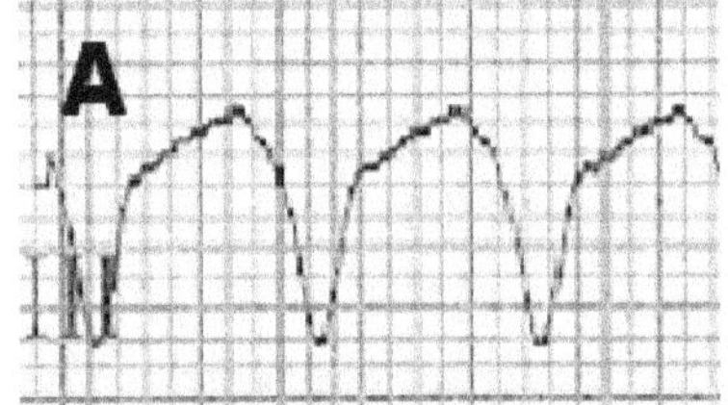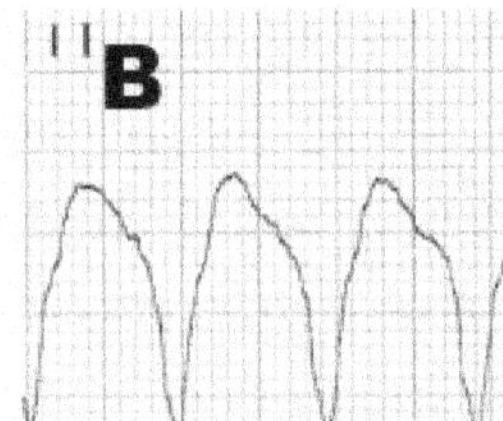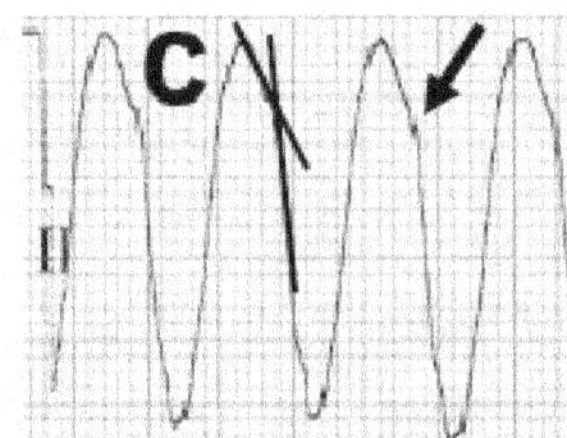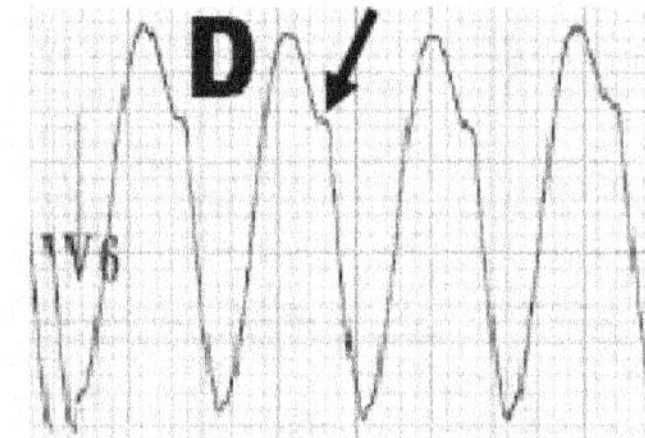

Figure 4-13

The QS complexes are among the most confusing (Figure 4-13). Sometimes they look almost like a sine wave, and other times you think there just might be a tiny r wave at the very beginning. Sometimes the distinction between a QS complex and the other deflections is simply a *change in the slope of the lines*, as in Figure 4-13C (arrow). Sometimes there is a *tiny notch at the beginning of the QS complex* that tips you off about where the baseline is and where the QS begins, as in Figure 4-13D (arrow).

The morphology of Figure 4-13D has created some heated arguments about whether it represents a **QS complex** or an **rS complex**. Let's look at another <u>real</u> rS complex with a very tiny r and compare them (Fig. 4-14).

PEARL | When you see that a QRS consists only of two deflections – an upright deflection and a negative deflection – you should *automatically* know that one of them is a T wave. *There must always be a T wave!*

Figure 4-14A is a true rS complex. In this example, you can see *both the upslope* and *downslope* of the tiny r wave. In Figure 4-14B, there is no upslope at all. Always remember that each deflection of the QRS complex (Q, R, and S) is a **vector** whose axis can be easily determined separately. A vector is defined by **amplitude** and **direction**. Its position *above* or *below* the baseline indicates its *direction* (*toward* or *away from* the recording electrode). Its *amplitude* is the *area enclosed within the deflection*

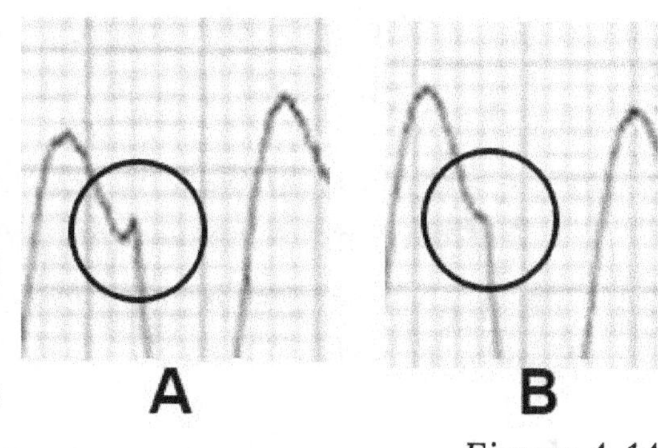

Figure 4-14

– i.e., **a deflection must enclose a measurable area**. Therefore, it must have three sides: an *upslope*, a *downslope*, and the *baseline if* **positive** or a *downslope, an upslope*, and *the baseline if* **negative**. Figure 4-14B should be considered a QS complex (the Brugadas even implied so in their classic paper which introduced their algorithm).

The QS morphology can be the most confusing. Study this section well. The most common mistake is to assume any change in slope at the onset of the QS wave represents an r wave. **It must contain an area to be a vector and, therefore, a deflection.**

Morphology #4 – The Problematic Q's

Sometimes Q waves can be very tiny and difficult to see and sometimes they can be accompanied by other notches and perturbations of the QRS complex that create confusion about exactly which deflections *are* – or *are not* – present. Here are some examples:

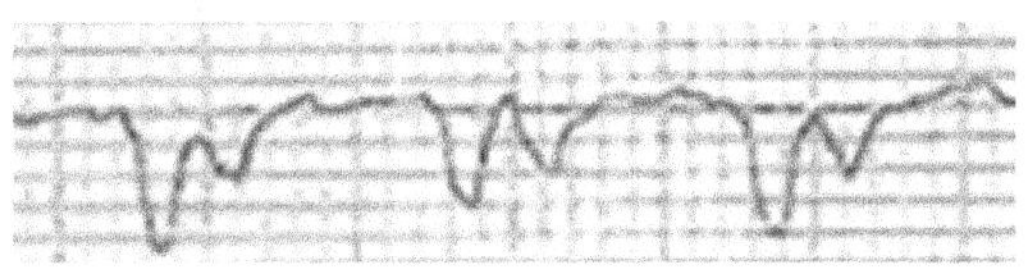

Figure 4-15

Figure 4-15 is a QS wave. I know it looks like a *triphasic* QRS, but the middle deflection never makes it above the baseline. **An R wave *must* be above the baseline. There is no such thing as a negative R wave.**

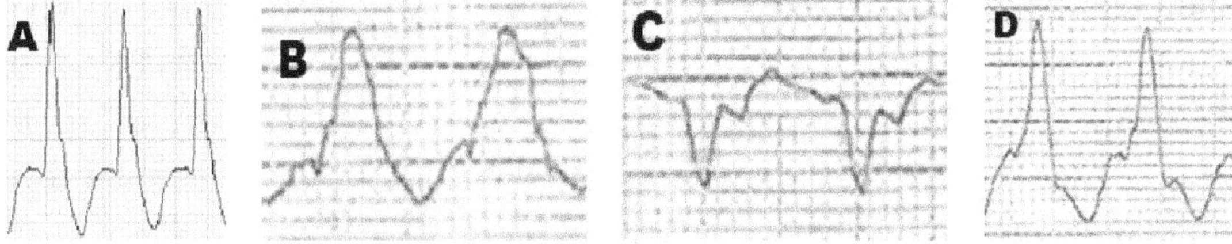

Figure 4-16 Examples of q waves.

Fig. 4-16A is a qR wave. The q is very tiny, but it's there. This should not be considered a monophasic R.

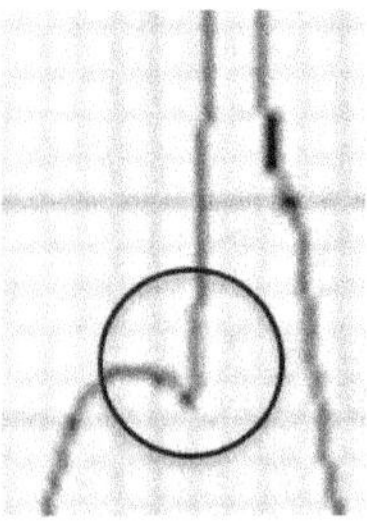

Here is a section of Figure 4-16A enlarged (Figure 4-17). The area in the circle always reminds me of a "potential space." Study Figure 4-16 for more examples:

When you aren't certain if a tiny initial deflection at the beginning of the QRS complex represents a q wave, look at the leads that follow to see if there is a progressive development of a q or Q.

Figure 4-17

PEARL | About 80% of wide complex tachycardias are VT, which means that about 70% of wide complex tachycardias are due to *scar-related VTs*. Most scar-related VTs are due to old myocardial infarction scars and most MIs occur in the left ventricle. What this means is: *that the majority of ventricular tachycardias that you will see will have an RBBB-like morphology in Lead V1. Since the majority of* idiopathic VTs occur in the right ventricle, *if you see an RBBB-like morphology in Lead V1 – think scar-related VT. If you see an LBBB-like morphology in Lead V1 think of two possibilities: benign idiopathic VT or lethal arrhythmogenic cardiomyopathy.*

Let's look at two deflections from wide complex tachycardias and determine the QRS morphology in Lead V1. Please use a magnifying lens if necessary.

Figure 4-18 is an **rS complex from Lead V1 with a notch in the upslope of the S wave.** It's important to note any notches in the R or S waves because that suggests a previous myocardial infarction and thus, a further indication of an ectopic origin (i.e., ventricular tachycardia). The scars left by an infarction provide an excellent substrate for a reentrant tachycardia.

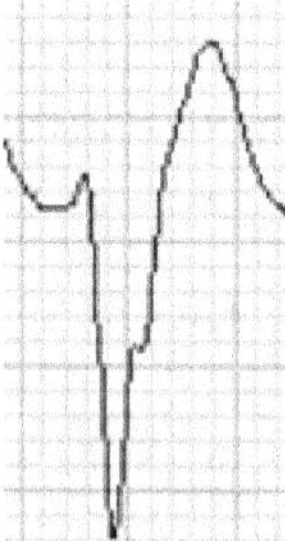

Figure 4-18

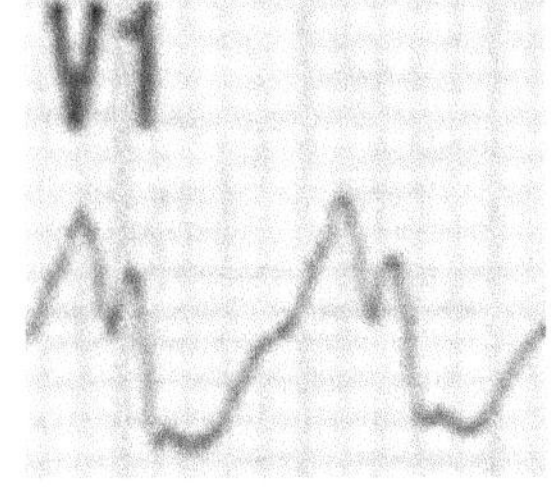

Figure 4-19

Figure 4-19 is a **monophasic R with a notched peak of the R wave.** Since this is from Lead V1, we are very interested in which peak is taller – the right or the left. In this case, the left peak is taller which is *very* suggestive of *ventricular ectopy* since it would be *extremely* unusual – if not impossible – for this to occur during a supraventricular rhythm with a right bundle branch block. If the right peak were taller *it wouldn't tell us anything* because ventricular ectopy (i.e., ventricular tachycardia) *can also present with a taller right peak* ("rabbit ear").

TIP | A taller LEFT rabbit ear rules <u>in</u> ventricular tachycardia, but a taller RIGHT rabbit ear does NOT rule it out!

Don't believe me? Look below... these are *all* from ventricular tachycardias (Figure 4-20):

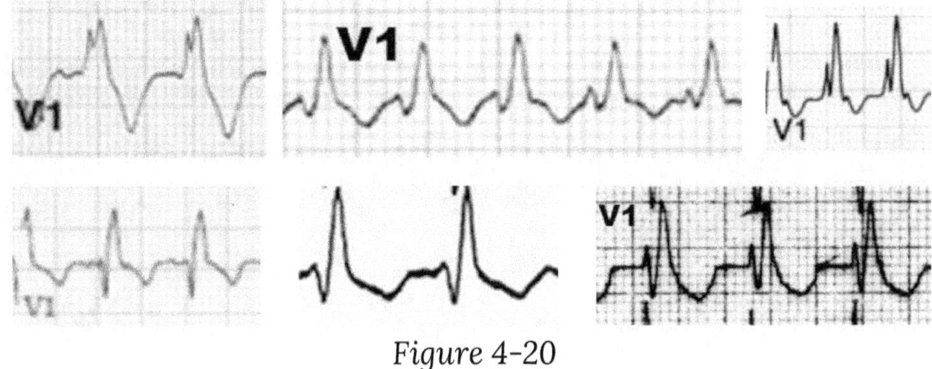

Figure 4-20

PEARL | Dr. Henry Marriott was the first to talk about the R wave peaks of RBBB-like morphologies in Lead V1 during wide complex tachycardias. Legend says that an ICU nurse had noticed it and drew his attention to it, calling the peaks "rabbit ears." While Dr. Marriott was the first to discuss the importance of a taller left peak, he was also the first to point out that ventricular tachycardias were *just as apt to have a taller right peak* – just like aberrant conduction. However, his words were quickly misinterpreted to imply that a taller right "rabbit ear" indicated aberrant conduction and ruled out ectopy. Dr. Marriott *never* said that!

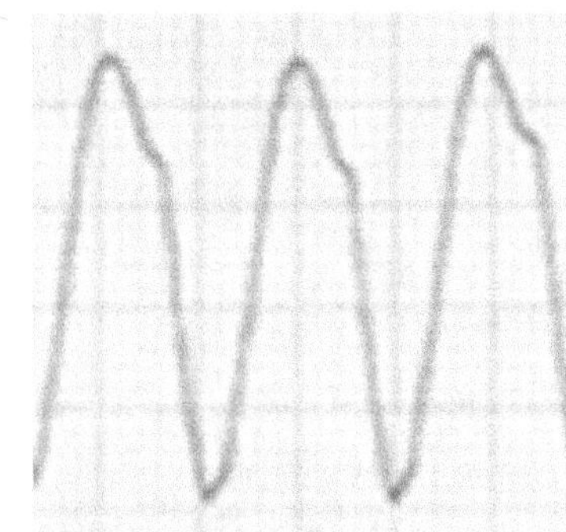

Figure 4-21

Figure 4-21 is not so easy, is it? This is a monophasic complex (no, that's *not* a tiny r wave before the negative deflection!), but is it a monophasic R wave with an inverted T wave – or is it a monophasic QS wave with an upright T wave? Here's a very important pearl:

PEARL | Repolarization is normally much longer than depolarization, but that isn't always evident during ectopic ventricular rhythms like VT in which a QRS may obscure the downslope of a T wave.

This complex (Figure 4-21, above) is a QS with an upright T wave.

TIP | It is a general rule in electrocardiography that "repolarization is proportional to depolarization." The area enclosed by the QRS should approximate the area enclosed by the T wave. This is based on the idea that the amount of myocardium that is depolarized would be the same amount that is repolarized. It doesn't work out that way exactly – but it's close!

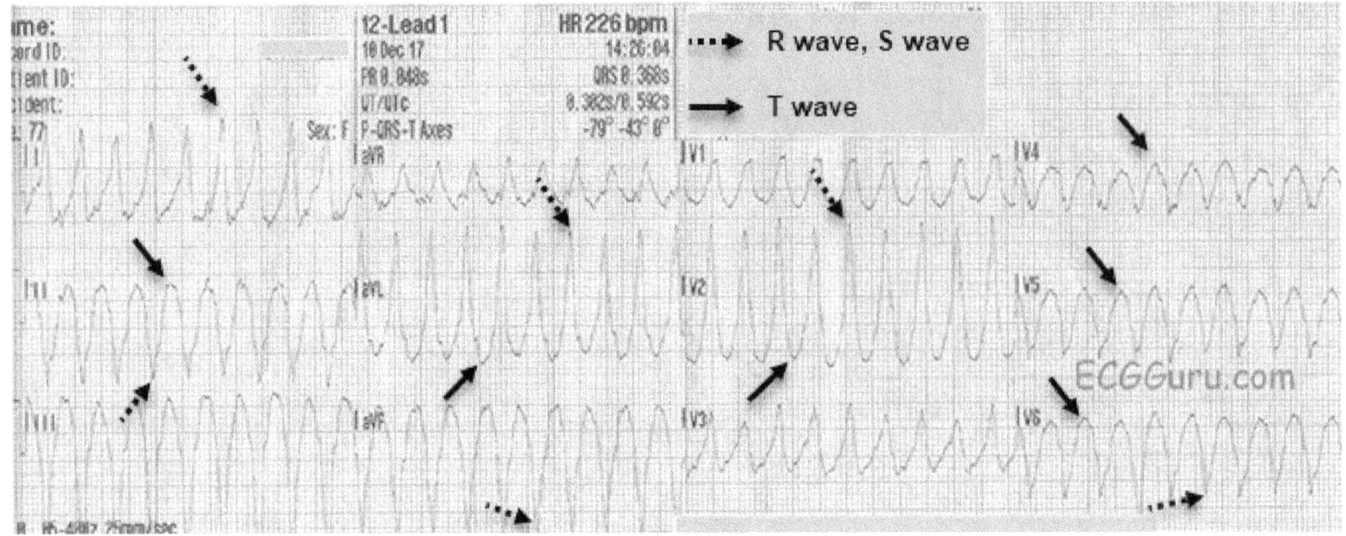

Figure 4-22

Here (Figure 4-22) is an excellent example of the difference in T waves (rounded, blunt) and R and S waves (sharper, more peaked). The dotted arrows indicate peaked R and S waves and the solid arrows indicate T waves (upright and inverted). This also demonstrates the finding that sometimes the "blunt" peak (T wave) can be a bit "sharper" and the "sharp" peaks (R and S waves) can be a bit more "blunt." The variation is subtle but not unusual.

These morphologies are *extremely common* in wide complex tachycardias, so learn them well and become very familiar with them! This book was written to enhance your ECG skills to the level that you will immediately recognize these deflections and not waste time trying to determine what they represent.

PEARL | A recurring theme in this book is that by studying the same examples again and again you will develop a greater familiarity with the morphologies faster. A pianist doesn't learn a concerto by playing a different piece of music every time he sits down to practice. You aren't going to develop a rapid recognition of these deflections by constantly looking at new ones *before* developing your expertise.

Chapter 5

QRS Morphology Recognition Practice

Determining Individual QRS Morphologies

ECG #1

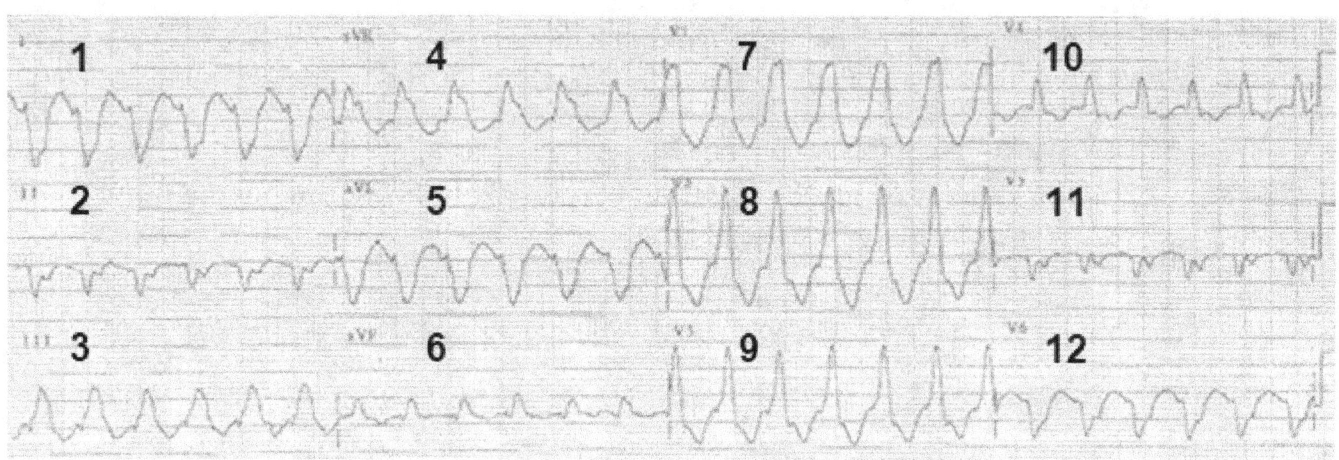

Indicate the QRS morphology for each Lead (numbered 1-12. Indicate the bundle branch morphology in Lead V1 (**RBBB-like** or **LBBB-like**).

❑ **RBBB-like**   ❑ **LBBB-like**

1 _____	4 _____	7 _____	10 _____
2 _____	5 _____	8 _____	11 _____
3 _____	6 _____	9 _____	12 _____

ANSWERS

1 – rS	4 – qR	7 – MR	10 – MR
2 – QS	5 – rS	8 – MR	11 – QS
3 – qR	6 – qR	9 – MR	12 - QS

MR = Monophasic R

ECG #2

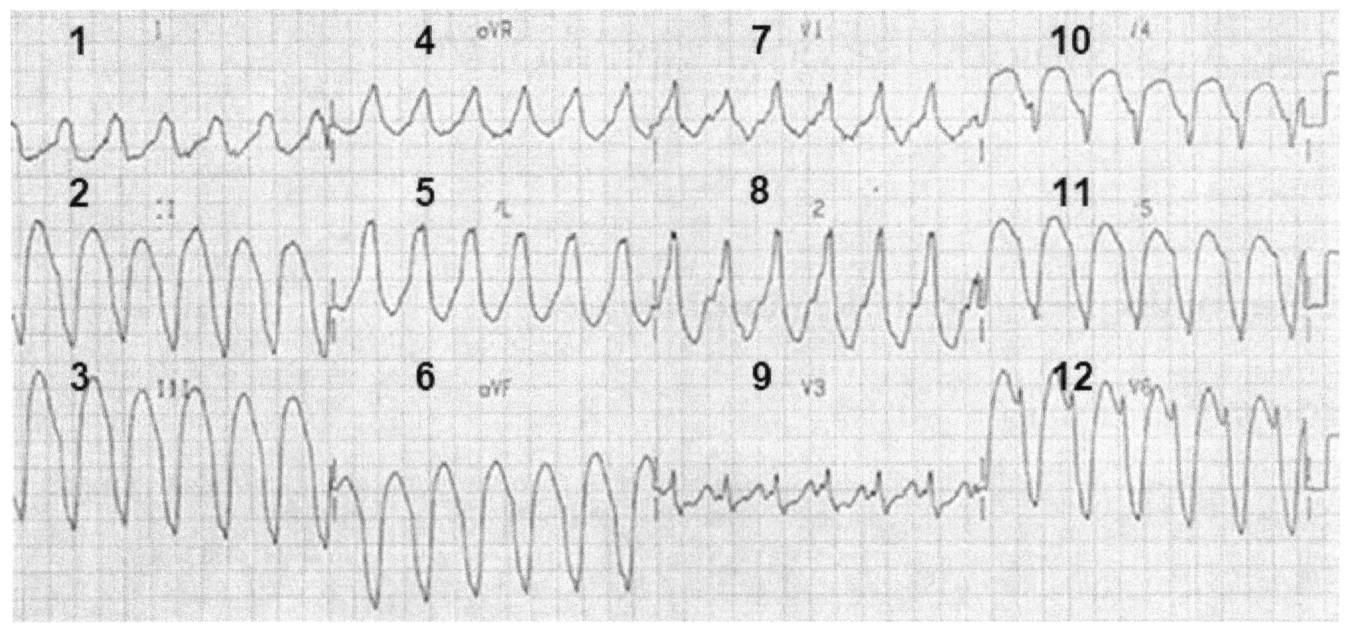

Indicate the QRS morphology for each Lead (numbered 1-12. Indicate the bundle branch morphology in Lead V1 (**RBBB-like** or **LBBB-like**).

❏ **RBBB-like**　　❏ **LBBB-like**

1 _____　　4 _____　　7 _____　　10 _____

2 _____　　5 _____　　8 _____　　11 _____

3 _____　　6 _____　　9 _____　　12 _____

MR = Monophasic R

1 – MR	4 – MR	7 – MR	10 – QS
2 – QS	5 – MR	8 – MR	11 – QS
3 – QS	6 – QS	9 – Rs	12 - rS

ANSWERS

ECG #3

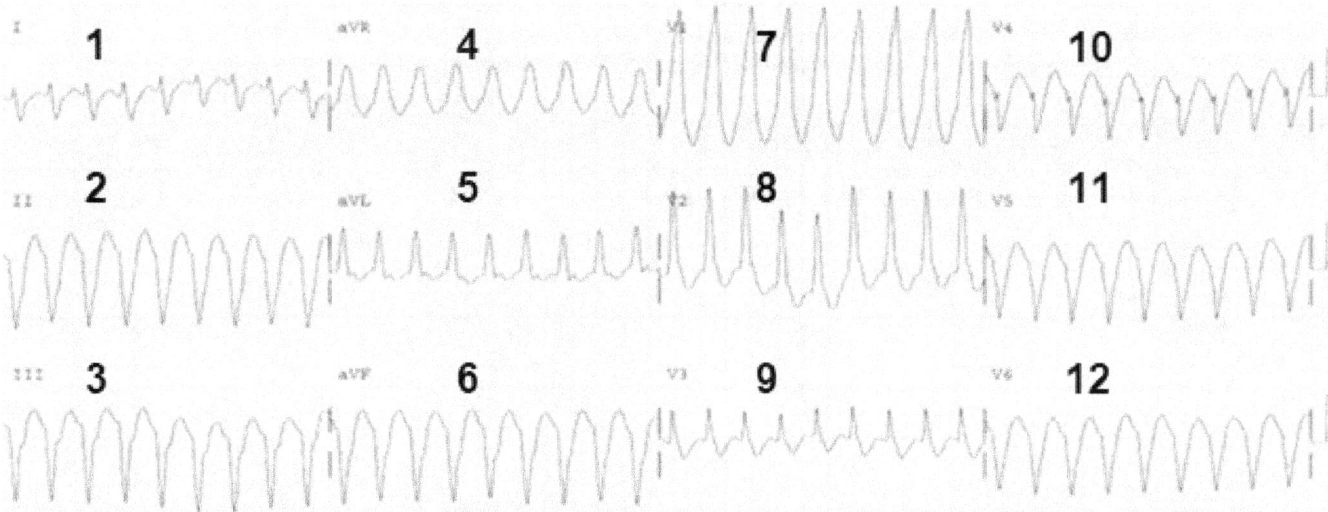

Indicate the QRS morphology for each Lead (numbered 1-12. Indicate the bundle branch morphology in Lead V1 (**RBBB-like** or **LBBB-like**).

❑ **RBBB-like**   ❑ **LBBB-like**

1 _____   4 _____   7 _____   10 _____

2 _____   5 _____   8 _____   11 _____

3 _____   6 _____   9 _____   12 _____

ANSWERS

MR = Monophasic R

1 – rS	4 – MR	7 – MR	10 – rS
2 – QS	5 – MR	8 – MR	11 – QS
3 – QS	6 – QS	9 – MR	12 - QS

ECG #4

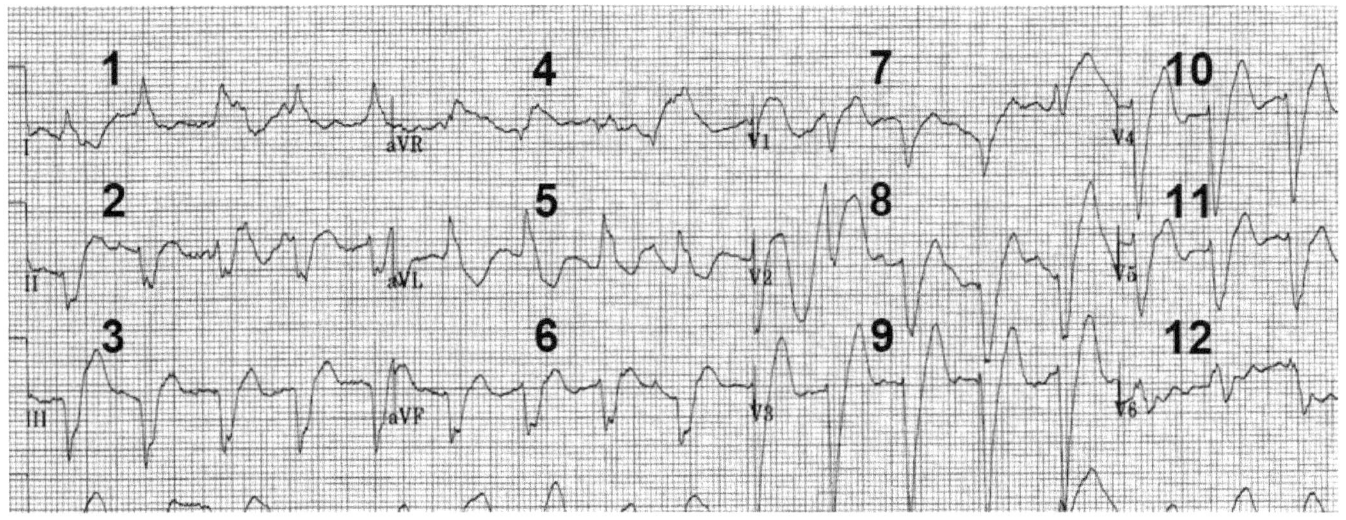

Indicate the QRS morphology for each Lead (numbered 1-12. Indicate the bundle branch morphology in Lead V1 (**RBBB-like** or **LBBB-like**).

❏ **RBBB-like**   ❏ **LBBB-like**

1 _____	4 _____	7 _____	10 _____
2 _____	5 _____	8 _____	11 _____
3 _____	6 _____	9 _____	12 _____

ANSWERS

1 – MR	4 – ?	7 – QS	10 – rS
2 – rS	5 – MR	8 – rS	11 – rS
3 – QS	6 – QS*	9 – rS	12 – rS

MR = Monophasic R

*It *could* be an rS.

ECG #5

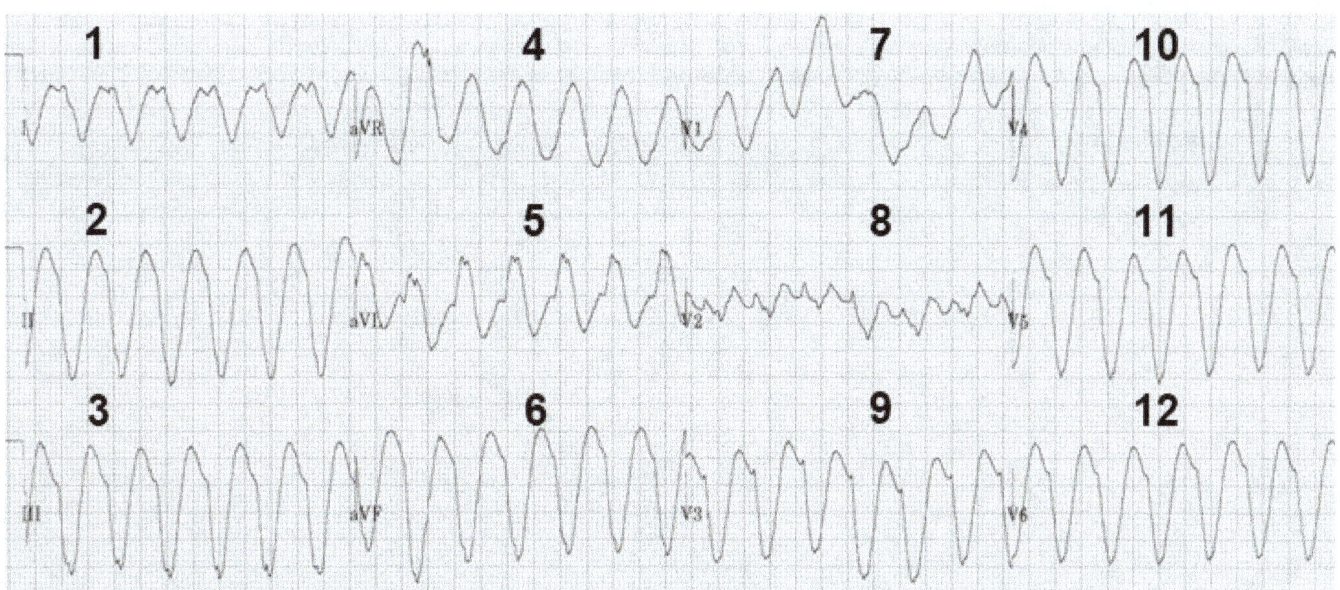

Indicate the QRS morphology for each Lead (numbered 1-12. Indicate the bundle branch morphology in Lead V1 (**RBBB-like** or **LBBB-like**).

❑ **RBBB-like**   ❑ **LBBB-like**

1 _____   4 _____   7 _____   10 _____

2 _____   5 _____   8 _____   11 _____

3 _____   6 _____   9 _____   12 _____

MR = Monophasic R

1 – rS	4 – MR	7 – MR	10 – QS
2 – QS	5 – MR	8 – rS	11 – QS
3 – QS	6 – QS	9 – rS	12 - QS

ANSWERS

Chapter 6

Localizing the Origin of a Ventricular Rhythm

We are going to assess four ECGs with wide complex tachycardias and see how much we can learn about them in just a matter of seconds. If you are still having difficulty recognizing the various morphologies, go back to Chapters 4 and 5 and review them. I can't impress on you enough that practice and familiarity will make this much, much easier for you.

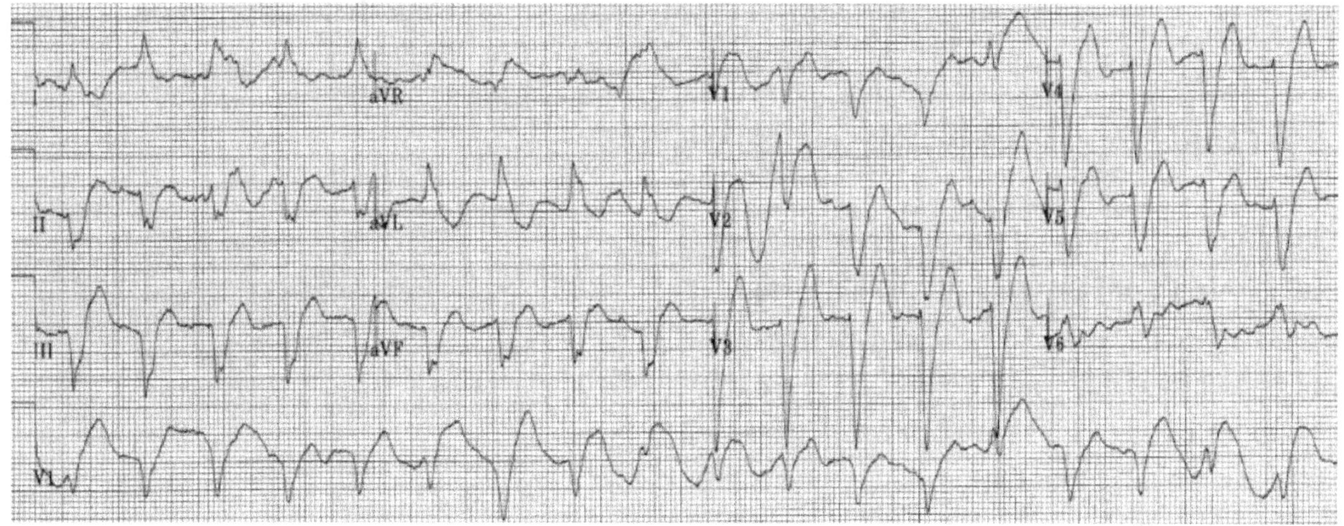

Figure 6-1

PEARL | Reviewing the *same* abnormal morphologies again and again will improve your recognition of them. It creates a familiarity with the forms that you may not achieve by looking at a lot of different morphologies. However, looking at different morphologies will eventually expand your knowledge and experience.

My approach with every wide complex tachycardia (and a stable patient) is very methodical. Let's take this step by step...

1

Always look at Lead V1 first to determine which ventricle is the source of the rhythm – whether it is aberrant or ectopic. If the QRS is POSITIVE, the origin is in the LEFT ventricle; if

NEGATIVE, the origin is in the RIGHT ventricle. LBBB-*like* means RIGHT ventricle; RBBB-*like* means LEFT ventricle. This QRS (Figure 6-1) – bizarre as it is – is NEGATIVE, so the site of origin of the tachycardia is in the right ventricle. If the QRS happens to be RBBB-*like*, then note the height of the R wave peaks: is there a taller left peak (left "rabbit ear")? If so, think "VT!"

2

Next, we want to know in which part of the ventricle the origin is located – the upper part (*outflow tract*) or the lower part (*apex*). Always remember TWO things:

OUTFLOW TRACT – GOOD!

APEX – BAD!

(I didn't know how to make it any clearer than that.)

> **PEARL |** Nothing *good* comes out of the APEX!

But how do we know if the origin is in the outflow tract or the apex? We use the *inferior leads* (Leads II, III, and aVF). At this point, most journal articles and textbooks begin talking about inferior and superior axes which tell us – in a most "roundabout" way – where the ectopic pacemaker is located.

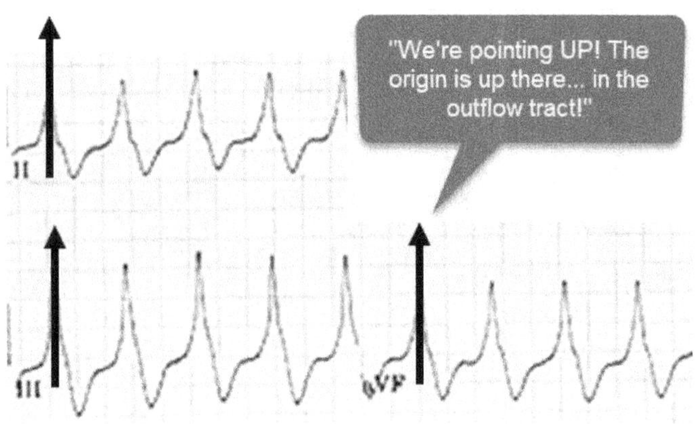

Figure 6-2

> **Roundabout |** Indirect, confusing and unnecessarily complex

There is a much easier way to use the inferior leads and it requires no thought at all: *just let the QRS complexes in the inferior leads <u>point</u> to the origin of the tachycardia. If there are tall R waves in the inferior leads, they are pointing UP to the superior part of the ventricle – the outflow tract. On the contrary, if there are deep S waves in the inferior leads, they are pointing DOWN to the lower ventricle, i.e. the apex.* This concept is equally applicable to both the right and left ventricles.

Now, don't misinterpret what I am saying. Tall R waves in the inferior leads indicate an impulse that is traveling downward TOWARD the aVF electrode on the left foot. But if the impulse is traveling DOWNWARD, then its origin must be located UPWARD... and **it's the location of the ORIGIN of the impulse that we are interested in – not its destination!**

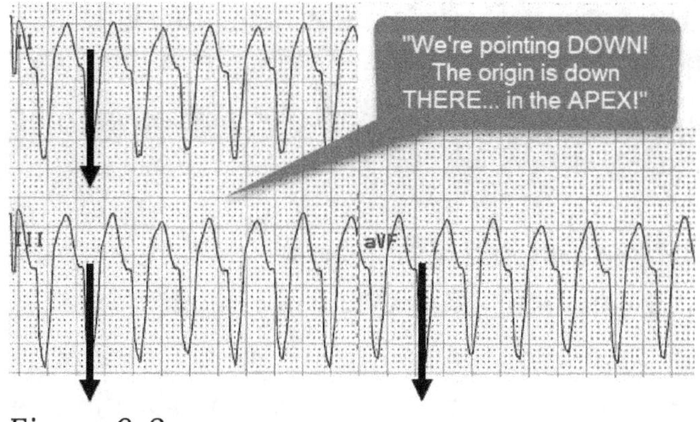

Figure 6-3

If the QRS complexes in the inferior leads are all deep S waves pointing DOWNWARDS, the ectopic pacemaker is located in the apex of the ventricle. This is NOT good news for the patient.

3

We can still go a bit further with this. It's possible we can determine *where* – within the apex – the ectopic focus is located: *free wall* or *septum?* This is where the *precordial transition* helps us. Impulses originating in the mid-to-lower right ventricle will have *late* precordial transitions – usually from Lead V4 through V6 and sometimes beyond.

Where is the transition on this ECG (Figure 6-1)? The QRS in Lead V6 appears roughly equiphasic, so in this case, the transition *point* and the transition *lead* are about the same! The transition *point* is where the R/S ratio = 1.0, i.e., the R wave height equals the S wave depth. The transition *lead* is the first lead with an R/S ratio ≥ 1.0. In most cases, the transition point falls *between* leads, so *for practical reasons*, we use the concept of the transition *lead*. The precordial transition on this ECG indicates an origin in the free wall of the right ventricle.

PEARL | Origins on or around the septum are closer to conducting fibers, so the QRS complexes tend to be thinner. Origins in or near the free wall of either ventricle are much further removed from conducting fibers, so the QRS complexes will tend to be wider.

Another PEARL | The further to the *right* the ectopic focus, the further to the *left* the precordial transition (and *vice versa*). An ectopic focus located on or very near the right side of the septum will have a precordial transition around V4. An ectopic focus located further to the right on the right ventricular free wall will have a transition around V6 or beyond. (Need to review? Revisit Chapter 1, Figure 1-30.)

Let's review...

1. Locate the ventricle with the ectopic focus.

2. Determine if the origin of the dysrhythmia is in the upper ventricle (outflow tract) or lower ventricle (apex).

3. If the precordial transition is around V4, the ectopic focus is on or near the right side of the ventricular septum. If the precordial transition is further to the left (i.e., later), the ectopic focus is in the right ventricular free wall. (The precordial transition is going to give us a little *surprise* in the next ECG!)

OK… look at the 12-lead ECG once more (Figure 6-1). You should be able to see that the ectopic focus is located in or near the free wall of the right ventricular apex. This is usually home to a very dangerous condition known as *arrhythmogenic cardiomyopathy* (formerly: arrhythmogenic right ventricular cardiomyopathy). In this condition, the ventricular myocardium is gradually replaced by islands of fat and fibrous tissue – the perfect substrate for dangerous scar-related ventricular tachycardias.

Let's look at another ECG (Figure 6-4)…

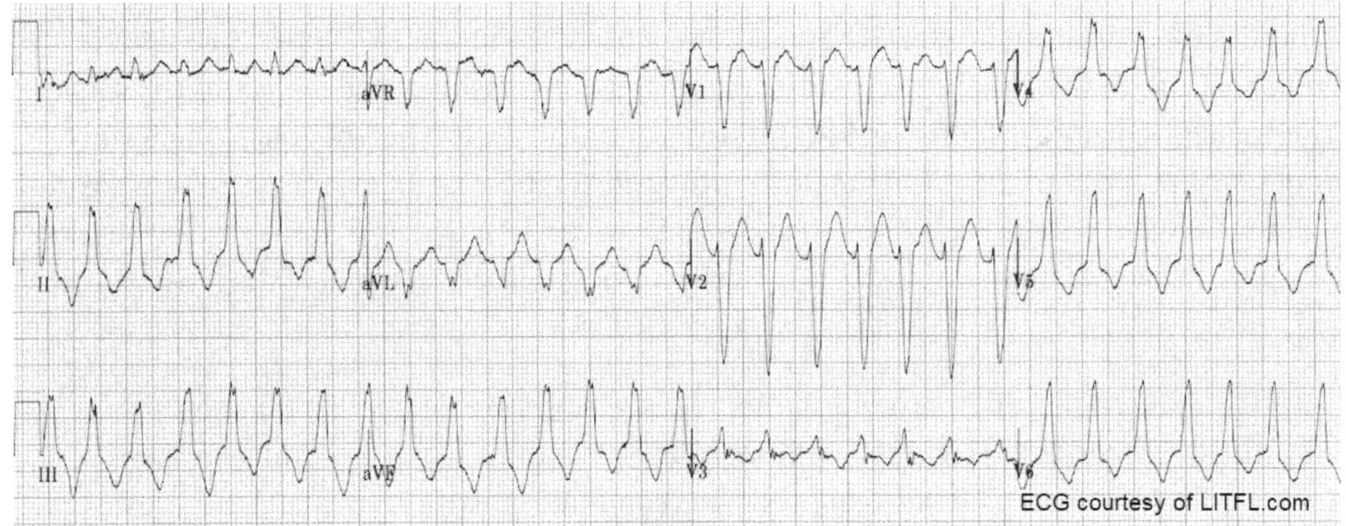

Figure 6-4

1. In which ventricle is the origin located?

2. Where in the ventricle – upper (outflow tract) or lower (apex)?

3. Is the ectopic focus near the septum or more laterally in the free wall?

This tachydysrhythmia is a ventricular tachycardia. But doesn't it look more like a regular left bundle branch block (LBBB)? Note the morphology of the first part of the QRS – smooth straight lines. Also, note the width (duration) of the QRS complexes – 120 msec! That is *not* wide for ventricular tachycardia! This tachycardia developed in or very, very near conducting tissue. Rather classic!

Discussion...

1. There is a LEFT bundle branch block pattern – quite classic – so the ectopic focus is in the right ventricle.

2. All the QRS complexes in the inferior leads are tall R waves pointing UP to the upper part of the right ventricle – *the outflow tract*. The ectopic focus is in the outflow tract (and that's *good* news for the patient!).

3. The precordial transition has occurred between Leads V2 and V3. Wow! What a surprise! That's *very early* for an impulse originating in the right ventricle. Most precordial transitions involving a focus in the right ventricle begin around Lead V4 and point further on to the left. But remember from your anatomy lesson in Chapter 1: the upper part of the right ventricular outflow tract is no longer separated from the left ventricular outflow tract by the thick, muscular septum. In the uppermost portion of both outflow tracts, the septum is reduced to a relatively thin, membranous wall (Figure 6-5). It is in this part of the outflow tract that the right ventricular outflow tract wraps around the base of the aorta and becomes *more leftward* than the left ventricular outflow tract. That's right! At this point, the RVOT is on the *left* and the LVOT is on the *right*. Now it's a bit more understandable why the precordial transition of an ectopic focus in the upper RVOT (white "X," Figure 6-5) may look more like it's originating in the left ventricle based on the precordial transition.

The black arrows (Figure 6-5) demonstrate the thinning of the interventricular septum as it curves to the left with the leftward extension of the right ventricular outflow tract. The uppermost part of the RVOT is to the left of the lower RVOT (and also much of the LVOT), which likely contributes to the uncharacteristically *early* precordial transition for a right-sided ectopic focus.

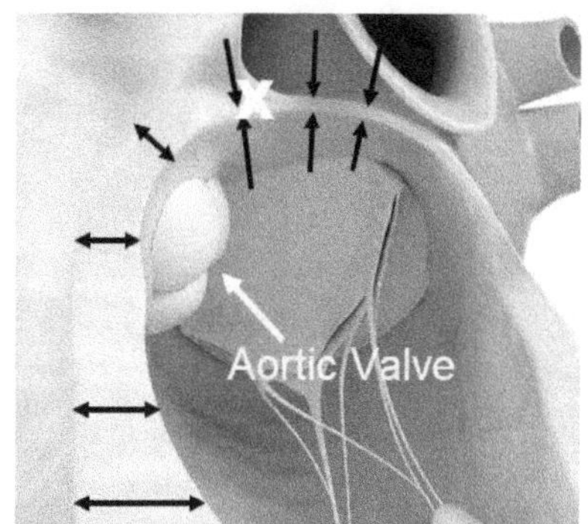

Figure 6-5

PEARL | It always helps to know the anatomy of the heart. Do you recall which structures the upper, basilar area of the septum is near? How about the end of the bundle of His just before it divides into the right and left bundle branches? An impulse there can immediately enter one or both bundle branches causing near-simultaneous activation and resulting in a narrower QRS complex. What else is very close? The annulus of the aortic valve. Aortic valve calcifications or para-aortic abscesses can easily disrupt AV conduction at this point by causing pressure on the His bundle.

Here are two more 12-lead ECGs that you can use for practice...

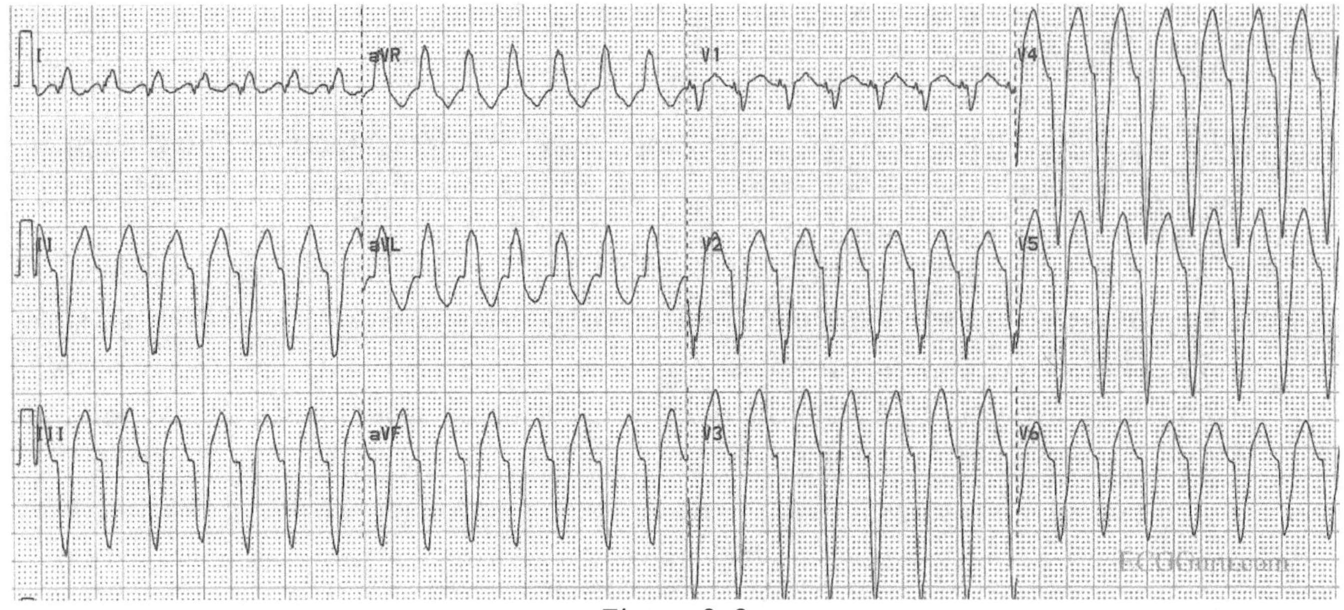

Figure 6-6

1. In which ventricle is the origin located?

2. Where in the ventricle – upper (outflow tract) or lower (apex)?

3. Is the ectopic focus near the septum or more laterally in the free wall?

Use the space below to record any notes.

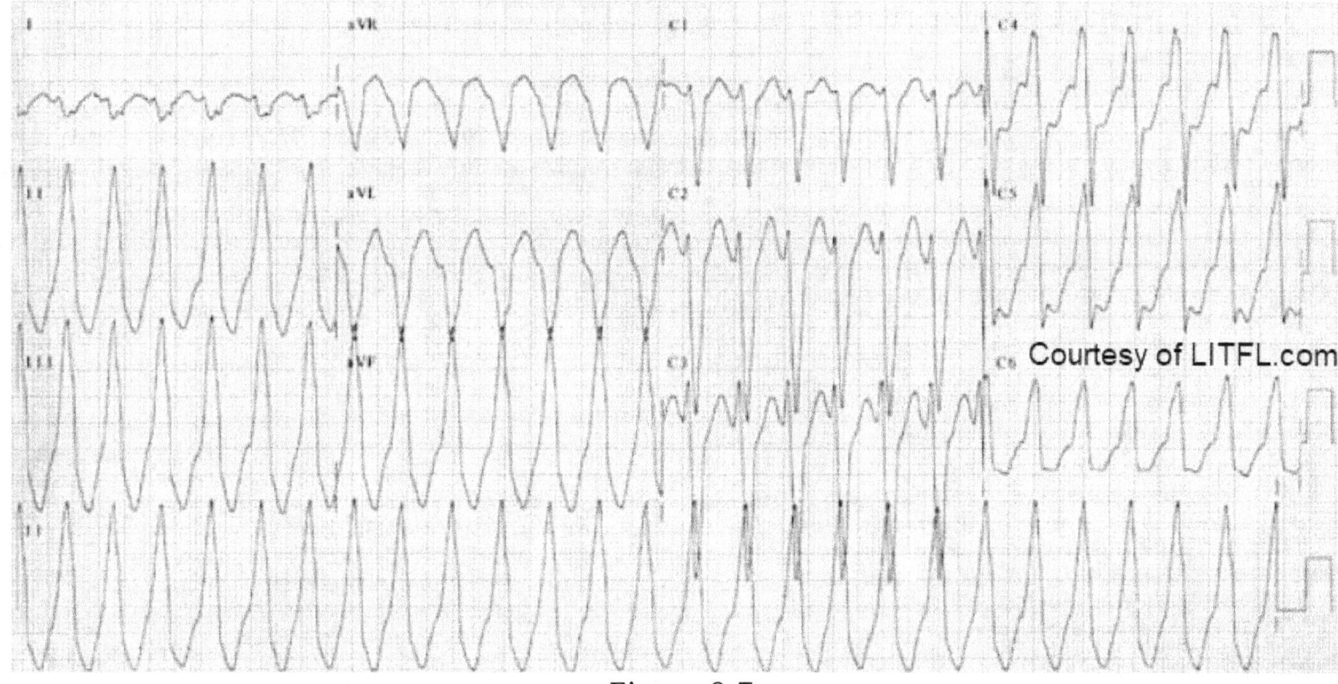

Figure 6-7

1. In which ventricle is the origin located?

2. Where in the ventricle – upper (outflow tract) or lower (apex)?

3. Is the ectopic focus near the septum or more laterally in the free wall?

Use the space below to record any notes.

Chapter 7

Demonstrate Your Knowledge and Progress

Here are a few questions and tasks just to see how much you have learned so far.

For each of the snippets, designate whether the arrow is pointing to an **R wave**, an **S wave**, or a **T wave** (T waves may be inverted or upright).

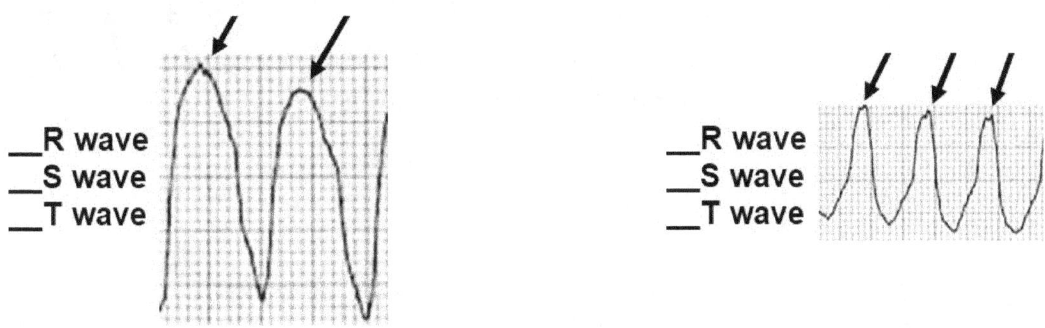

Figures 7-1 and 7-2

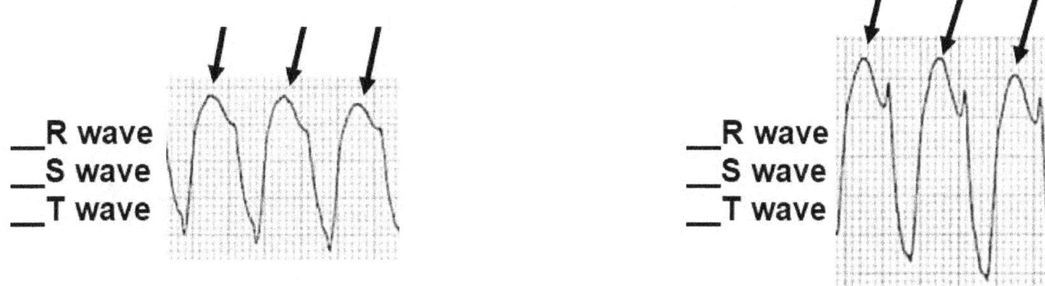

Figures 7-3 and 7-4

Figures 7-5 and 7-6

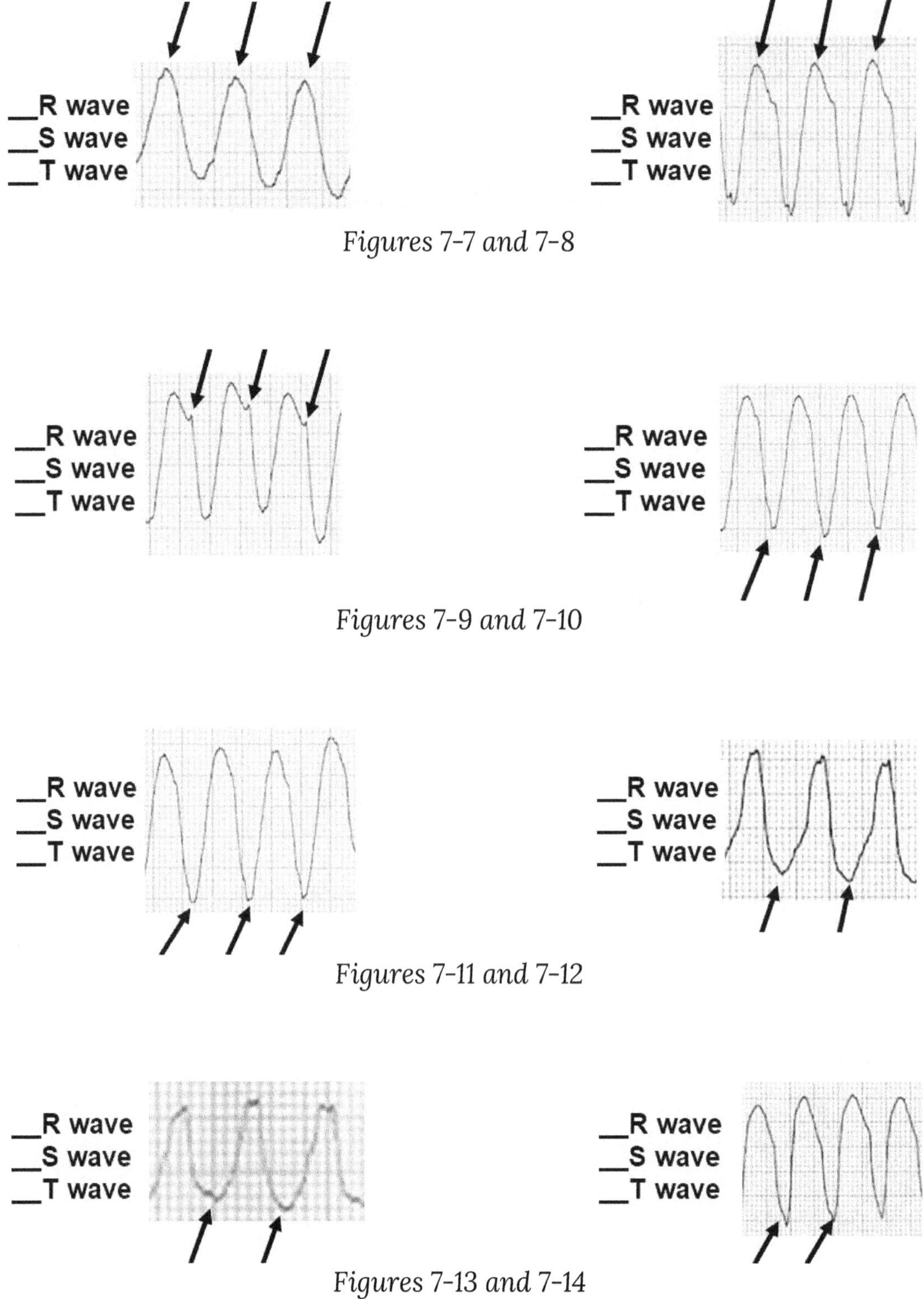

Figures 7-7 and 7-8

Figures 7-9 and 7-10

Figures 7-11 and 7-12

Figures 7-13 and 7-14

(Figure 7-15) Is there an S wave present in this snippet?

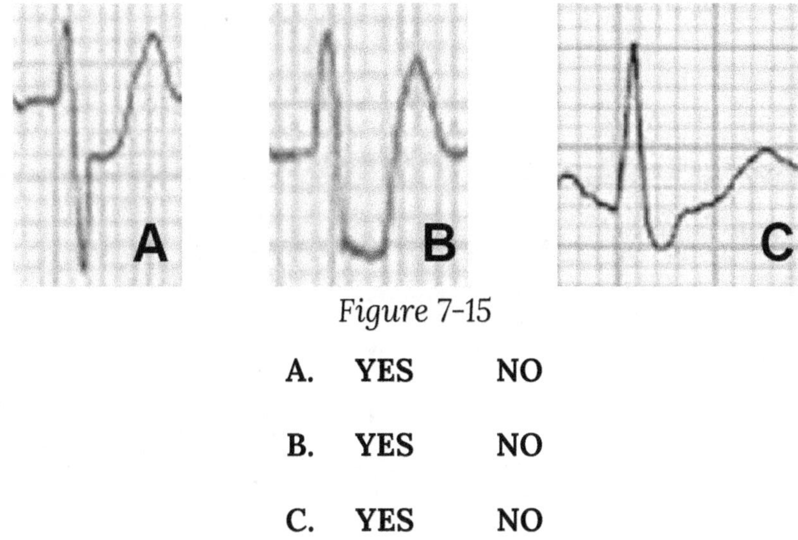

Figure 7-15

A.   YES   NO

B.   YES   NO

C.   YES   NO

(Figure 7-16) Is the arrow indicating an S wave or a T wave?

This is Lead V1 and it is from a ventricular tachycardia. Do you notice anything else unusual about this snippet?

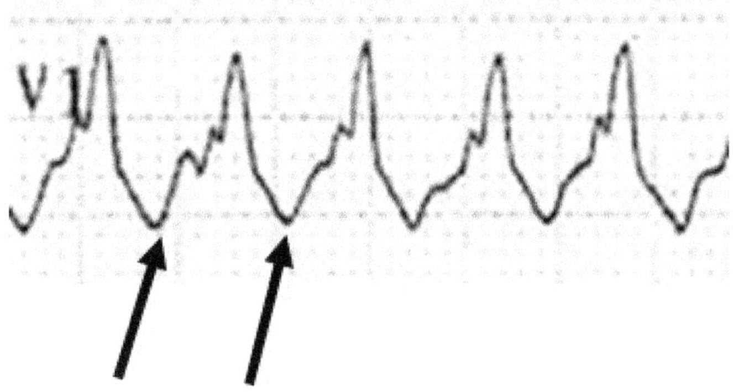

Figure 7-16

Select the correct QRS morphology.

A. Monophasic R
B. Monophasic QS
C. rS
D. rSR'

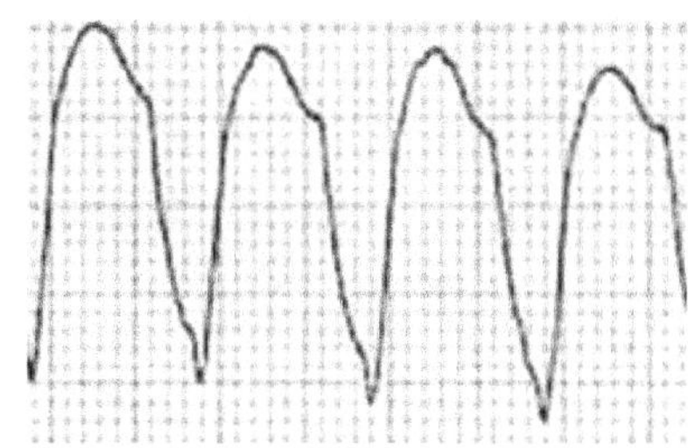

Figure 7-17

A. Monophasic R
B. Monophasic QS
C. rS
D. rSR'

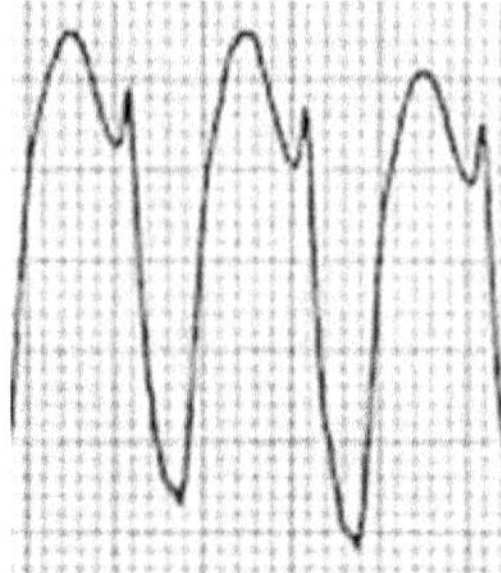

Figure 7-18

A. Monophasic R
B. Monophasic QS
C. RS
D. rSR'

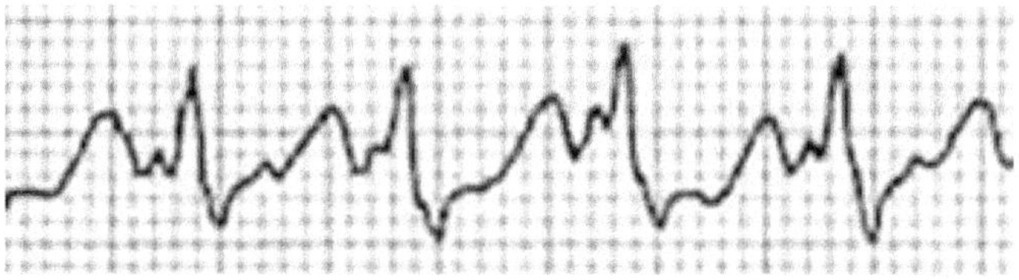

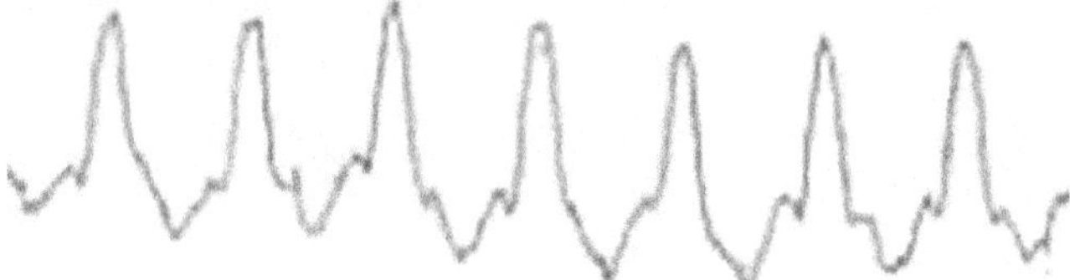

Figure 7-19

A. Monophasic R
B. qR
C. RS
D. RsR'

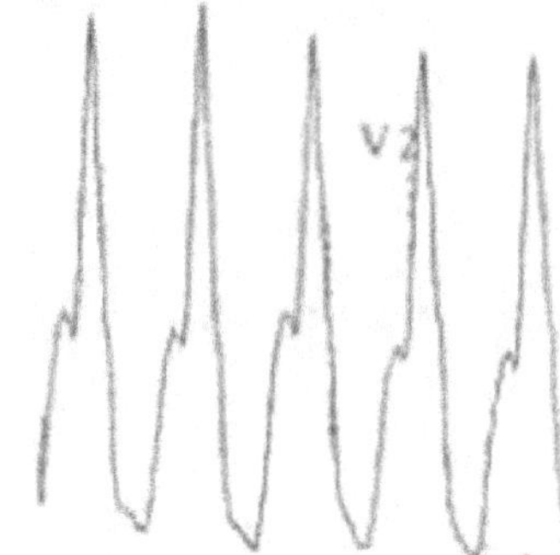

Figure 7-20

A. Monophasic R
B. Rs
C. qRS
D. qR

Figure 7-21

What is the morphology of this QRS? What other valuable information does it provide?
A. Monophasic R
B. rS
C. Rs
D. qR

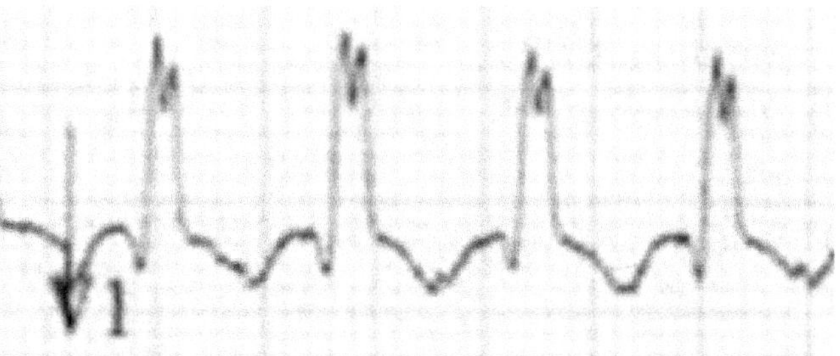

Figure 7-22

What is the morphology of the QRS complexes in the following snippets?

A. Monophasic R

B. Monophasic QS

C. RS

D. Rs

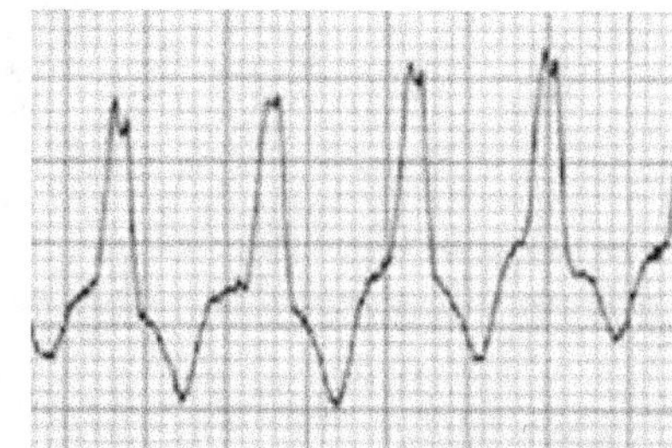

Figure 7-23

A. Monophasic R

B. Monophasic QS

C. RS

D. Rs

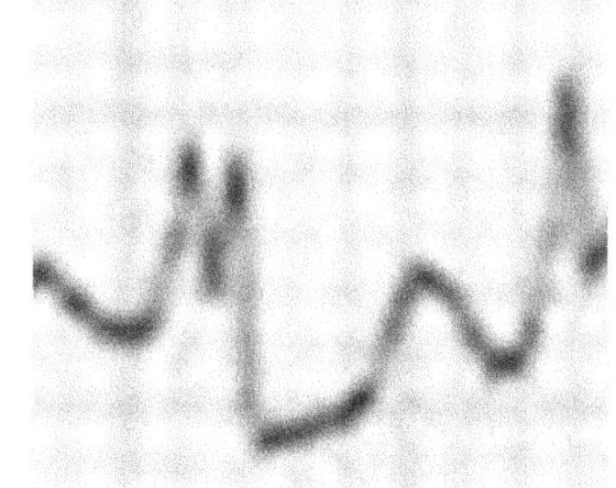

Figure 7-24

A. Monophasic R

B. Monophasic QS

C. RS

D. Rs

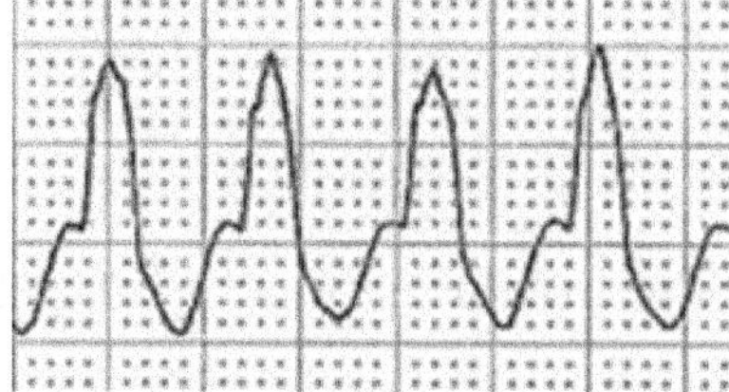

Figure 7-25

Answers

7-1: T

7-2: R

7-3: T

7-4: T

7-5: R

7-6: r

7-7: R

7-8: T

7-9: r

7-10: S (QS)

7-11: S (QS)

7-12: T

7-13: T

7-14: T

7-15: A – YES; B – NO; C – YES

7-16: T (Probable P wave at first arrow; VT with taller right peak in V1)

7-17: B

7-18: C

7-19: C

7-20: B

7-21: D

7-22: D (Taller left peak)

7-23: A

7-24: A[*]

7-25: A (Evidence for small q is not consistent)

*The presence of a deep notch in an R wave does not create a second R wave. Although some authors may refer to the second peak as an R', it is still a *notched monomorphic R wave.*

The notch between the two peaks must return completely to the baseline for the second peak to be considered a true R' wave. The notch does not have to extend *below* the baseline, however; there is no requirement for an S wave between the two deflections.

A Bit More About QRS Morphology

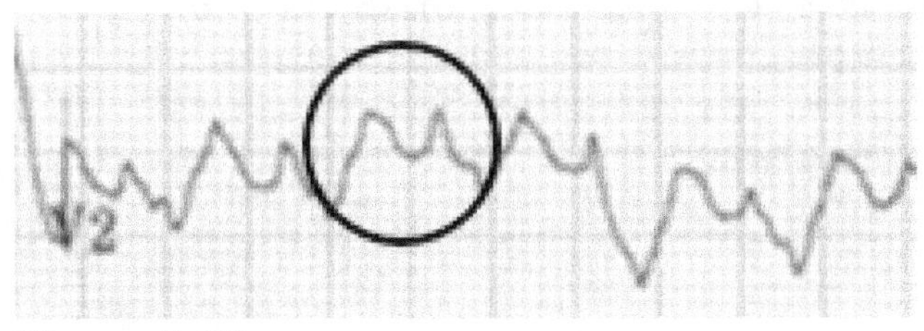

Figure 7-26

Let's look at Lead V2 (Figure 7-26). What are some hints about this lead that would help us decipher it more easily? Generally, there are only two sizable *positive* deflections in a tracing of a wide complex tachycardia: the R *wave and an upright T wave*. Of course, you will occasionally see P waves, but they will be very small and very infrequent.

> **PEARL |** *The T wave is usually wider at the level of the baseline than the R wave or QS wave.*

If you see positive deflections of two different widths, try interpreting with the idea that *the narrower positive deflection is the R wave*. In this lead, we see positive deflections of two different widths: one is wide and the other is narrower and more pointed. Let's assume the narrower one is the R wave and the wider one is the T wave. We are going to check ourselves by using our straight edge and a little common sense. By now you should be able to easily see the tiny r wave in Lead V3 of Figure 7-27 (below).

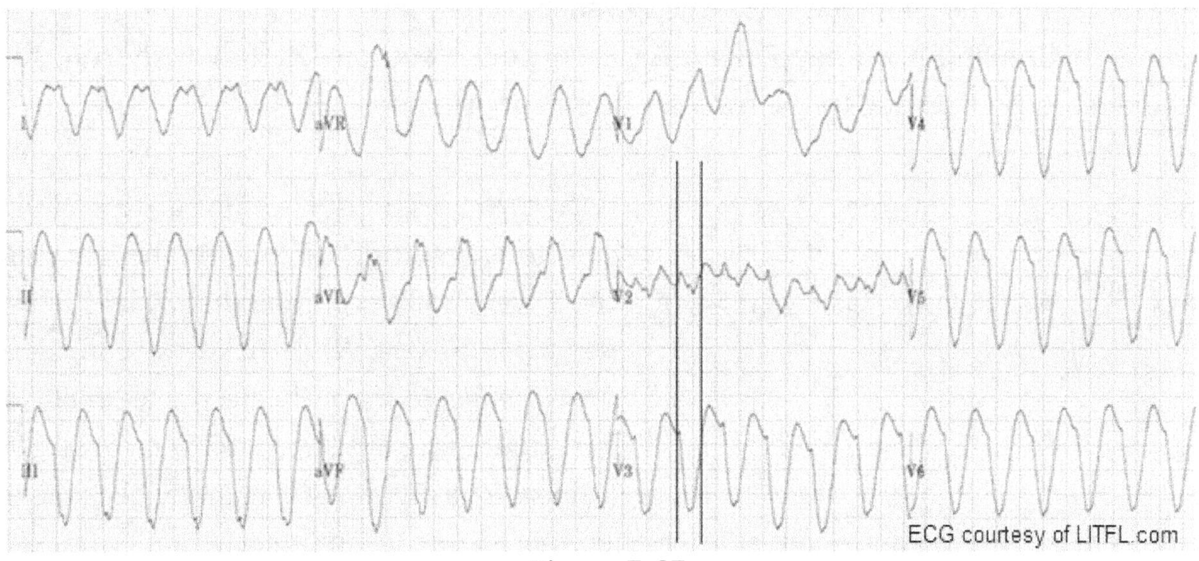

Figure 7-27

Align your straight edge with the beginning of that r wave and follow it to Lead V2 to see where the QRS complex starts. We now have to determine where the QRS complex *ends*. To do this, we will *make a general assumption* that the end of the QRS complex in Lead V3 is *directly across the baseline* from that little r wave. The reason I say "general" assumption is that this is without considering the possibility of ST elevation or depression. Mark that point near the end of the upslope of the S wave, then move your straight edge over there to find the end of the QRS complex in Lead V2. Were we correct in assuming the more narrow deflection was indeed an R wave? We chose correctly and the lines even indicate an RS complex.

There's also an *intuitive* way to determine this...

There are TWO positive (upright) deflections on this snippet (Figure 7-28) – one is WIDE and the other is visibly NARROWER. When the two upright deflections appear next to each other, the WIDE one always precedes the NARROW-ER deflection with no intervening *negative* deflection. But when the NARROWER deflection precedes the WIDE deflection, it is always separated from the WIDE deflection by a *negative* deflection. The WIDE deflection is a T wave and the NARROWER deflection is an R wave.

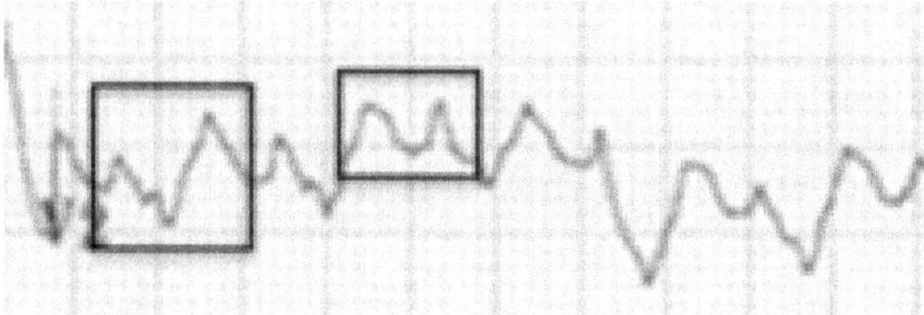

Figure 7-28

> **PEARL |** During a wide complex tachycardia, both *supraventricular tachycardia with aberrancy* and *ventricular tachycardia*, have *repolarization abnormalities.* Therefore, there cannot be two R waves immediately adjacent to each other (except for a *rare RR'*) and there cannot be an upright T wave following an R wave without an intervening S wave. Although that is common – even usual – during sinus rhythm, it doesn't happen during a ventricular ectopic rhythm or aberrantly conducted rhythm due to the repolarization abnormality.

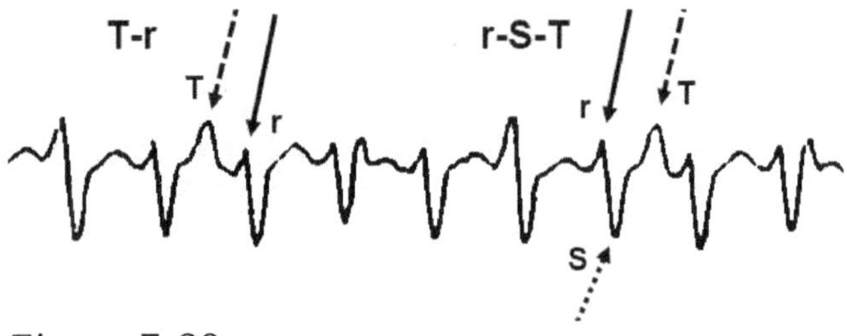

Figure 7-29

If the two upright deflections do appear adjacent to each other, the one on the left *must* be the T wave followed immediately by the R wave (Figure 7-29, **T-r**). While an R wave can encroach on a T wave, *when a T wave immediately follows an R wave during ventricular tachycardia, it must have an opposite polarity* because of the required repolarization abnormality. If not, then there *must* be an intervening S wave (Figure 7-29, **r-S-T**). Exception: acute ischemia may result in a primary repolarization abnormality in which the T wave will have the same polarity as the last deflection of the QRS complex.

> **PEARL |** Under most circumstances, the earlier the precordial transition, the further to the left the ectopic focus is located. Ectopic foci in the upper part of

the right ventricular outflow tract can have uncharacteristically early precordial transitions (Lead V3 or between Leads V2 and V3).

Chapter 8

Confusing and Problematic QRS-T Morphologies

The "Terrible Twelve"

The "Terrible Twelve" are twelve of the most common and sometimes most problematic QRS morphologies that you will encounter in wide complex tachycardias. Study them closely so that when you encounter them on an ECG you will not have to stop and try to decipher what they are. The more familiar you become with these iconic morphologies, the more rapidly wide complex tachycardias will resolve from what initially appears to be nothing but chaos and confusion.

1. (Figure **8-1**) This morphology looks almost like a sine wave. But it's either a *monophasic R wave with an inverted T wave* or a *monophasic QS wave with an upright T wave*.

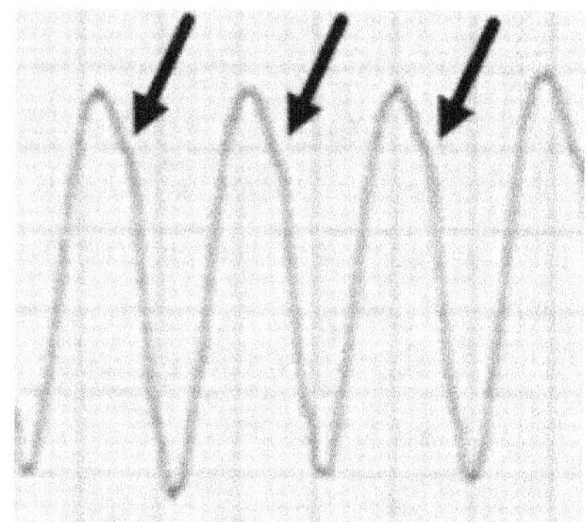

Figure 8-1

> **PEARL |** Ectopic ventricular beats and aberrantly conducted beats *always* have repolarization abnormalities, so the T wave is always opposite the last major deflection of the QRS.

> **TRICK |** It is best to try to define the T wave first. Remember: a QRS complex does not have to have an R wave or an S wave, but *it must be followed by a T wave*. There will ALWAYS be a T wave.

> **PEARL |** T waves tend to have more rounded peaks (or nadirs) than R waves or QS waves.

The deflections at the bottom of this ECG snippet (Figure 8-1) appear to have a subtle but sharper nadir than the peak of the upright deflections. So these are monophasic QS waves with upright T waves. Look closely... do you see how the tops of these deflections are slightly more rounded than the bottoms?

Now where is the baseline? About 4 or 5 small squares from the top you should see a subtle change in slope in each descending line (arrows). Connect these areas and you will have found the (presumed) baseline.

2. (Figure **8-2**) I will tell you that this QRS con- 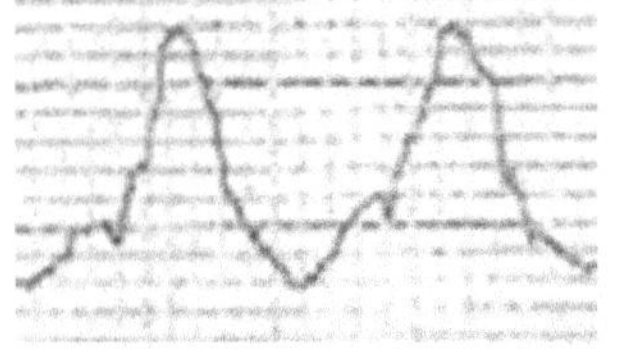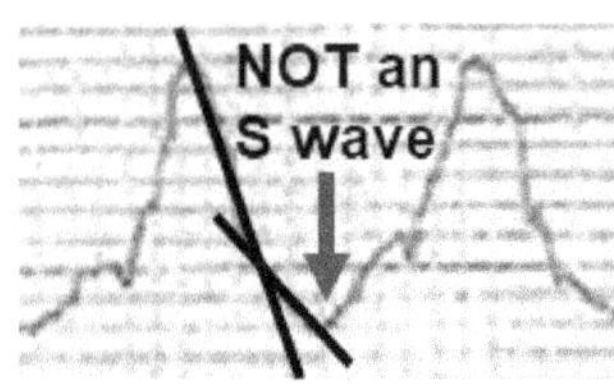
sists of a small q wave and a very wide R wave.
The T wave is inverted. To find the baseline, just
connect the tops of all the little q waves. That
portion below the baseline is not an S wave – it's

Figure 8-2

an inverted T wave. There are only two *major*
deflections of this QRS complex (not including the small q wave) and one of them *must* be
a T wave. When ectopy originates outside the conducting system, the QRS will be followed
by a repolarization abnormality. That means that if the QRS is a monophasic R wave, then
the T wave will be *inverted*; conversely, if the QRS is a monophasic QS wave, then the T
wave will be *upright*. While this is certainly characteristic of ventricular tachycardia, it is
also characteristic of antidromic conduction through an accessory pathway and SVTs with
aberrancy. So, the presence of a repolarization abnormality does not help in distinguishing
VT from SVT with aberrancy.

Also, note how *wide* and *bizarre* these monophasic R waves appear in Figure 8-2! Those
impulses originated far *outside the conduction system.*

3. (Figure **8-3**) This morphology causes a lot of con- 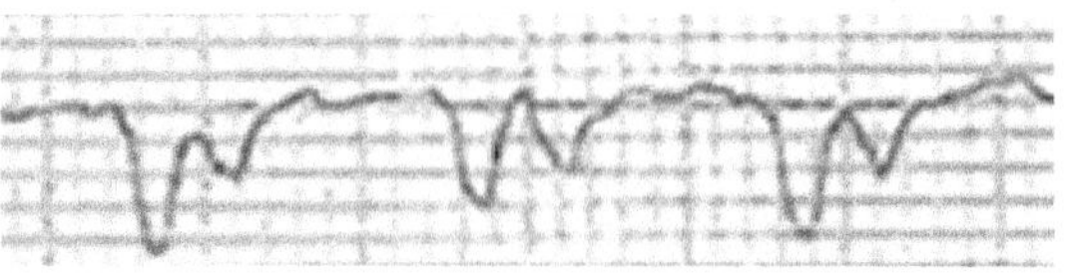
fusion for some. What is it? Let me tell you what it is
not: it is *not* a QS wave followed by an inverted T wave.
It is simply a *notched* QS. What makes this even more
confusing is a T wave that is almost isoelectric. If you

Figure 8-3

look at the baseline following the third QS you will see a small T wave. There is a little bit of
baseline wander in this snippet, but the notch never actually breaches the baseline.

> **TIP |** An S wave is not a separate deflection from an R wave – they *both* are record-
> ings of the *same* depolarization impulse. The difference is not in the deflections –
> the difference is in the perspective of the recording electrodes.

4. (Figure **8-4**) This morphology causes most of its confusion during the first step of the Brugada Algorithm. Is this an rS or a QS complex? The response to the first step ("Is there a lack of RS complexes in all precordial leads?") depends on how you identify this complex. Here's how you determine the answer: remember that each deflection on an ECG – including each deflection *within* a QRS complex – each Q, each R, and each S – is a *vector*. A vector must have *direction*, in this case its *polarity* – positive (upright) or negative (inverted). It must also have *magnitude* – the "area

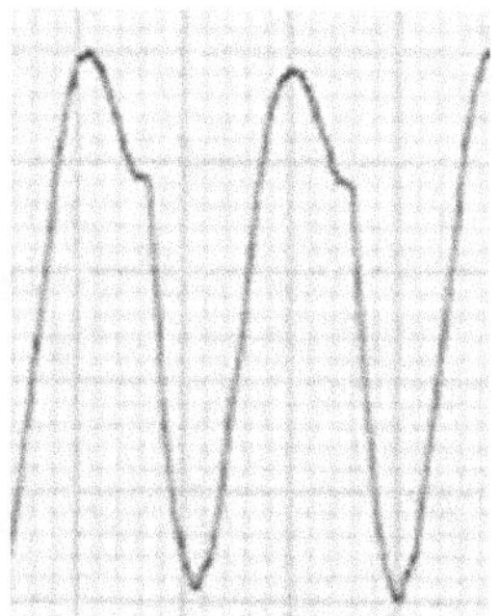

Figure 8-4

within the *deflection*" which consists of its *upslope*, its *downslope*, and the *baseline*. In this snippet, if we enclose the large *negative* deflection using the baseline, we see a considerable amount of area within that deflection. OK... now try doing that with what appears to be an r wave just before the negative deflection. You can't. There is no upslope to that bit of irregularity near the baseline. Therefore, *it is not a vector* and, consequently, *it is not an r wave*. What you are seeing in this snippet is a QS wave. But be very careful here! Let's take a look at a similar QRS morphology:

5. (Figure **8-5**) This may look very similar to you, but it looks very different to me! This is a true rS complex. Look at the tiny r waves just before the deep S waves. They all have an upslope and a downslope even though they are very small. If the baseline were to act as the third side (base) then there would be a definite area enclosed there. That means it is a *vector* and, consequently, a *true deflection*.

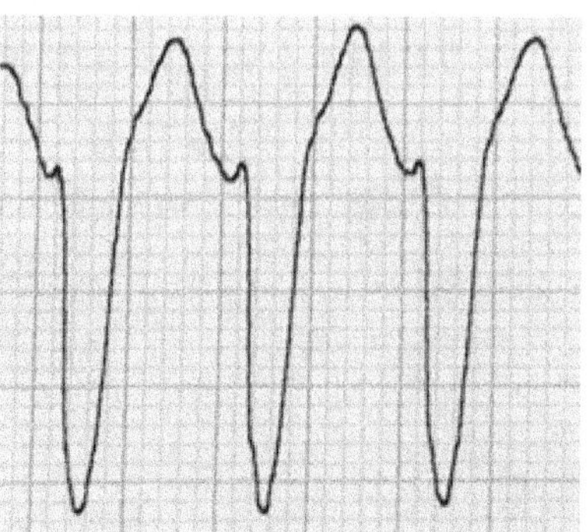

Figure 8-5

Here are the differences enlarged (Figure 8-6)...

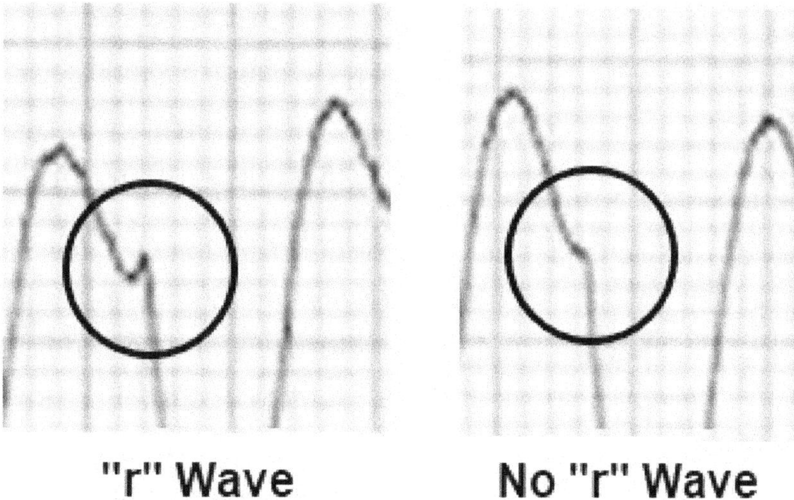

Figure 8-6

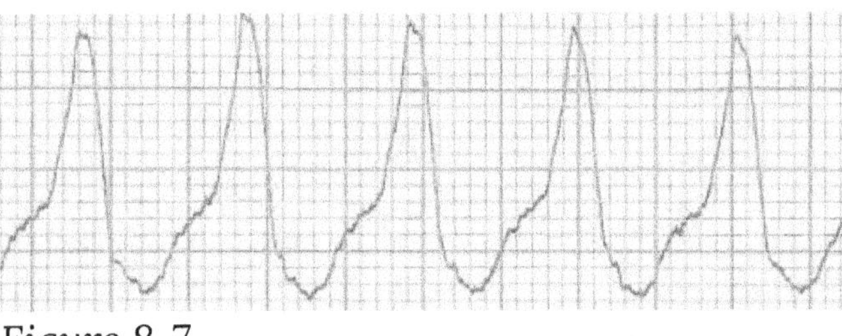

Figure 8-7

6. (Figure **8-7**) This QRS morphology should be very obvious to you by now but a lot of people still fail to recognize it. This is a *monophasic R wave with an inverted T wave.* That negative deflection is *not* an S wave. If that were an R wave and an S wave – how many deflections would be present? There would be TWO deflections present – the R wave and the S wave. But aren't we forgetting something? Where is the T wave? Remember: you don't have to have an R wave and you don't have to have an S wave, but you must *always* have a T wave.

TIP | The S wave is normally the last deflection of a QRS complex. If you think you see an "S wave," then you *must* identify the T wave that follows it!

PEARL | While a T wave cannot interrupt an R wave, an R wave can interrupt a T wave leaving it only partially visible. That's why some QS waves appear huge while the T waves appear disproportionately small – it's because you aren't seeing all the T wave!

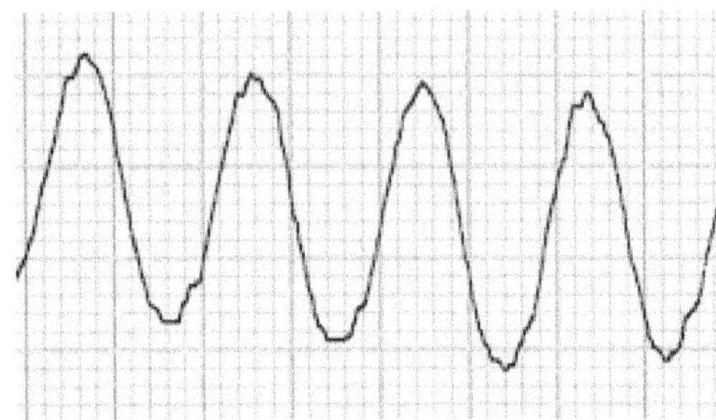

Figure 8-8

7. (Figure **8-8**) OK... what's the first thing we look for when deciphering these difficult QRS morphologies? T waves! And where is the T wave in this snippet? The very first thing that should have caught your eye here is that there are only TWO deflections – so one of them MUST be a T wave! That just leaves two choices: a monophasic R wave with an inverted T wave or a monophasic QS wave with an upright T wave.

Now let's look closely at these two deflections. Remember that T waves are usually more rounded at their peak or nadir. So which deflection is more rounded? It's a very close call, but the negative deflection is more rounded; therefore, I would consider this a monophasic R wave with an inverted T wave. The peak of the upright deflection is bifid (two small peaks). I cannot tell you what that represents other than that the peak of a monophasic R wave with an LBBB-like morphology is frequently notched. T waves do not manifest *consistently* bifid peaks during wide complex tachycardias. They can, however, present with *occasional* bifid peaks when AV dissociation is visible and there is a P wave hiding in there. LQTS 1 and hypokalemia can also present with bifid T waves, but only during sinus rhythm – not during a polymorphic ventricular tachycardia (more about *that* later).

> **TRICK: "The 4 mm Rule" |** Here's a trick I devised years ago. It has never been validated, but it has certainly helped me to determine the morphology of a biphasic wide complex QRS. I call it the "4 mm Rule." Count down 4 mm (that's 4 small squares) from the peak of the upright deflection and 4 mm up from the nadir of the inverted deflection. Assess the widths of the deflections at that point. The wider one is more likely to be from the T wave.

For some of these rhythms, it is obvious that the patient will be very unstable. Of course, electrical cardioversion will be the first step after a very brief assessment of the patient. However, if a 12-lead ECG has already been recorded, you should be able to interpret it quite well.

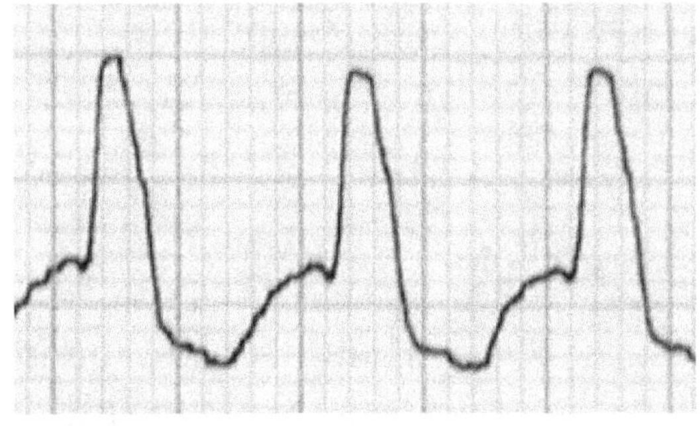

Figure 8-9

8. (Figure **8-9**) This is not a monophasic R wave – it is a qR complex with a depressed ST segment and an inverted T wave. A q wave is a Q wave no matter its size. While the size of a Q wave is used to distinguish septal q waves from pathological Q waves (during sinus rhythm), size never disqualifies a q wave from being designated as a q wave. And it is *never* "OK" to intentionally overlook a small q wave for the purpose of considering a QRS complex as a monophasic R wave. In sinus rhythm, a qR complex in Lead V1 may indicate a critical right ventricular strain. During a wide complex tachycardia, however, a qR complex in Lead V1 may indicate a specific type of left ventricular outflow tract tachycardia. Here is another example of a qR complex:

This one (Figure **8-10**) is a bit more obvious but often dismissed or overlooked because of the irregularity in the recorded tracing. These are qR complexes. Know them when you encounter them! You should not have to spend any time analyzing them.

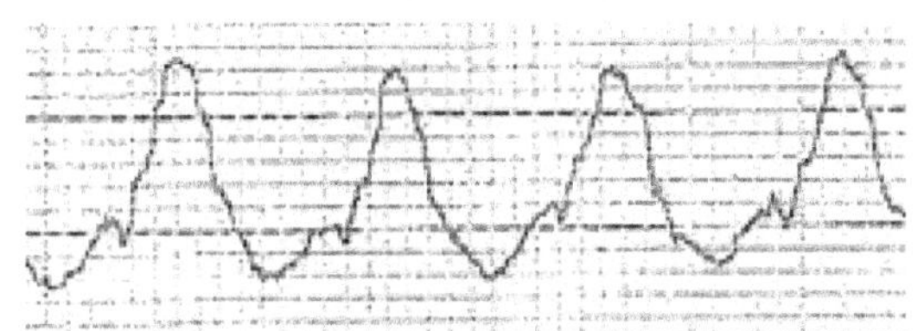

Figure 8-10 (same as Figure 8-2)

> **TIP |** Although during sinus rhythm a tiny q wave in Leads I, aVL, V5, and V6 may indicate normal initial conduction in the left ventricle, that does not apply to ectopic ventricular rhythms. Any Q wave is abnormal.

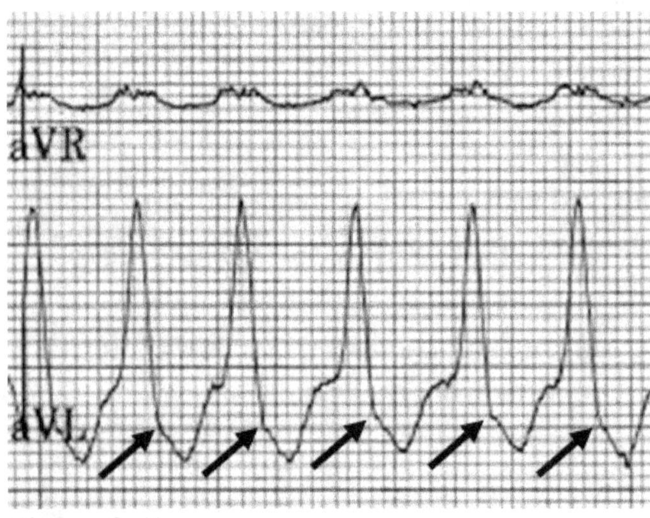

Figure 8-11

9. (Figure **8-11**) Once again, there is an impossible-to-identify QRS morphology in Lead aVR, so we are going to have to depend on the QRS complexes in Lead aVL to help us out. The onset of the QRS in Lead aVL is obvious. But this time the end of the QRS in Lead aVL is also clearly visible. This snippet of aVL represents a morphology that can be very confusing if you don't know what to look for and how to interpret it. This is an R wave followed by an inverted T wave.

The arrows indicate the end of the QRS and the beginning of the T wave – *below* the baseline. If this were sinus rhythm, we would be very concerned about an ST depression of 3 mm (normally, we only allow 1 mm of ST depression at the onset of a secondary repolarization abnormality). However, this ST depression occurred *during a tachycardia* and it is never advisable to diagnose ischemic ST depression *during* a tachycardia. Such ST depressions often resolve the instant the tachycardia is terminated. Note the abrupt change in slope at that point.

This is a very complex morphology (aVL) with a lot of teaching points.

First, at times there appears to be a small q wave adjacent to the R wave; but this is not found consistently because in some complexes, in the same lead, the "q" wave is not there at all and its morphology is not reproduced in others. I suspect that it is just an artifact and would not consider it a deflection.

Second, just because the downslope of the R wave goes beneath the baseline does not automatically make it an S wave. Remember: *all deflections* – including S waves – *are vectors*. For an S wave to qualify as a true deflection, it must satisfy the rules for vectors:

    1. it must have *direction* (its polarity) and

    2. it must have *magnitude* (an area within the deflection).

For a deflection to be considered an S wave, *it must at least begin its ascent to the baseline before the onset of the T wave* (Figure 8-12). This will provide an area within the deflection which will satisfy the second rule for vectors. It does not have to reach the baseline before merging into the upstroke of the T wave (which *can* begin below the baseline).

Sometimes S waves can be *slurred* and look very similar to the inverted T wave in this snippet of Lead aVL (Figure 8-11).

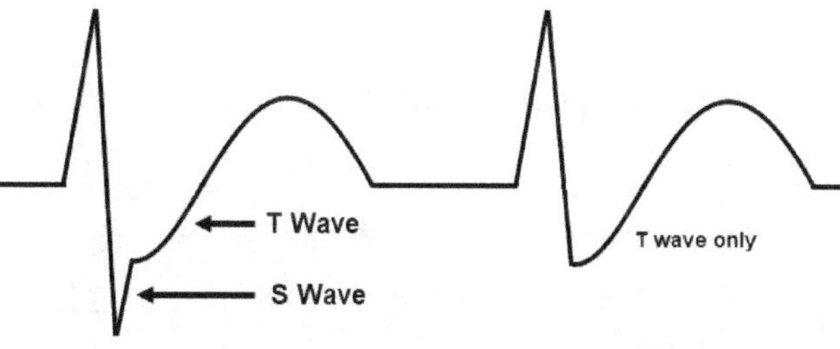

Figure 8-12

PEARL | For a deflection to be considered an S wave, it must at least begin its ascent to the baseline before the onset of the T wave. This will provide an area within the deflection.

Here is an example:

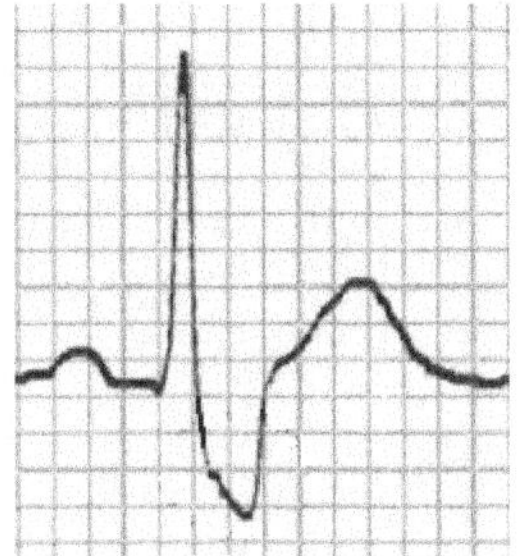

Figure 8-13

10. (Figure **8-13**) In this snippet, which looks very similar to those in the snippet of Lead aVL above, notice how the change in slope is not abrupt but rather gradual – a smooth curve. This is typical of a *slurred S wave*. And, of course, *there is an obvious T wave following it.* The presence of a P wave tells us that this is not an ectopic ventricular rhythm, but it's the QRS morphology that is important here!

PEARL | Don't confuse S waves with the ST segment. The ST segment begins at the *end* of the QRS – whether it's an R wave or an S wave. The S wave is *never* part of the ST segment. The ST segment represents Phase 2 of the action potential which is *repolarization;* an S wave represents Phase 0 – *depolarization!*

Compare Figure 8-13 above with the snippet in Figure 8-14. You should be able to identify the onset of the QRS as well as its end (you've seen this snippet before, but we are going to take a much closer look now!). Here's the difference: the inverted T wave looks very much like the slurred S wave above. How do we know that it's not an S wave? Because there is no clear indication of an S wave turning upward toward the

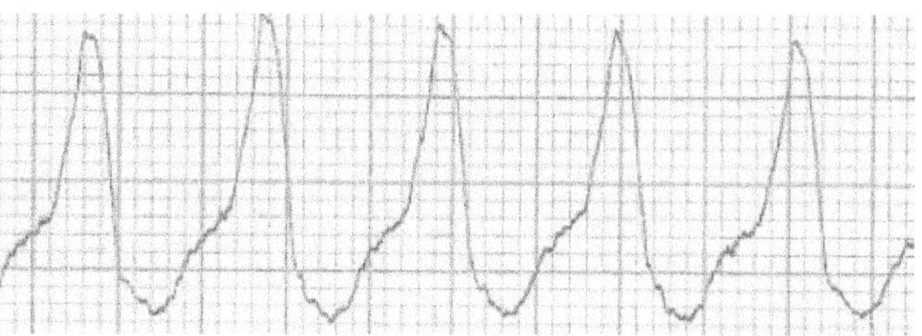

Figure 8-14

baseline. There is only one inverted deflection turning upward to the baseline. Once again, ask yourself, "How many deflections are present?" There are just TWO deflections present so one of them MUST be a T wave. Which is it – the *inverted* deflection with the *rounded* nadir or the *upright* deflection with the *pointed peak?* T waves are more likely to be rounded at their peaks or nadirs, so the inverted deflection is the T wave and the upright deflection with the pointed peak is a monophasic R wave. (Remember the 4 mm Rule.)

PEARL | Since the S wave is *generally* the last deflection of the QRS, *if you think you are seeing an S wave then you MUST identify the T wave following it!*

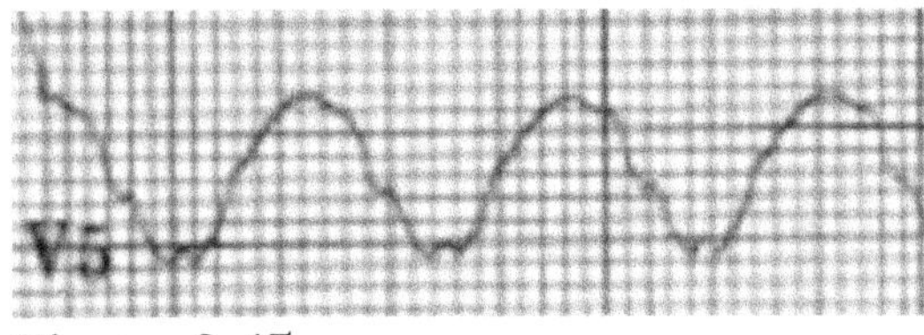

Figure 8-15

11. (Figure **8-15**) Another sine wave morphology that looks more like a true sine wave than anything we've seen so far! Again, you would seek help from the leads printed above and below V5. But there's a special message this snippet is sending us, and while we look for the baseline at the top or bottom of a deflection, some-times it is located in the middle! If you look in the middle of the downslope of each QRS you will see a small notch that appears consistently in the same location. Our best option would be to connect those notches with a line and designate that line as the baseline, at least initially.

PEARL | Don't diagnose ventricular flutter from a single lead rhythm strip un-less the ventricular rate is above 250 beats/minute and preferably close to 300/minute. Some of the "sine wave" appearing deflections are from ECGs in which other leads had relatively well-formed QRS complexes. Ventricular flutter will look about the same in every lead. The rhythm in Figure 8-15 may look very ominous... but the heart rate is only 130. It's possible other leads may have well-formed QRS complexes (Yeah, I agree... probably not!); but it's always best to see the 12-lead ECG before making a decision.

REMEMBER! | A heart rate of 130 does *not* rule out **hyperkalemia** as a cause of the wide complex tachycardia!

12. (Figure **8-16**)

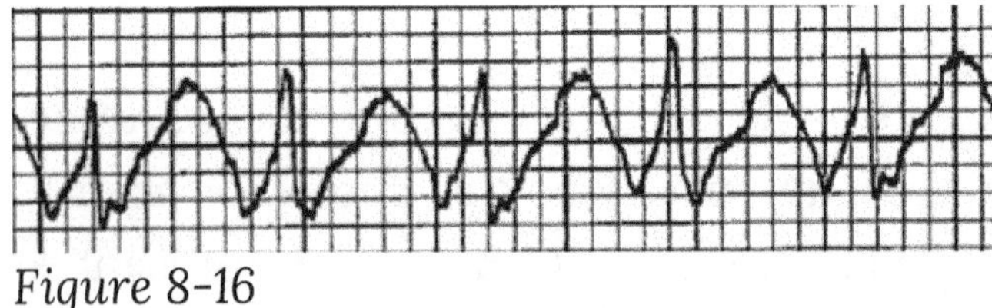

Figure 8-16

You will see this QRS morphology occasionally and there's no need to waste time trying to decide if it is a QRS followed by an upright T wave or an RS with the appearance of a Q wave caused by the fact that the QRS complex begins on the end of the T wave. Neither lead gives us a solid hint regarding the location of the baseline. Fortunately, I have another ECG with the same morphology in which there is a momentary pause in the tachycardia (Figure 8-17) that gives us an answer:

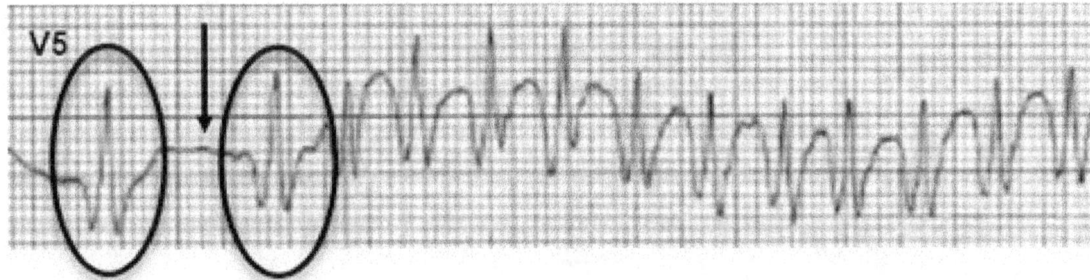

Figure 8-17

This pause has *multiple teaching points*:

First, these are NOT capture beats. A capture beat must appear BEFORE the next expected QRS based on the tachycardia rate. In other words, **the QRS of the capture beat must terminate an R-R interval that is SHORTER than the R-R interval of the predominant rhythm**, i.e., the tachycardia.

Second, the arrow is pointing to a sinus P wave that has conducted.

Third, we can see that the QRS complexes during the pause in the tachycardia are the same as the QRS complexes during the tachycardia itself.

Fourth, the morphology is indeed a true qRs, and

Fifth, it should now be apparent that the baseline may shift during a tachycardia (like THIS one, Figure 8-18). Let's take a closer look:

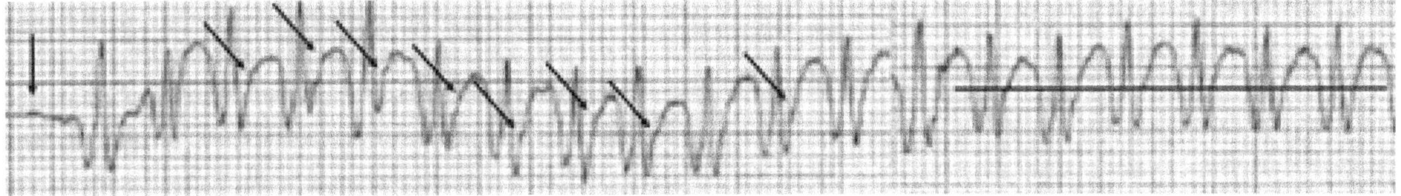

Figure 8-18

QRS complexes that look the same during the tachycardia as they do in sinus rhythm are very supportive of an SVT with aberrancy, but they can also occur during a bundle branch tachycardia (Chapter 18). But there's one last thing to think about: the little notches that the arrows are pointing to in Figure 8-18 – could they also represent retrograde P′ waves? Quite possibly!

> **PEARL |** P waves or P′ waves seen during a wide complex tachycardia are often much, much smaller than you would expect. Sharpen your eyes and look for them very carefully!

Let's take a closer look (next page):

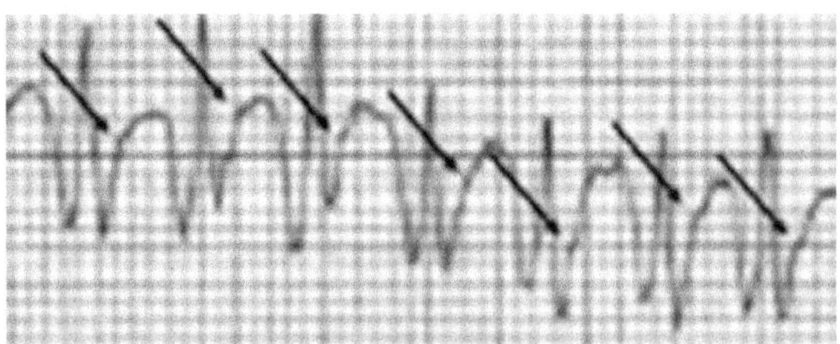

Figure 8-18 enlarged

TIP | Bundle branch tachycardia is the only ventricular tachycardia that may present with the same bundle branch block morphology as in sinus rhythm.

The Faux Twins

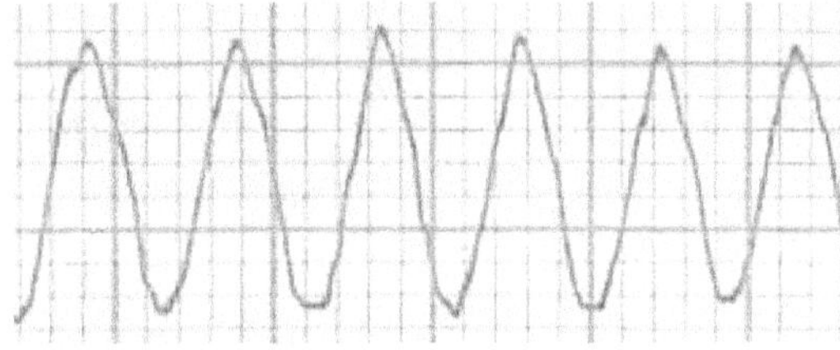

Figure 8-19

Look at this snippet on the left (Figure 8-19). How quickly can you determine the morphology here? Is it a QS complex with an upright T wave or a monophasic R wave with an inverted T wave? If it is a bit of a struggle for you now, don't worry. I think it will be easier by the time you finish this section – The Faux Twins! Two QRS-T morphologies will need some extra practice. These *look the same* – yet they are *quite opposite!* And when confronted with a wide complex tachycardia, you shouldn't have to spend much time trying to decipher and label these deflections.

Some of these snippets are – I admit! – from cases that would likely require *immediate cardioversion*. DON'T SKIP OVER THEM! Use them to sharpen your eyes to these morphologies.

Faux Twin #1

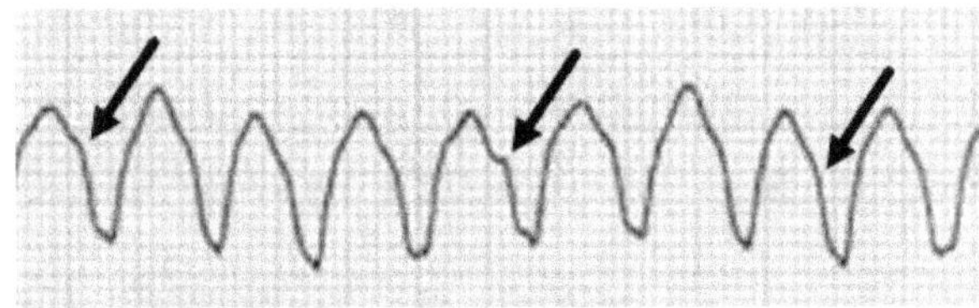

Figure 8-20

(Figure 8-20) Is this a monophasic R with an inverted T wave or a QS with an upright T wave? On close inspection you will see some "notching" or a slight *change in the slope* of the line (arrows) just before the onset of the negative deflection – most obviously just before the first and fifth negative deflections (but it's in all the others, too). Begin by assuming that's the baseline. It appears to wander a bit, doesn't it? That's not unusual and is something you should get used to seeing. Let's look at another view of this same snippet (Figure 8-21) in which I've invoked the 4 mm Rule:

As you can see, the upright deflection at 4 mm from the apex is visibly wider than the inverted deflection at 4 mm from its nadir. According to the 4 mm Rule, the T wave is wider than a monophasic R or a QS complex at the 4 mm level. That's because repolarization takes a lot longer than depolarization, even under *normal* circumstances.

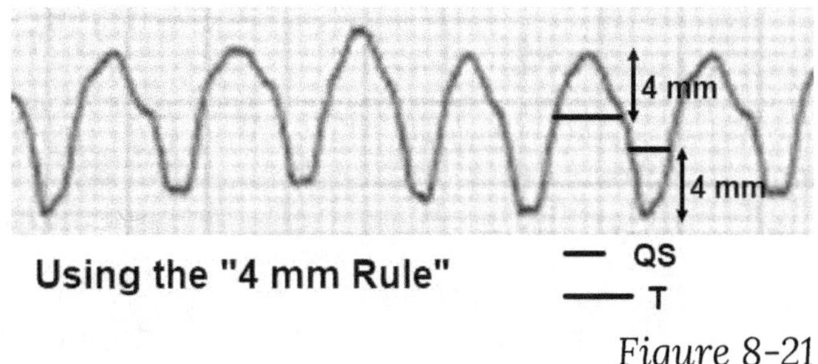

Figure 8-21

Consider the **4 mm Rule** as a *suggestion* of mine – it has never been formally validated.

> **PEARL |** It has been my experience that you will improve your skills faster by studying the same ECGs and rhythm strips over and over again. That creates a *familiarity* with the subject matter faster.

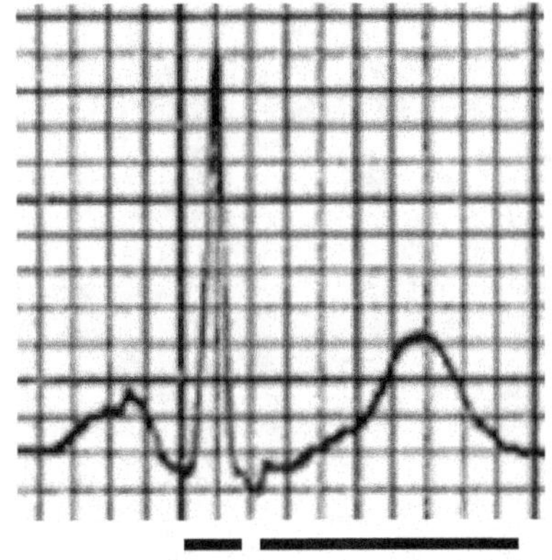

Figure 8-22

Here (Figure 8-22) is a QRS-T from a normal ECG. Look at the difference in width between depolarization and repolarization demonstrated by the two lines. The difference is less during an ectopic tachycardia – *but it's still there!* Depolarization occurs over *rapidly conducting fibers; repolarization is by cell-to-cell conduction.*

Getting back to our rhythm strip (Figure 8-20 or 8-21), you should also have noticed that the nadir of the inverted deflection is just a bit sharper than the apex of the upright deflection. That's because R waves and S waves have a more abrupt change in polarity than T waves.

(Figure 8-20) These are QS *complexes* followed by *upright T waves*. Look at these examples very closely. Satisfy yourself that you can quickly locate the base of each deflection and then compare them in your mind. It helps tremendously if you can quickly identify any baseline. Can you see the subtle change in slope at the beginning of *every* QS?

> **PEARL |** You can often see the difference in depolarization and repolarization by observing the angle formed at the peak or nadir. The deflection with the widest angle is usually the T wave. I often use this to validate my impression.

Faux Twin #2

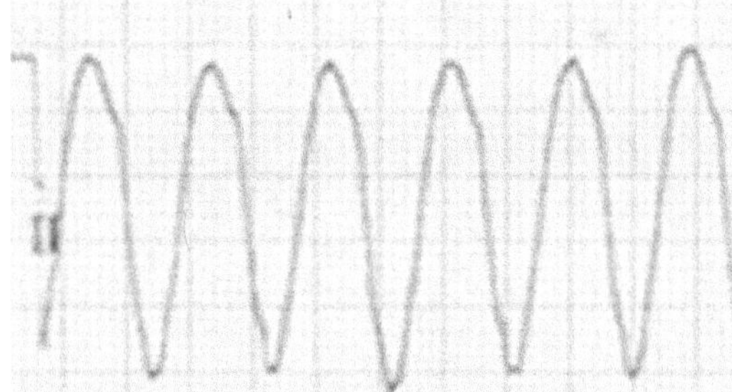

Figure 8-23

(Figure 8-23) First, note that this is a *monomorphic* ventricular tachycardia (that will be important in a moment). It is also monophasic because there are just two deflections present, and you already know that one of them *must* be a T wave! Now try to locate a "presumed" baseline. The baseline is a lot more subtle here but that's what this workbook is about – *to train you to see the subtleties!* If you locate the baseline you will immediately see a very obvious contradiction to what I said in earlier chapters. *The T waves are much smaller and appear to have a more narrow base than the QS waves.* (You should have been able to note the sharper nadir of the QS deflections as distinguished from the more rounded apex of the T waves (Figure 8-24, below). Are the T waves really that small (circle), or is that an illusion caused by something else?

There is an even faster approach to take with this type of deflection. The arrows in Figure 8-24 indicate a change in slope which strongly suggests the onset of a deflection. As you can see, there are just two deflections present – a positive deflection and a negative deflection. The possibilities here are a monomorphic R wave which is being partially obscured by an inverted T wave, or a QS wave which is partially obscuring an upright T wave.

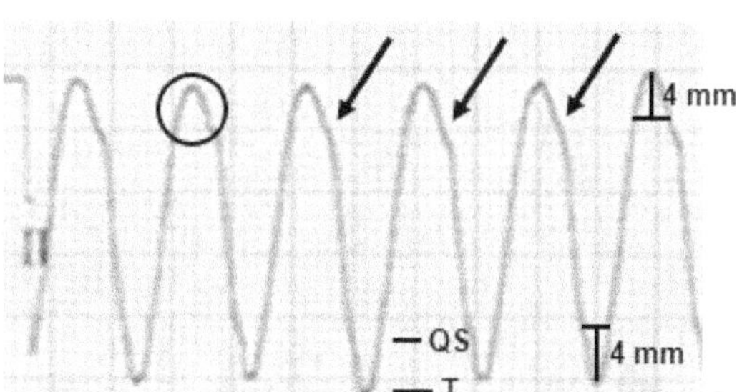

Figure 8-24

By invoking the 4 mm Rule, one can see that the inverted deflection is a QS and the upright deflection is a T wave.

> **PEARL |** T waves do *not* cover up or otherwise obscure any part of a QRS complex! Never!

So, Faux Twin #2 demonstrates QS complexes with upright T waves.

Faux Twin #3

Here we have two *faux twins* in the same rhythm strip (Figure 8-25). This is a short snippet of a polymorphic ventricular tachycardia that degenerated into ventricular fibrillation (more on *that* later).

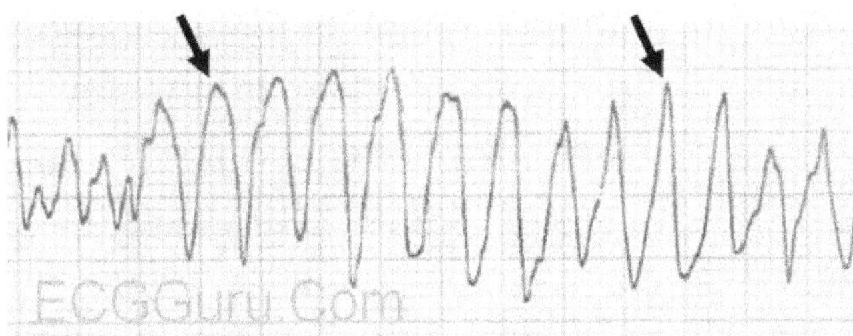

Figure 8-25

The first arrow (left) indicates the T wave of a *monophasic QS complex* while the second arrow (right) indicates the peak of a *monophasic R wave*. The axis has shifted so much that the polarity at the end of the episode is opposite the polarity at the beginning. As you can see, the spindle-shaped morphology of this episode is becoming less organized as the rhythm transitions to ventricular fibrillation (not seen in this snippet). Here is another similar-appearing example (Figure 8-26):

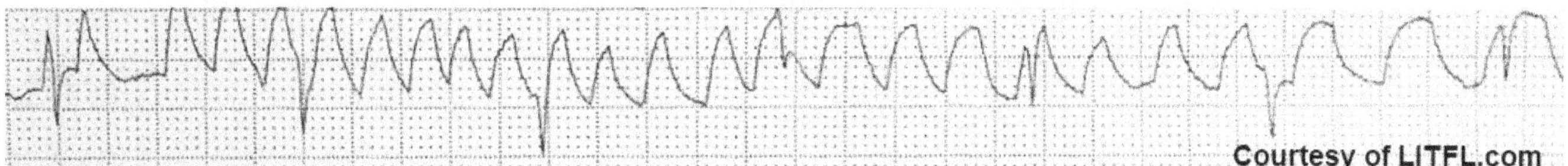

Figure 8-26

If you look closely, you will see that there are very narrow complexes appearing at very regular intervals. Hints that this "tachycardia" is an artifact include: 1) the patient looks fine despite a horrible-looking rhythm, 2) the "tachycardia" is not present in all the leads and 3) the narrow-complex rhythm is unaffected by the other "ventricular" activity. This is just a motion artifact. Keep this in mind!

TIP | During a wide complex tachycardia, q waves (in Lead V6 with LBBB-like morphology) and notching of the R waves or S waves *may* indicate previous infarctions. QS complexes generally do not! A QS complex indicates a focus that is likely in the periphery of the ventricular wall. This is discussed in Chapter 1.

Faux Twin #4

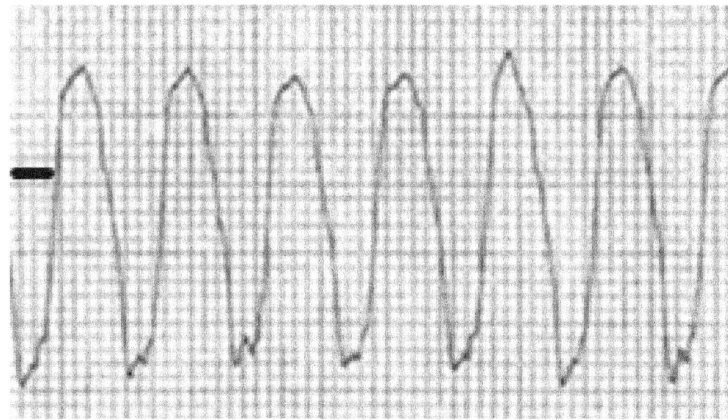

Figure 8-27

(Figure 8-27) This is another very subtle distinction between *depolarization* and *repolarization*. There is no good hint regarding the location of the baseline. I have drawn a short black line at the approximate level that I perceive some changes in slope that could indicate a baseline – but I cannot be certain. What do you think? You must be able to detect very slight changes in slope in these deflections because sometimes that is all you will have to formulate your opinion. In the Masterclasses we call these "Eye Exercises."

In this snippet, we are also forced to confront subtlety in another method for distinguishing depolarization from repolarization: it appears that both deflections have pointed tips (apex and nadir). Here is the subtle distinction: the nadirs are consistently pointed but the apices are less pointed and more rounded than the nadirs… but still, *a very subtle distinction.* Try using the 4 mm Rule.

These are QS complexes with upright T waves.

PEARL | When there are only TWO deflections, one of them MUST be a T wave! Comparing the QRS complex with the lead above and/or below may add clarity to the determination of the morphology.

FYI | Have you ever wondered why many of the depolarizations are so large yet the T waves are comparatively much smaller? Shouldn't they at least be somewhat proportional? As the cycle length (another term for "R-R interval") decreases, depolarization begins to invade the terminal part of the previous repolarization (T wave) more and more, hiding it from view. That T wave is there and it really is wide. You just can't see it because it is hidden by the R or QS wave.

Faux Twin #5

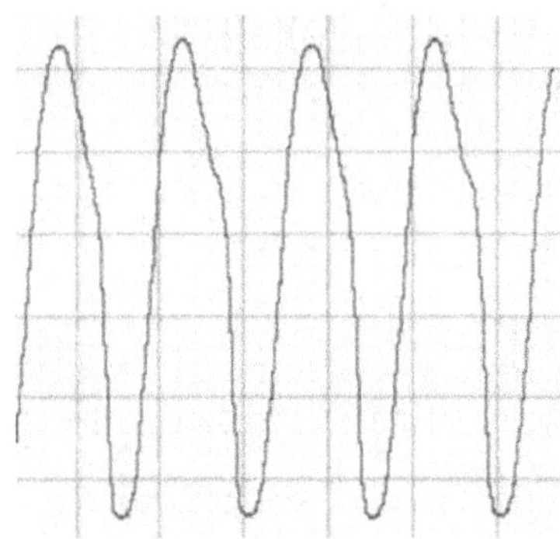

This (Figure 8-28) might have been difficult for you at the beginning of "Faux Twins," but it should be easier for you by now. First, *look for a possible baseline.* If it isn't obvious, then *look for a subtle change in slope occurring at about the same place in each deflection.* If you still don't see it, look about a third of the way down from the peak (apex) of the deflections. There (*probably*) is the baseline. Only two deflections are present – one upright, one inverted. You already know that one of them has to be a T wave – but which one? In this snippet, the apices and the nadirs look almost the same! The 4 mm Rule can't help us very much here. What do we do now?

Figure 8-28

TIP | We can depend on a secret that I learned a long time ago: *the change in slope just before the onset of a negative deflection which you have trained your eyes so well to recognize often marks the onset of depolarization!* So, we have some very large QS complexes followed by upright T waves.

PEARL | QS waves represent depolarization as much as monophasic R waves. It's just a different view of the *same* depolarization. It's all Phase 0 of the action potential!

TIP | Why the concern over locating a baseline? Is it really necessary? Establishing a baseline is the first step to identifying whether a deflection is an R wave or an S wave. Remember: there is no such thing as a negative R wave or a positive S wave. Just because there may be a downward notch in an otherwise monophasic R wave doesn't make it an S wave. S *waves must enclose a negative area that exists only below the baseline.*

This snippet (Figure 8-28) demonstrates a ventricular tachycardia that is *regular, monophasic, very wide,* and with QRS complexes that are *not well-formed.* This is quintessential scar-related *ventricular tachycardia* and *very, very dangerous!*

Faux Twin #6

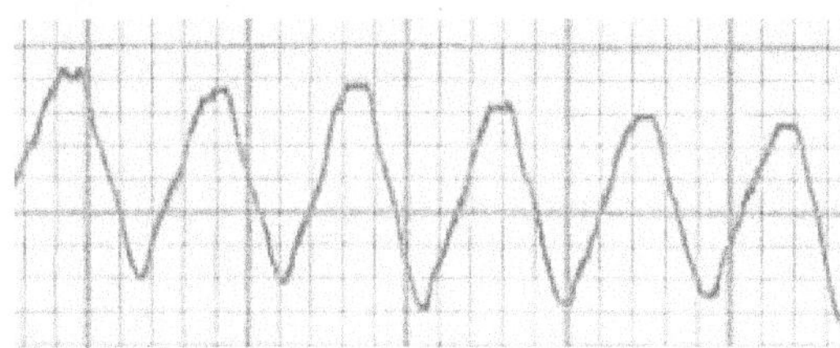

Figure 8-29

(Figure 8-29) First, look for a possible baseline. If it is not obvious (and this one isn't), then look for a *subtle change in slope occurring at about the same place on each deflection.* You should have been able to determine an estimated baseline by now. If not, then look at my estimation of the baseline in the next figure:

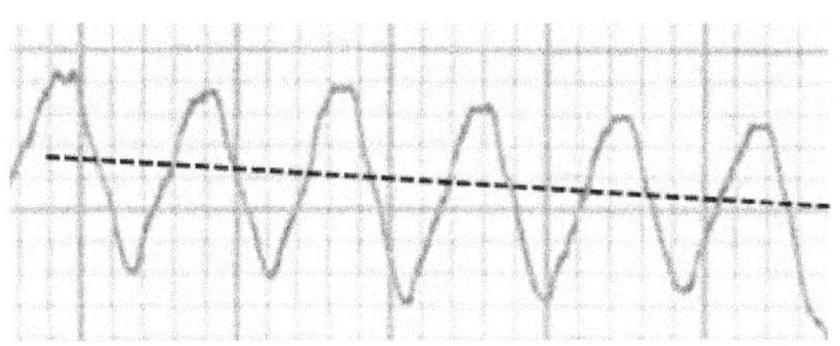

Figure 8-30

If you were not able to locate a possible baseline, compare the two figures and sharpen your eyes to the subtle change in slope. As you see, my estimated baseline (Figure 8-30) slopes downward because the real baseline is wandering a bit. *Never assume that the baseline will be perfectly horizontal.*

It should be very apparent that the apices are wider and more rounded than the nadirs, which are also rounded but much more narrow – one could even say "peaked."

I included this snippet just for the "Eye Exercise." These are QS complexes with upright T waves. At a rate of approximately 300/minute, I would call this ventricular flutter and cardiovert immediately. With an ECG like this, I can't imagine the patient being "stable."

Faux Twin #7

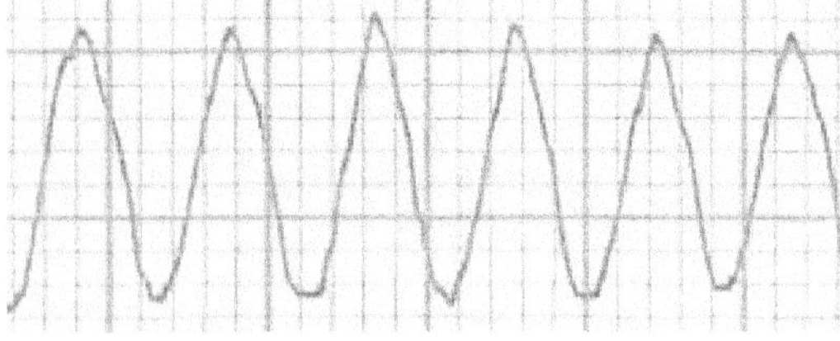

Figure 8-31

This should be getting easier for you by now. If not, go back over the previous "Faux Twins." Try to find a baseline by recognizing very subtle changes in slope (Figure 8-31). If that doesn't help, then compare the morphology of the apices with the nadirs. Is one more or less rounded than the other? What do you think of this Faux Twin?

The peaks are sharp and the nadirs are very rounded. These are monophasic R waves with inverted T waves.

There is one other confounder that could present with wide, rounded depolarizations (QS or monophasic R waves) and narrow, peaked repolarizations (T waves): HYPERKALEMIA! Always keep that diagnosis in your thoughts when seeing very wide QRS complexes and a "slow VT" (N.B., what you are seeing here is NOT "slow VT"). Hyperkalemia can be seen in rates compatible with the lower range for ventricular tachycardia, around 100 – 130 beats/minute. Always be alert to this!

Faux Twin #8

(Figure 8-32) This should be easy for you by now! First, locate a prospective baseline. You will have to depend on *subtle changes in slope* to locate it, but there they are – in exactly the same place on each deflection. Next, compare the morphologies of the peaks and nadirs. The peaks are very rounded and the nadirs are quite sharp. If you measure the base of the negative deflections at the baseline and compare it to the base of the upright deflection at the baseline, you can easily see that the bases of the upright deflections are definitely wider than the negative (inverted) deflections. The 4 mm Rule can be easily visualized without having to specifically measure for it.

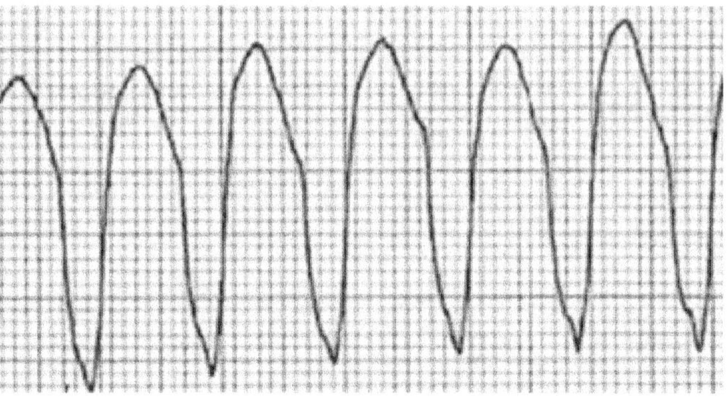

Figure 8-32

These are QS complexes with upright T waves.

PEARL | Observing the width of the QRS is how we measure the conduction velocity – the wider the complex, the slower the conduction. The heart rate has nothing to do with conduction velocity in the His-Purkinje system. It *can*, however, affect the conduction velocity in the AV node.

Chapter 9

Recognizing AV Dissociation, VA Association and VA Dissociation

ATTENTION! *There is a lot of information in this chapter because it discusses one of the most important tasks in electrocardiography: establishing the presence of AV or VA dissociation during a wide complex tachycardia. Plan on reading through this more than once and referring back to it frequently.*

Before beginning, you must understand that the AV node is a TWO-WAY street. It allows impulses to travel from the *atria to the ventricles*, but it also allows impulses to travel from the *ventricles to the atria*. This is very important because, in your search for AV dissociation, you will also be searching for VA dissociation and will often be as concerned about the R-P′ interval as the P-R interval.

A classic Mobitz I AV block presents with the P-R interval gradually increasing in duration until a P wave fails to conduct causing a QRS complex to fail to appear. The SAME THING can happen in the *opposite* direction also, during VA conduction. Mobitz I VA block will present with a gradually increasing R-P′ interval until a ventricular impulse fails to cross through the AV node into the atria and the P′ fails to appear. A block in the AV node will terminate any reentrant tachycardia that depends on the AV node as part of its circuit, and that includes AVNRT and AVRT. Remember that ventricular tachycardia does NOT depend on the AV node as part of its reentrant circuit – so ventricular tachycardia will persist despite a Mobitz I, Mobitz II, or even third degree AV or VA block. If a wide complex tachycardia persists despite a Mobitz I or a Mobitz II VA block, then it *must be ventricular tachycardia* – an antidromic AVRT would have been terminated once the retrograde P′ wave disappeared.

AV Dissociation | Presence of autonomous pacemakers in the atrium (usually the SA node) and in one of the ventricles – an *accelerated accessory ventricular pacemaker* if the sinus rhythm is normal or *ventricular escape beats* if the sinus rate is much slower than normal.

Because the pacemakers are firing at different rates, there will usually be no association between the P waves and the QRS complexes which are characterized by varying PR intervals. Since AV dissociation does NOT require an AV block, occasional atrial impulses will successfully cross the AV node and excite ("capture") the ventricles. These are called *capture beats* and **they always appear early** – before the next expected ectopic beat.

> **PEARL |** The fact that a sinus impulse makes it through the AV node to the ventricles does NOT make it a capture beat. Many ventricular tachycardias are paroxysmal and will frequently stop spontaneously, allowing sinus impulses to control the ventricles, at least for a few beats. Those are NOT capture beats. Capture beats MUST interrupt the ectopic ventricular rhythm by appearing BEFORE the next expected ectopic QRS. If it's not EARLY – it's NOT a capture beat and it only proves that there is no fixed bundle branch block! It does NOT prove an acceleration-dependent block or a ventricular tachycardia!

A capture beat is proof of AV dissociation and in the presence of a wide complex tachycardia, a very high likelihood of ventricular tachycardia. If the sinus-conducted impulse happens to overlap one of the ventricular-generated beats, the two beats will merge and produce a QRS that is an intermediate blend of the two impulses. Those are called *fusion beats*. Just think of them as capture beats that collided with a ventricular beat. They, too, are indicative of AV dissociation and a high likelihood of ventricular tachycardia. Can you find the capture beats in the rhythm strip below (Figure 9-1)? (Answer: #1, #5, and #9 because they appeared early, interrupting the ventricular rhythm)

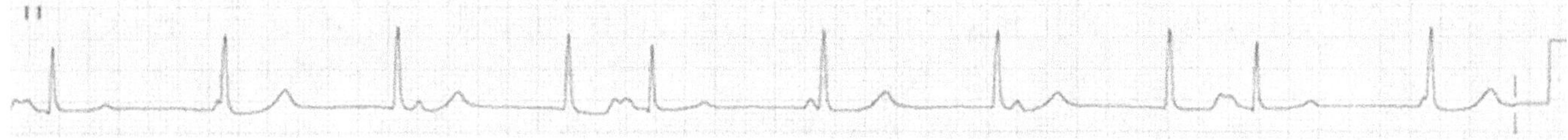

Figure 9-1

Understanding Ventriculoatrial (VA) Conduction

Many people who read ECGs are not familiar with *ventriculoatrial* (VA) conduction. There's nothing difficult about it because it is just the *opposite* of AV conduction! During AV conduction a P wave is produced in the atria, it then crosses through the AV node using the FAST pathway – which takes a small amount of time – and then it excites the ventricles and produces a QRS complex. Because it uses the FAST pathway (under NORMAL circumstances), the PR interval is not very long – up to (and including) 200 msec. But what if the sinus impulse were to use the SLOW pathway instead? What would the ECG look like then? Well, there would still be a sinus P wave followed by a QRS complex – but now the PR interval may be 400 msec or even longer. There would also be a greater separation between activations of the two chambers (atria then ventricles).

TIP | Blocks in the AV node can be *unidirectional* (antegrade or retrograde) or *bidirectional* (blocked in *both* directions). Unidirectional blocks are not uncommon.

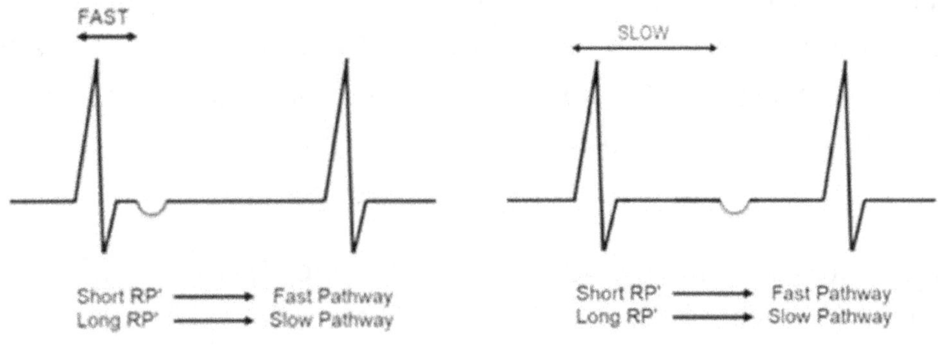

Figure 9-2

OK, so what happens during VA conduction? Instead of a P wave activating the ventricles, there is a QRS complex activating the atria. We know that an impulse traveling through the AV node from the atria to the ventricles takes from 120 msec to 200 msec. How long does it take for a ventricular impulse to cross through the AV node and create a P′ wave? It takes roughly the same amount of time, though there may be a little more variability in the RP′ times. The reason for that is that under normal circumstances, the sinus impulse normally takes the FAST pathway. Its recovery from refractoriness is timed so that the impulse arriving from the SA node finds it ready to conduct. However, conduction from the ventricles to the atria is never a normal event, so the ventricular impulse may take either the FAST or the SLOW pathway. It just depends on which one is ready to conduct when the ectopic ventricular impulse arrives.

If an ectopic ventricular impulse travels up the FAST pathway and then activates the atria, the retrograde P′ wave will appear very close to the ectopic QRS complex (Figure 9-2). However, if the FAST pathway is refractory and the ectopic ventricular impulse travels up the SLOW pathway, the retrograde P′ wave will be much further removed from the end of the ectopic QRS complex.

During a Mobitz I **AV** block, the P-R intervals grow longer and longer. During a Mobitz I **VA** block, the R-P′ intervals grow longer and longer. Both conductions eventually fail. In the case of a Mobitz I AV block, a QRS complex fails to appear; in the case of a Mobitz I VA block, a retrograde P′ wave fails to appear.

If you are looking for P waves or P′ waves to diagnose AV or VA dissociation to prove a ventricular tachycardia, you should thoroughly understand exactly WHAT you are looking for and WHY you are looking! As an esteemed colleague of mine once asked, "Why bother looking for P waves during a wide complex tachycardia if you have no idea what the P waves mean should you find any?" Let me clearly and unequivocally explain P waves and P′ waves to you so you will be well-informed should you locate any P waves during a wide complex tachycardia!

There are two types of P waves you might find: *upright* P waves and *inverted* P waves. *All* upright P waves come from the atria! *M*ost inverted P′ waves come from below the AV node (and it's still called the "AV node" no matter which direction the impulse is traveling!) A very small number of inverted, retrograde P′ waves *may* originate in the lower right atrium – but they are very scarce. Don't worry about them for now.

TIP | Don't waste your time trying to *memorize* which leads should have upright P waves and which leads may have inverted P′ waves.

Just read what I am about to explain to you very carefully and you will understand P waves very thoroughly. You shouldn't have to memorize anything!

PEARL | If you *understand* something, you won't have to memorize it.

Sinus P waves will always be positive and upright in the inferior leads (II, III, aVF) because all the inferior leads have their positive pole on the left foot. An impulse traveling *downward* from the SA node toward the positive pole of the inferior leads will inscribe a positive deflection – an upright P wave – in those leads. Any impulse, ventricular or atrial, that is traveling *upward* and therefore away from their positive pole will appear as a negative and inverted deflection *in the inferior leads*. So any inverted P′ waves in the inferior leads are retrograde and coming from below the AV node – most likely the ventricles.

IMPORTANT! | Retrograde P′ waves are NOT inverted in ALL leads! This is a common misconception that many beginners have. Retrograde P' waves will be upright in those leads that have their positive poles in superior locations: mainly Leads aVL and aVR. That is because the retrograde P′ waves are traveling *upward* – *toward* their positive poles.

Retrograde P′ waves will always appear upright in Lead V1 – though they are typically a lot smaller than the normal P waves. Retrograde P′ waves may be either upright or inverted in Leads V5 and V6. It depends on whether the electrodes for those leads were placed in the proper positions on the chest wall; if placed too low (and they frequently are), they may act like inferior leads and manifest inverted P′ waves.

OK… great! You've found retrograde P′ waves in one or more of the inferior leads! So what does that tell you? So far… nothing! So many people studying ECG interpretation think that the issue of AV dissociation is solved simply by *finding* P waves. NO, IT'S NOT! That's just the beginning! What if you find retrograde P′ waves after *every* QRS? Doesn't that prove AV dissociation and therefore ventricular tachycardia? NO!… it is not diagnostic of AV dissociation nor does it prove ventricular tachycardia!

Using P and P′ waves to Diagnose AV and VA Dissociation

Here is *how to use the presence of P waves or P′ waves* – to diagnose AV dissociation or VA dissociation during a wide complex tachycardia:

Upright P Waves…

If you can locate more than one P wave, try to ascertain a rate (atrial rate, P-P interval). Ideally, it will be much slower than the ventricular rate. P waves that are upright in Leads II, III, and aVF are likely sinus P waves. If the P waves are upright in the inferior leads and appear at a rate that is different than the ventricular rate– AV dissociation is present. AV dissociation is NOT 100% proof that the wide complex tachycardia is ventricular tachycardia, but the other possible rhythms range from very infrequent to quite rare.

Inverted P′ waves…

If you find P′ waves that are inverted in the inferior leads, they are likely being transmitted by impulses from the ventricles to the atria. These inverted P′ waves can appear in THREE ways:

1. After every ventricular QRS complex at a fixed, constant R-P′ interval (VA association);

2. At increasing R-P′ intervals following the ventricular QRS complexes until a P′ fails to appear (2nd degree Mobitz I VA block); or,

3. After every ventricular QRS complex at a fixed, constant R-P′ interval with an occasional missing P′ (2nd degree Mobitz II VA block).

The 2nd degree VA blocks are both 100% evidence of ventricular tachycardia. The VA association proves nothing.

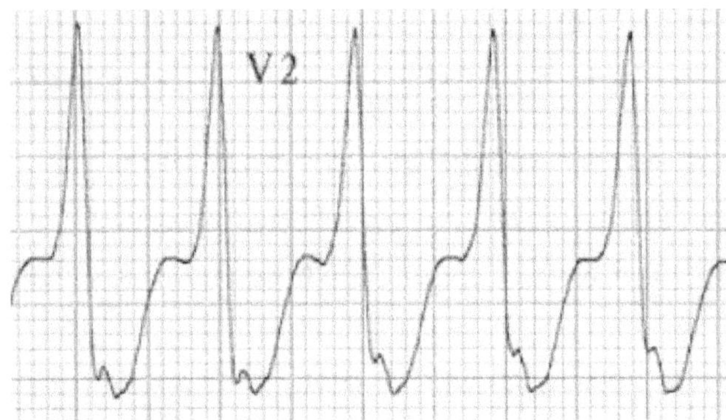

Figure 9-3

Keep reading... there's a lot more on how to find and recognize P waves and P′ waves, including more to learn in Chapter 24.

VA Association | VA association occurs when there is a separate pacemaker firing in the ventricle that is faster than the SA nodal rate. Impulses from the ventricle can cross through the AV node in a retrograde manner and then excite the atria, producing a retrograde P′ wave that is typically located at the same R-P′ interval following each ventricular depolarization (QRS complex).

This is fairly common in ventricular tachycardia (Figure 9-3) but *it does NOT prove that a wide complex rhythm is ventricular tachycardia – an antidromic AVRT can do the same thing!*

VA Dissociation | Similar to VA association except the fixed relation between the QRS and retrograde P′ wave (constant R-P′ interval) is not present. It most commonly presents as a retrograde VA block of some sort (Mobitz I or Mobitz II). *VA dissociation is <u>proof</u> of ventricular tachycardia!*

So, why is VA *dissociation* proof of ventricular tachycardia while VA *association* is not? What are two rhythms that would commonly result in VA association? Ventricular tachycardia and antidromic AVRT. If there is any kind of block in the AV node, how would that affect a ventricular tachycardia focus? It wouldn't because the source of the VT would never be affected by anything happening in the AV node – it's totally independent of conduction through the AV node. On the other hand, how would an antidromic AVRT be affected by a retrograde block in the AV node? It would immediately be terminated! So the fact that a wide complex tachycardia persists despite an obvious retrograde block in the AV node (Figure 9-4) tells you that the rhythm *must* be ventricular tachycardia. Therefore, VA *dissociation DOES prove that the wide complex rhythm is indeed ventricular tachycardia!*

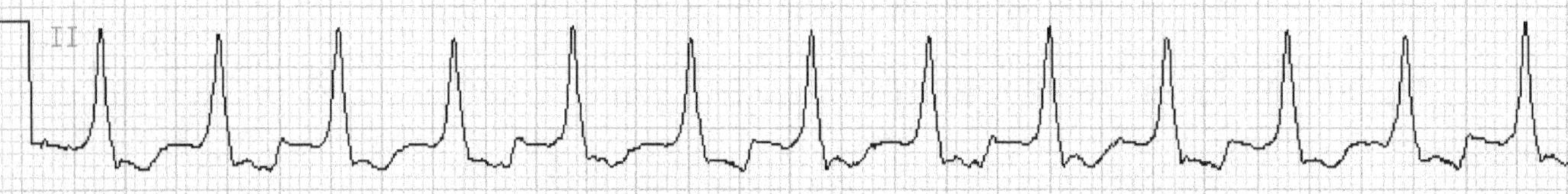

Figure 9-4

Is AV Dissociation Really 100% Specific for Ventricular Tachycardia?

Many authors of textbooks and articles will tell you that AV dissociation *proves* ventricular tachycardia – that it is 100% conclusive. Sorry, but that's simply *not true!* While it *strongly suggests* ventricular tachycardia, AV dissociation may also be present in wide complex tachycardias due to:

1. AVNRT with an upper common pathway block and aberrant conduction

2. junctional tachycardia with aberrant conduction

Both these dysrhythmias are very infrequent, so when AV dissociation is present on an ECG with a wide complex tachycardia, *you should pay very close attention!* But, sorry – it only proves that two pacemakers are competing with each other. It doesn't necessarily tell you where the second one is located.

Finding P Waves in a Wide Complex Tachycardia (WCT)

But to diagnose AV dissociation or VA dissociation, one must be able to locate and recognize P or P′ waves during a wide complex tachycardia. Let's look at an example:

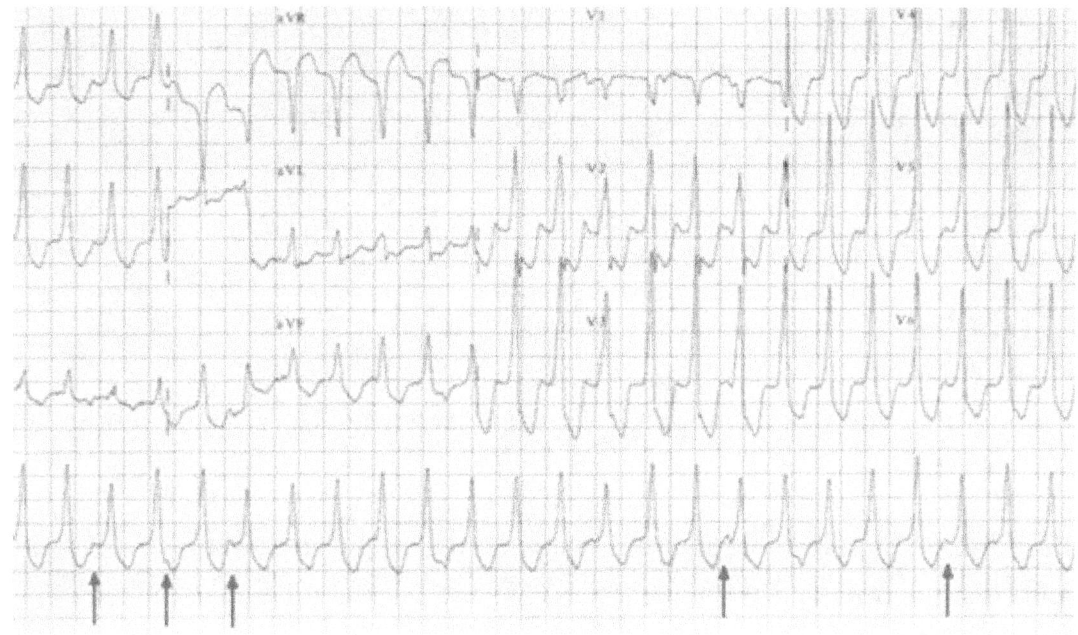

Figure 9-5

See how many other P waves you can find on this tracing (Figure 9-5). I very quickly found 17 more without including the rhythm strip at the bottom of the tracing. You should find at least that many or even more. *P waves in a wide complex tachycardia will be on the baseline or the T wave. They do not noticeably distort the QRS.*

But what about the ones that are not so obvious? They are a lot more subtle, but with a little practice and some eye training, they become much more apparent. There are a few examples in the tracing above (Figure 9-5). Look at Leads V4 through V6. Each R wave has a short, nearly isoelectric segment just in front of it. There are four QRS complexes in those leads. Look at the second one, comparing the short preceding segment with the other three. There is a tiny bump there making it different than the others. That is a P wave and it is present in the second complex of all three leads. P waves are usually found in the ST segments and T waves. T waves, however, sometimes manifest the presence of a P wave by deforming the peak of the T or by increasing (or decreasing) the amplitude of the T wave. Let's look at some more (Figure 9-6)...

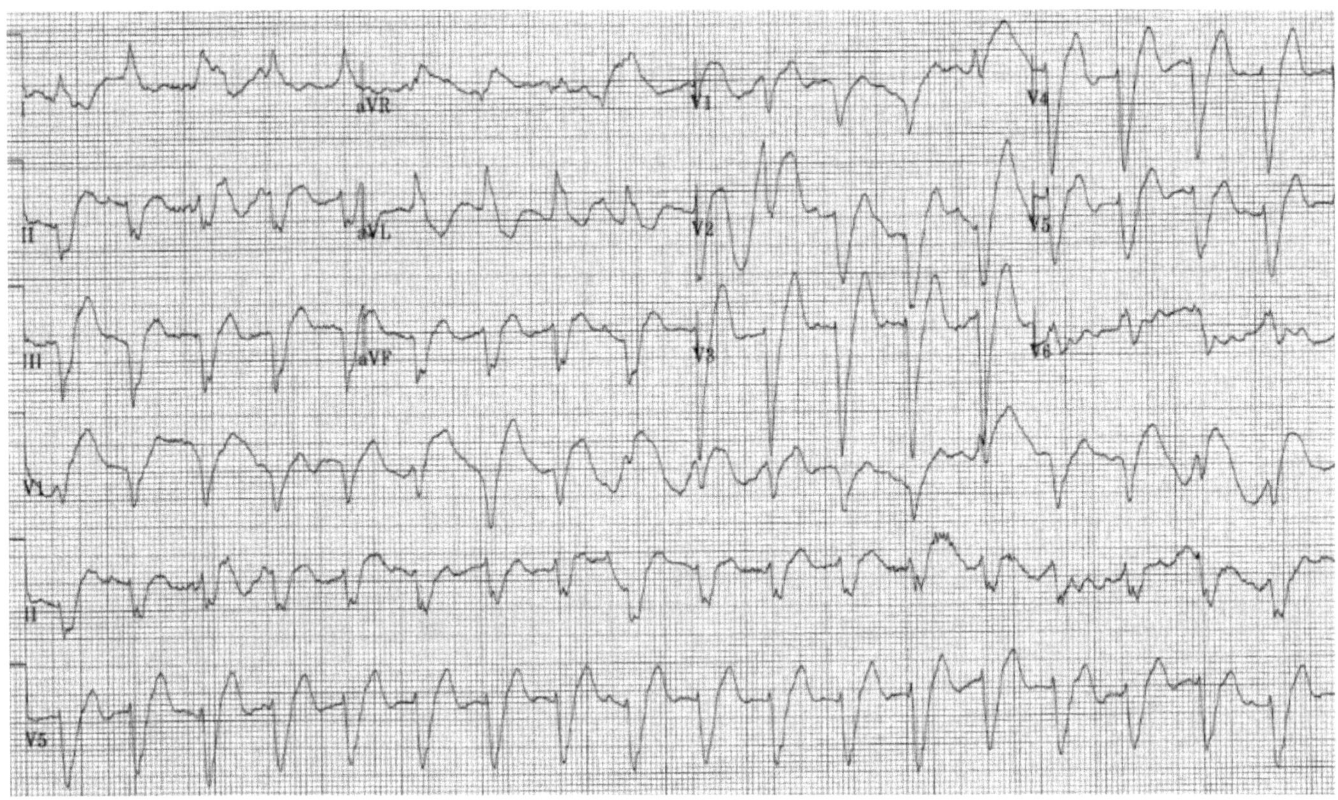

Figure 9-6

With AV dissociation, you will be looking for upright P waves. Don't worry about retrograde atrial ectopics for now.

With VA dissociation, you will be looking for inverted P′ waves (remember: if it did not originate in the sinus node, it's a P′).

There are P waves throughout this tracing: some appear as bumps and others as subtle deformities of the T waves.

Find a P wave of either type that you are certain is indeed a P wave, then find the very next one. Measure the distance between them and start mapping out P waves with your ECG calipers and see if your calipers coincide with the deflections you thought were P waves. If the measured P-P interval is rather slow (long), calculate half that distance and readjust your calipers – sometimes you can only see every second or third P wave, so you have to adjust your calipers accordingly to check that possibility.

Look at this tracing (Figure 9-7) and see how many signs of AV dissociation you can find...

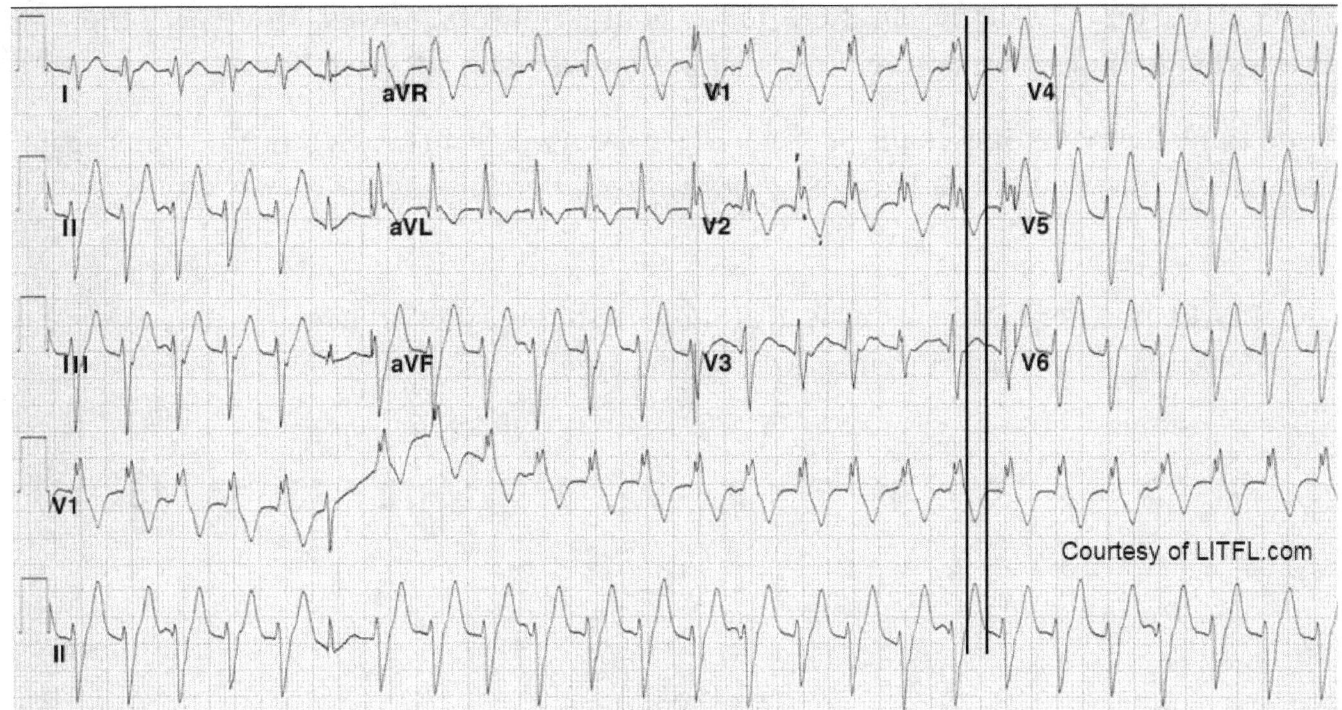

Figure 9-7

Now let's tackle a collection of very subtle, hidden P waves...

Eye Exercise: Finding Subtle P Waves

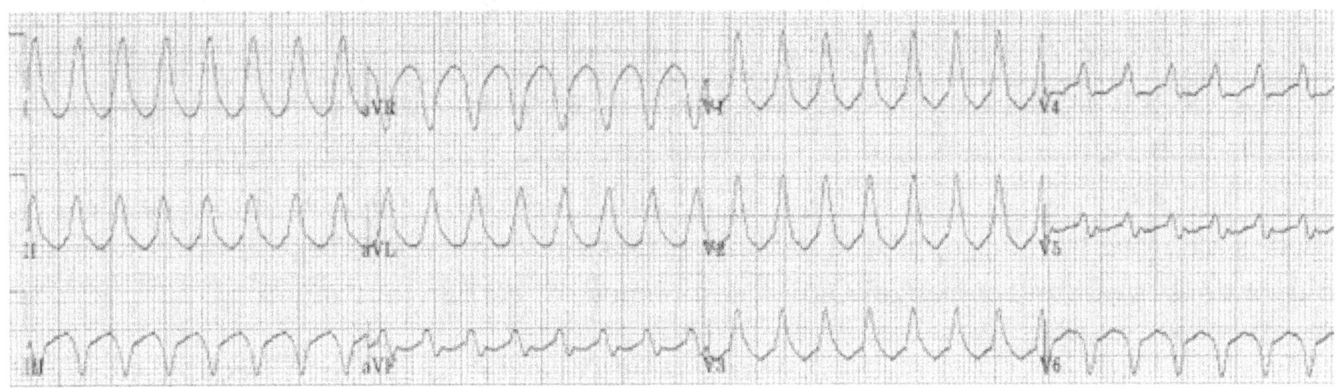

Figure 9-8

Do you see any very subtle P waves in the above tracing (Figure 9-8)? Look closely and use a magnifying lens.

TIP | If you are serious about interpreting ECGs and rhythm strips at an advanced level, there are TWO things you will need: good quality ECG calipers and a small pocket-sized magnifying lens. An additional helpful item would be a 6" transparent plastic ruler to use as a straight edge that you can see through.

Concentrate on very subtle variations in the contour of the T waves. There are other interesting findings on this tracing, but right now we're on a P wave hunt.

If you think that your only chance of finding P′ waves will be in Leads II or V1 – think again. Here are TWO IMPORTANT PEARLS to remember when looking for P or P′ waves:

PEARL | 1) They can be in *any* lead and 2) whether upright or inverted, they may be *much, much smaller* than you'd ever imagine!

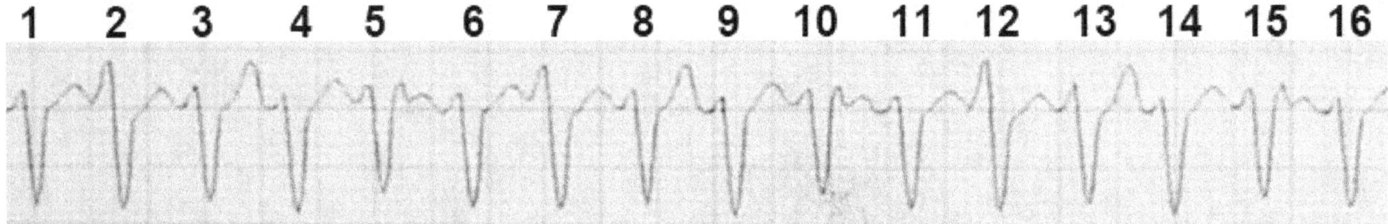

Figure 9-9

When searching for P waves to prove AV dissociation, you must look first at the QRS complexes, but you are *not* looking for P waves yet. You are looking for a *normal QRS* – a QRS complex that *begins normally* and *ends normally*. You will use that "normal" QRS to compare with other QRS complexes and *especially the baseline surrounding them*. In Figure 9-9, look at QRS complexes #1, #4, #6, #9, #11, #14 and #16. They all look the same – they have the same initial r wave and the same J point (end of the QRS). And they all have essentially the same T wave. Any one of these QRS-T complexes can be your point of reference. Now let's look at #2 – OK... that R wave is very different! Why is it so large? Something has *added positive voltage* to that deflection! What could it be? Of course... there's a P wave that has *appeared immediately before* that r wave. Take another look at one of your "point of reference" QRS-T complexes to refresh your memory.

Now let's look at #3... Look at that T wave! What caused it to suddenly become so large? Of course, there's an upright P wave hiding in there. How do I know it's an *upright* P wave? Because that T wave has gotten larger, that means some *positive voltage*, i.e., an *upright* P wave, *has been added to it.* (In Chapter 24 you will see the effect of *negative* voltage on a T wave.)

Now let's look at #5... Is that an r′ ("r prime") there at the end of the QRS? It isn't on any of the "point of reference" QRS-T waves. Of course, it's not an r′ - it's a P wave. Now YOU find all the other examples throughout this strip.

Here (Figure 9-10) are some P′ waves from Figure 9-8...

Note the *consistent* R-P′ intervals and note especially how *very small the P′ waves are!* When looking for P waves, remember that TWO types of P waves may – or may NOT – be helpful during a wide complex tachycardia: the *upright P wave in the inferior leads* and the *inverted P wave in the inferior leads.* Look for P waves first in the inferior leads; if you don't see any, then look in *all* the other leads.

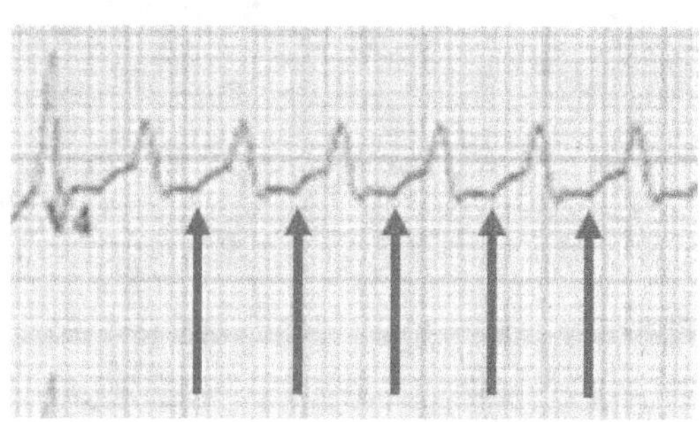

Figure 9-10

It is not unusual for some ECGs to have visible P waves only in Lead V3, for instance. They can hide in *any* lead!

> **PEARL |** P waves that are *upright in the inferior leads* (II, III, aVF) originate from the upper atrium, most likely from the sinus node. Upright P waves in the *inferior* leads are *never* retrograde!

P′ waves that are *inverted in the inferior leads* are a bit more complex because they can arise in the *lower part of the right atrium,* or they can be *retrograde P′ waves coming from impulses originating in the junction or ventricle* and entering the right atrium retrograde via the AV node. Inverted P′ waves can also appear after every QRS in the presence of an *orthodromic* AVRT with aberrant conduction. There would have to be either a permanent or rate-related bundle branch block to make it a wide-complex tachycardia; it *could* happen, but that would be a very rare occurrence! However, you can frequently determine which retrograde P′ wave is due to a *low atrial* origin and which is due to an *ectopic ventricular* or *junctional* origin.

> **PEARL |** If the inverted P′ waves are of *low atrial* origin, they will appear at the rate of the low atrial pacemaker and will thus manifest AV *dissociation* with the ventricular complexes since they will have no relationship to each other. If the inverted P′ waves are of *ectopic ventricular* origin, then they will appear after *every* QRS complex at the same, fixed R-P′ interval.

This is called VA *association* because each retrograde P′ wave has a fixed association with the preceding QRS complex (Figures 9-3 and 9-10).

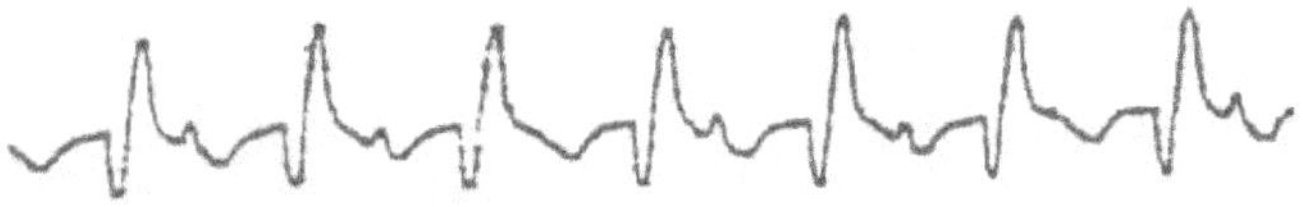

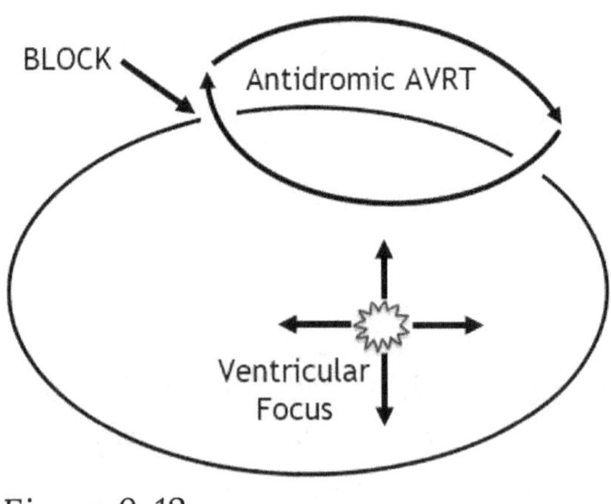

Figure 9-11

If the retrograde (inverted) P′ waves appear at slightly irregular R-P′ intervals, then there may be a retrograde block in the AV node (a *ventriculoatrial*, or VA *block*). If the R-P′ intervals gradually lengthen and then a retrograde, inverted P′ wave fails to appear, there is likely a *retrograde Mobitz I (Wenckebach) VA block* (Figure 9-11). If the retrograde P′ waves appear with every other QRS, there is likely a 2:1 VA block (Figure 9-4). Although a retrograde P′ wave that follows *every* QRS at a fixed R-P interval looks like it *should* indicate ventricular tachycardia... *it doesn't!* Orthodromic or antidromic AVRT can do the same (though only the antidromic AVRT will present as a WCT unless there is a pre-existing or rate-related bundle branch block). A retrograde VA block in the presence of a continuing, uninterrupted ventricular rhythm indicates VA *dissociation* and VA dissociation *does* indicate ventricular tachycardia!

Figure 9-12

But why does it indicate VT? If there is an antidromic AVRT (which is AV *nodal dependent*) and a Mobitz I or Mobitz II VA block suddenly occurs... what happens? The antidromic AVRT will quickly terminate! (Figure 9-12) Remember: that's how we stop AVRTs in any direction – we give adenosine which blocks the AV node *in BOTH directions* and the tachycardia is immediately extinguished! However, ventricular tachycardia will not terminate because *its existence does not depend on the AV or VA conduction through the AV node.*

So here are some PEARLS...

PEARL | If a P wave appears after each QRS (*inverted* in Leads II, III, aVF, *upright* in Leads aVR, aVL, V1) during a wide complex tachycardia, then consider it a retrograde P′ wave caused by each ventricular depolarization (QRS). It is NOT coming from the atrium! This is called VA association and it is NOT proof of ventricular tachycardia. I know... it looks like it *ought* to be, but trust me, it isn't!

PEARL | Just because retrograde P′ waves are inverted in the inferior leads does NOT imply they will be inverted in *all* the other leads. Retrograde P′ waves are always *inverted* (negative) in the inferior leads (II, III aVF) because the vector is traveling *away* from the positive pole for those leads (left foot). It will be upright in Lead V1, aVR, and aVL because the retrograde vector is traveling *toward* the positive poles of those leads. They are usually isoelectric (or nearly so) in Lead I because the upward vector is traveling *perpendicular* to Lead 1. If they can be seen at all in Lead I, they will be upright. Leads V5 and V6 can be variable, depending on whether the electrodes for those leads have been properly positioned.

More About AV or VA Dissociation

AV dissociation is one of the most misunderstood concepts in electrocardiography. To understand it, you must properly understand AV *association*. AV association implies that there is a relationship between the atria and the ventricles: the firing of one leads to the firing of the other. A similar situation – but in the opposite direction – is called VA *association*. *Whether you are going in or out of the room, you're still going through the same door.* With AV association, activation of the atria leads to activation of the ventricles. With VA association, activation of the ventricles leads to activation of the atria. VA association is, unfortunately, not a distinguishing factor since it can be present in both ventricular tachycardia and supraventricular tachycardia with aberrancy.

AV Dissociation by Usurpation

With AV dissociation *by usurpation*, the ventricular rate will be faster than the atrial rate – but the atrial rate will still be *within the normal range*. If the atrial rate could go faster, it would discharge the ventricles faster than the ventricles could discharge themselves and thus take control of the rhythm. AV dissociation by usurpation is *never* a good thing! AV dissociation during ventricular tachycardia is AV *dissociation by usurpation*.

AV Dissociation by Default

With AV dissociation *by default*, the sinus rhythm slows down to the point that an accessory escape pacemaker awakens and starts firing to preserve cardiac output. With AV *dissociation by usurpation*, the atrial rate is normal and the ventricular rate is abnormally fast; with AV *dissociation by default*, the atrial rate is abnormally slow and the accessory junctional or ventricular pacemaker begins firing to support the person's blood pressure and perfusion of vital organs. AV dissociation by default represents an escape rhythm and *it is a good thing!*

If the atrial rate is faster, but it is not discharging the ventricles, there can be only one explanation: there is a block in the AV node preventing those P waves from getting through and discharging the ventricles.

The presence of AV dissociation proves that the atria are not consistently discharging the ventricles because the atria and the ventricles are usually discharging at different rates. However, **AV dissociation alone is not proof of AV block!**

Capture Beats and Fusion Beats

Here is where a lot of the misunderstanding appears. Many people think that if they can simply see P waves amid a wide complex tachycardia, then ventricular tachycardia is present. Well, P waves can appear amid an aberrantly conducted supraventricular tachycardia as well. So obviously, there's more to it than just the *presence* of P waves in the tracing.

AV dissociation is present when a P wave manages to hurry through the AV node at just the right moment and then discharge the ventricles, creating a normal, narrow complex in the middle of a wide complex tachycardia. That is called a *capture beat*.

Capture beats are probably the second most misunderstood electrocardiographic phenomenon after AV dissociation. The sudden presence of a normally conducted beat in a wide complex tachycardia is not *necessarily* a capture beat nor does it *necessarily* suggest AV dissociation (and presumably, ventricular tachycardia). **Only a normally conducted beat that appears SOONER than the expected R-R interval of the prevailing ventricular rhythm, i.e. the wide complex tachycardia, can be called a capture beat**. Why? Because by occurring at a shorter R-R interval than the VT, the normal beat proves two things:

1. it proves that there is no *pre-existing bundle branch block*, because it simply could not be produced in the presence of a fixed bundle branch block, and

2. it proves that the conduction system is quite capable of producing a normal, narrow QRS complex at a rate that is even *faster* than the WCT. That rules out a *functional, rate-related bundle branch block* producing aberrant conduction. Therefore, the WCT has to be generated from within the ventricles.

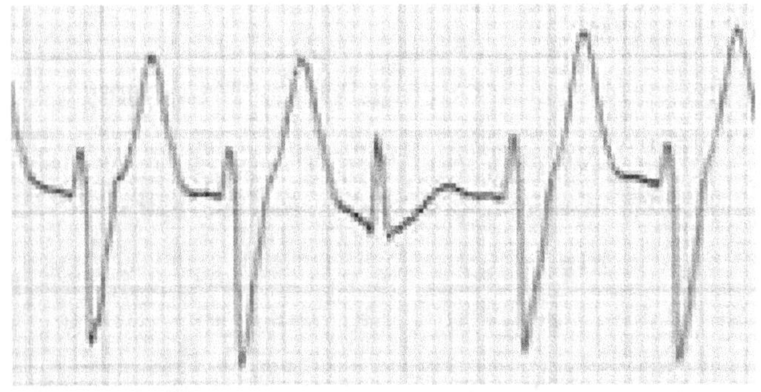

Figure 9-13

This (Figure 9-13) is an example of a capture beat. It appears slightly before an expected ventricular beat. (You will often need ECG calipers to see this.) Sometimes the early appearance of the capture beat can only be measured in milliseconds. If the narrow, normal complex appears *later* than the next expected wide complex, it only proves that there is *no pre-existing fixed bundle branch block*. It does not prove that there is no rate-related bundle branch block.

Another hint that AV dissociation is present is the appearance of a *fusion beat*. A fusion beat, as you may already know, is a hybrid between a normally conducted narrow complex and an ectopic wide complex. *The narrow beat will need to appear right at the time of the expected wide complex – or at least close enough for there to be an overlap of the QRS intervals.* A fusion beat also proves AV dissociation *in the context of a wide complex tachycardia* – but a fusion complex can occur with a sinus rhythm and a PVC, or a sinus rhythm and a ventricular parasystole.

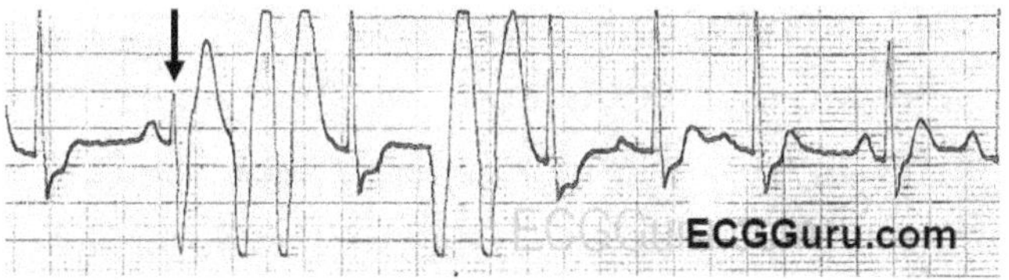

Figure 9-14

The arrow in this snippet (9-14) indicates a fusion beat. Note that it looks more like the beat following it. The PR interval is shorter, also. Identifying *this* QRS as a fusion beat is not difficult. How different a fusion beat appears depends on the contribution of the normally conducted beat. If the normally conducted beat arrives early enough, it will contribute more to the QRS and it will appear to begin like a normal, sinus-conducted beat. However, the more the ectopic beat dominates the depolarization, the more bizarre the depolarization will appear.

> **TIP |** Many fusion beats will look very similar to the ectopic rhythm and are often missed, making the recognition of AV dissociation somewhat problematic.

But you don't have to wait until a patient presents with a wide complex tachycardia and fusion beats to practice your skill at recognizing them. Just do an internet search for "wide complex tachycardia with fusion beats." (But be prepared for some incorrect examples!)

At left in Figure 9-15 is an actual capture beat occurring during ventricular tachycardia (the 6th QRS complex). These are *quite rare* – don't expect to see one on every tracing.

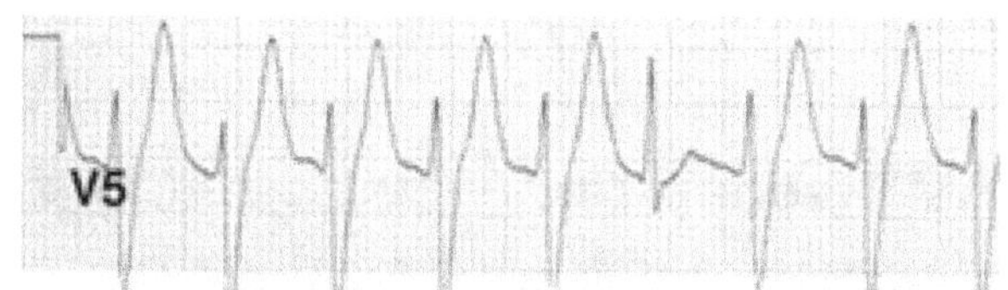

Figure 9-15 Courtesy of LITFL.com

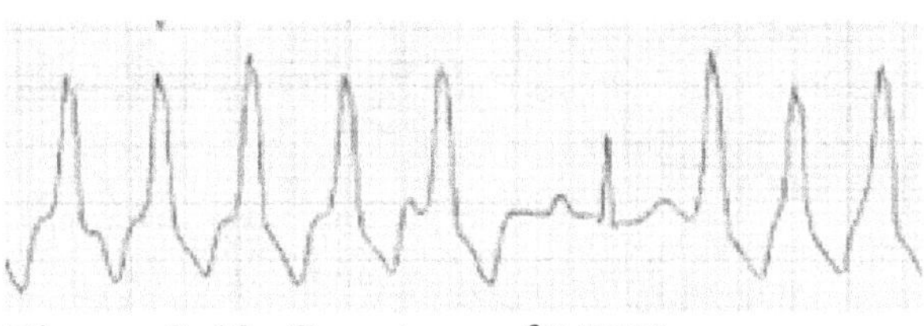

Figure 9-16 Courtesy of LITFL.com

In Figure 9-16, we see a normal beat that has captured the ventricles, but <u>it is not a capture beat</u>. It follows the preceding wide complex by an interval that is much longer than the R-R intervals of the WCT. The wide complex tachycardia *paused* just long enough to allow a sinus P wave to conduct. Wide complex tachycardias can do that. Ventricular tachycardias can do that, too. The term is *paroxysmal* which means start/stop, start/stop, etc. I reserve the use of the term *capture beat* to refer to sinus-conducted beats that end an R-R interval that is *shorter* than the prevailing rhythm (i.e., the wide complex tachycardia). Such beats indicate AV dissociation. A sinus conducted beat that appears at a *longer* R-R interval following a wide QRS complex *proves nothing* (see Figures 9-17 and 9-18) and should <u>not</u> be referred to as a capture beat!

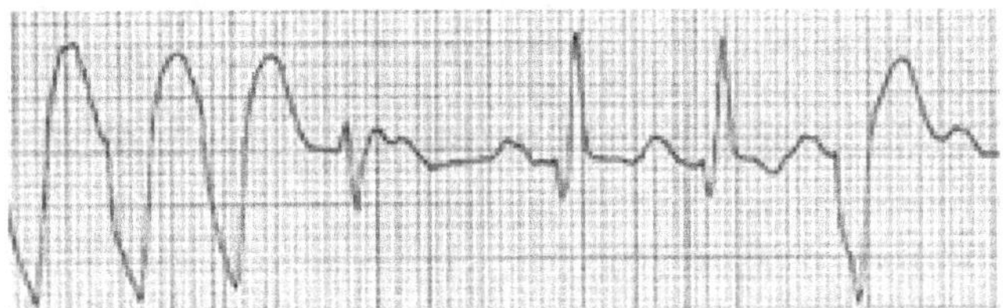

Figure 9-17 Courtesy of LITFL.com

In Figure 9-17, we see two wide complexes followed by a fusion beat which is intermediate between the ventricular ectopic beats and the normally-conducted sinus beats which, in turn, are followed by a ventricular ectopic beat. Let's keep this in perspective: **capture beats and fusion beats are rare**. Don't expect one in every tracing! Look for fusion beats at the beginning and end of the wide complex tachycardias – although they can appear just about anywhere. They are not as easy to spot because there is no eye-catching disruption in the ventricular rhythm. The rhythm is sometimes disrupted *slightly* – but usually so slightly that you won't notice it. Very often the shape and amplitude will be very similar to the ectopic beats, but just a little narrower.

These two sinus-conducted beats (Figure 9-18) with cross-marks are *not capture beats!* To be a capture beat – *which implies AV dissociation* – the sinus-conducted QRS must end an R-R interval that is shorter than the dominant rhythm, in this case,

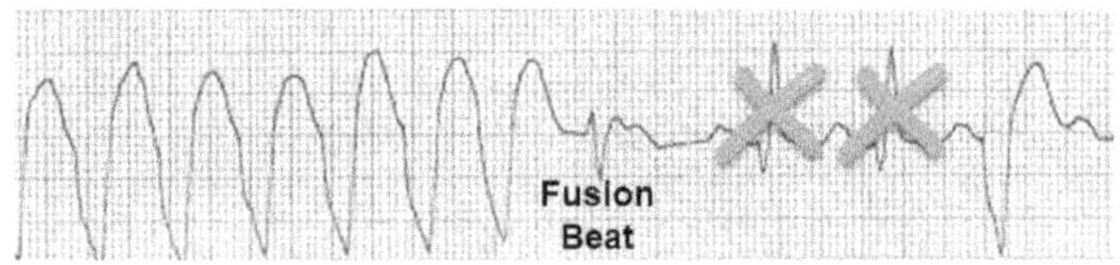

Figure 9-18 Courtesy of LITFL.com

the ventricular tachycardia. Unfortunately, fusion beats may not be so obviously different than the ectopic beats and sinus-conducted beats. Depending upon the exact moment the fusion occurs, the fusion beat may look a lot more like one of the other beats.

Let's practice!

AV Dissociation Practice: ECG #1

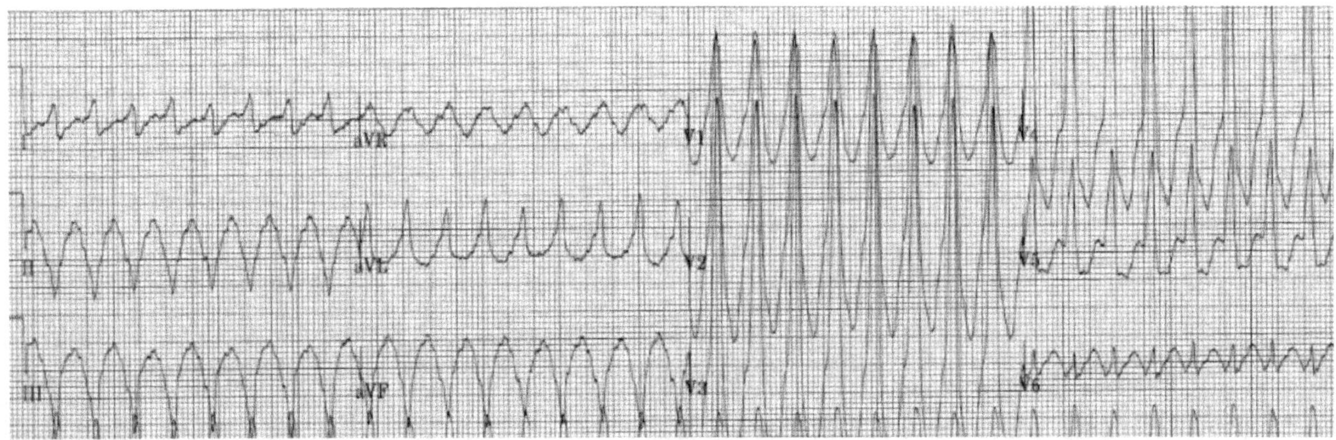

Figure 9-19

Can you find the evidence for AV dissociation in this tracing (Figure 9-19)? Take a look at Lead V5. What's happening there? Let's take a look at Lead V5 enlarged a bit (Figure 9-20)...

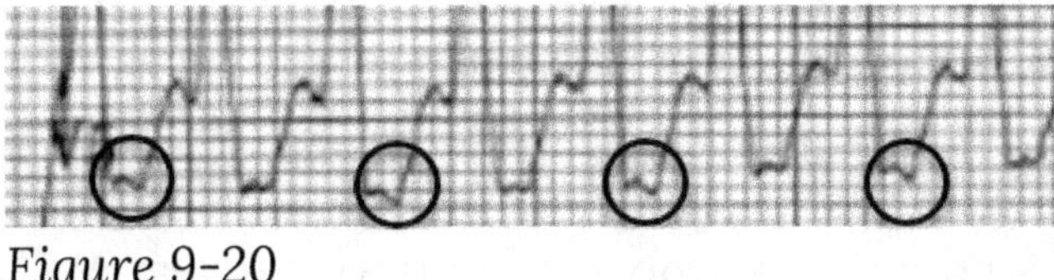

Figure 9-20

I've taken the liberty of circling a few examples of P' waves. When you spot a "hidden" P wave, check out the corresponding complexes in the leads above and below – some will be more obvious and some a lot more subtle, but both will hone your skill at detecting AV dissociation.

Figure 9-20 is an example of VA *dissociation*. The retrograde P' wave appears on every second beat. That indicates a 2:1 VA block and that *proves ventricular tachycardia.*

TIP | THREE VA blocks are detectable on an ECG: Mobitz I, Mobitz, II, and a 2:1 VA block. The 2:1 block is either a Mobitz I or a Mobitz II, but because there is no second P' to check for an increased R-P' interval, we must call it a 2:1 VA block.

AV Dissociation Practice: ECG #2

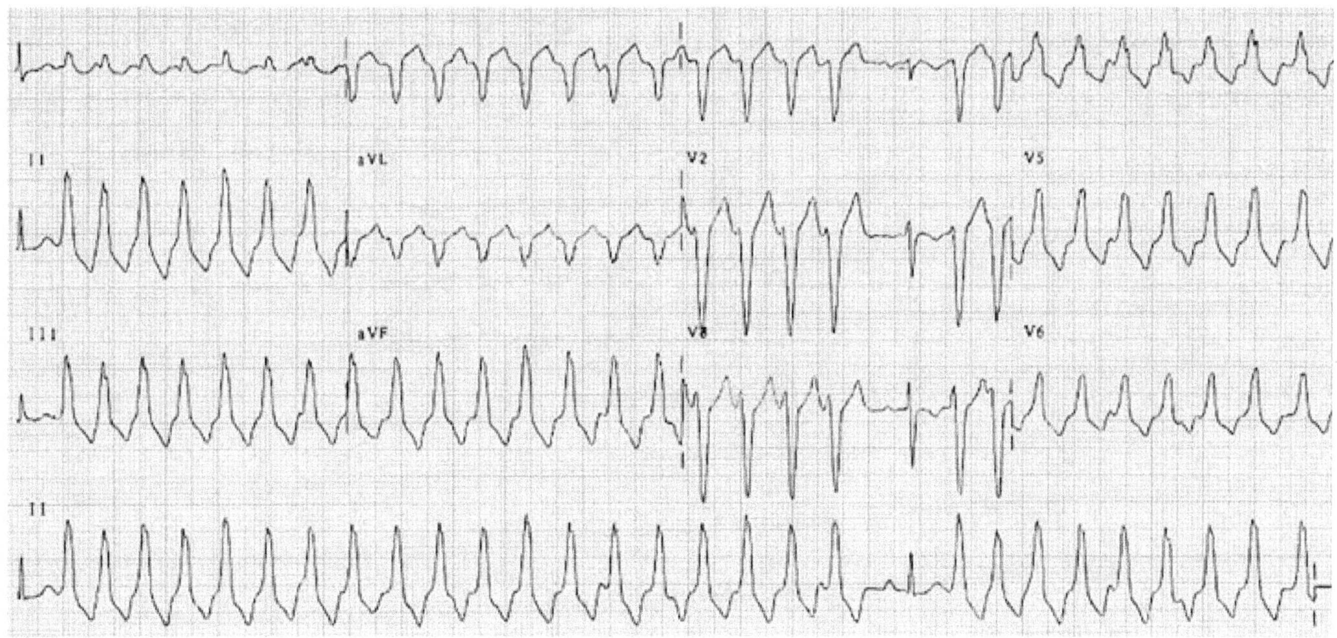

Figure 9-21

You've seen part of this ECG before (Figure 9-21): it contains a narrow complex that is *not* a capture beat. Even though there is no capture beat, there is still a lot of AV dissociation here. Study it carefully using your magnifying lens.

TIP | Start by focusing on the "shoulders" of the QRS complexes.

(Figure 9-22A) is a QRS complex with "normal shoulders." The shoulders are the part of the baseline just *before* and just *after* the QRS complex. You will learn more about "banks" and "shoulders" in Chapter 24, "More Practice with AV Dissociation."

(Figure 9-22B) demonstrates two consecutive QRS complexes whose shoulders suggest AV dissociation:

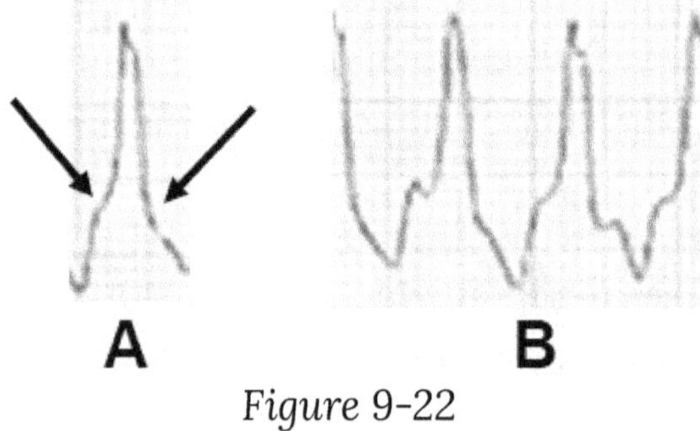

Figure 9-22

Recommended Reading:

Marriott HJL, Schwartz NL, Bix HH. Ventricular Fusion Beats. *Circulation*. 1962;26:880-884.

This is a classic paper. Read it carefully; I admit that it is easy to get confused as the discussion of fusion beats gets deeper. I'm sure you all recognize Dr. Marriott from his famous textbook. Dr. Bix, however, you may recognize from the famous "Bix rule": "When the ventricular rate is around 150/minute and the 'P waves' appear to be in the middle of the R-R intervals – always check for atrial flutter!"

Wang K, Benditt DG. AV dissociation, an inevitable response. *Ann Noninvasive Electro-cardiol*. 2011 Jul;16(3):227-31. doi: 10.1111/j.1542-474X.2011.00436.x. PMID: 21762249; PMCID: PMC6932318.

Chapter 10

How to Approach a Wide Complex Tachycardia

The "5 Step Start"

These are steps that I often take *before* beginning an algorithm or specific method. Some of the steps come from those same algorithms or methods. A few of the findings can essentially diagnose ventricular tachycardia while others simply provide information about the wide complex tachycardia that you will need for some algorithms and should be considered with other findings before making a diagnosis.

The question often arises, "*Must* I use an algorithm or method?" My answer is, "No, there's no rule or law that says you must... but until you have reached an expert level of ECG interpretation, I think you would be very foolish not to do so." And, as I have mentioned before, if you choose *not* to follow an algorithm or method and have a bad outcome, the situation may become very problematic for you. There are so many exceptions and nuances to these algorithms and methods that I would strongly recommend that you learn one or two of them quite well and use them. However, that does *not* prevent you from exercising your powers of observation, your knowledge, and your experience. You will learn my recommendations, tips, tricks, and – most importantly – caveats further on in this workbook.

> **PEARL |** While several findings can "rule in" *ventricular tachycardia*, SVT with aberrancy remains a diagnosis of exclusion.

Step 1 – Which Ventricle?

Whether the WCT is due to aberrantly conducted impulses originating in the supraventricular structures or whether it is due to impulses originating in the ventricle, they both have one thing in common: they are activating the ventricles *in succession – not simultaneously!* So, the first thing you must do is ascertain which ventricle the tachycardia source is activating first. We do this by checking Lead V1.

Lead V1 has the unique ability to distinguish right from left and we can almost always instantly determine which ventricle is activated first by the type of bundle branch block-*like* morphology present in Lead V1. Again, by bundle branch block-*like* we mean similar – but not necessarily *exactly* like – a classic bundle branch block. If the QRS is predominantly upright (positive), then it is right bundle branch block-*like*, and ventricular activation originated in the LEFT ventricle (LEFT – not right!). If the QRS is predominantly inverted (negative), then it is left bundle branch block-*like*, and ventricular activation originated in the RIGHT ventricle (RIGHT – not left!).

So, we always look at Lead V1 (and *only* Lead V1) first to learn which ventricle was activated first.

Step 2 – Outflow Tract or Apex?

OK… so you've determined which ventricle was activated first. *Where* in that ventricle did the activation begin? This is not a difficult question since we are going to divide the ventricles (both left and right) into two halves – upper and lower. The upper half we will refer to as **the outflow tract** and the lower half as **the apex**.

To determine whether the ventricular activation began in the outflow tract or the apex, we turn our attention to the *inferior limb leads* (Leads II, III, and aVF). If there is a *superior* axis, then the activation focus is located in the *apex* of that ventricle. If there is an *inferior* axis, the origin is located in the *outflow tract*.

A *superior* axis means the depolarization vector is traveling *upward*, from bottom to top, from *apex* to *outflow tract*. An *inferior* axis means the depolarization vector is traveling *downward*, from top to bottom, or from *outflow tract* to *apex*. This is very confusing – even for me! Just remember that **the QRS complexes in the inferior leads point to the *origin* of the impulse!**

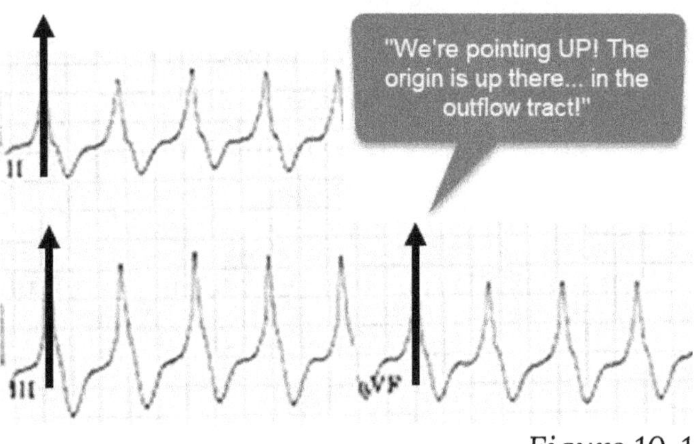

Figure 10-1

PEARL | The QRS complexes in the inferior leads always POINT TO WHERE THE IMPULSE ORIGINATED. Our concern is with where the impulse originated – not where it is going! Tall R waves in the inferior leads point UP to the outflow tract; rS complexes in the inferior leads point DOWN toward the APEX. Don't worry about "superior" and "inferior" axes. That's just too confusing!

Here is a practice example (Figure 10-3). Look at Lead V1 and determine *which ventricle* is activated first (because that is where the ventricular rhythm originated) and then check the inferior leads (II, III, aVF) to determine whether the impulse is originating in the *outflow tract* or the *apex*. Remember: **the QRS complexes in the inferior leads will *point toward the origin* of the impulse**.

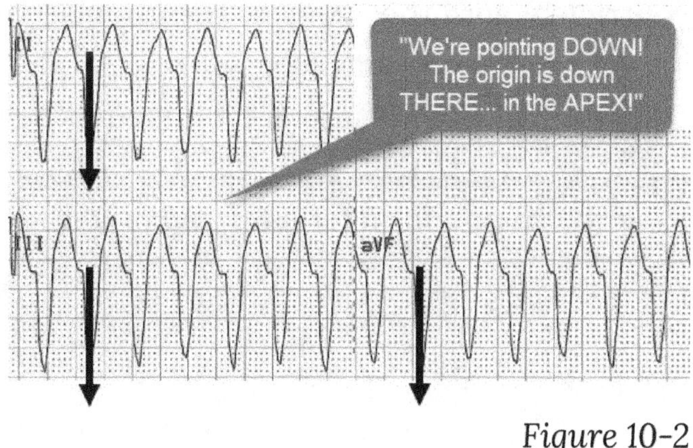

Figure 10-2

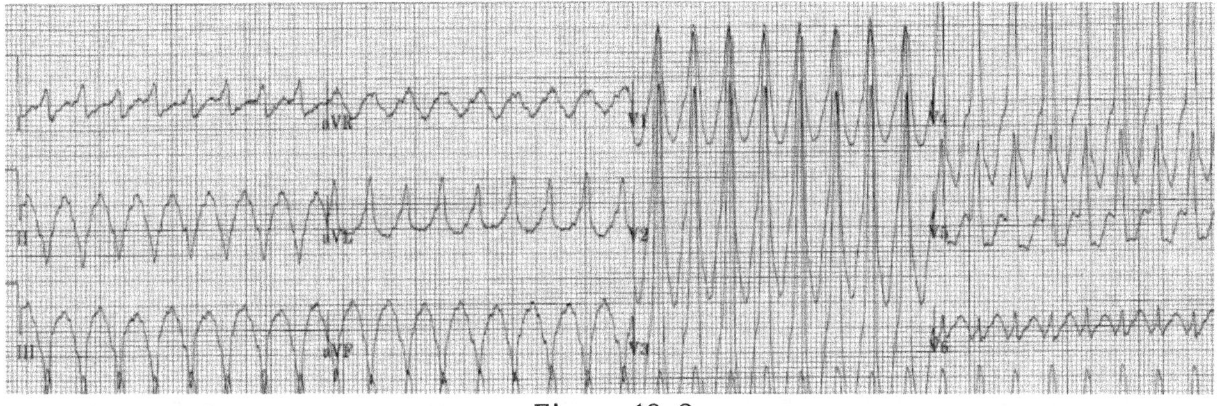

Figure 10-3

Now that wasn't so hard, was it? The QRS in Lead V1 had an RBBB-like morphology which tells us that the ventricular impulse originated in the LEFT ventricle. The QRS complexes in all the inferior leads were pointing downward (deep S waves) which indicated that the impulse was originating in the *apex* and traveling *upward* – a *superior axis*. Let's try another one...

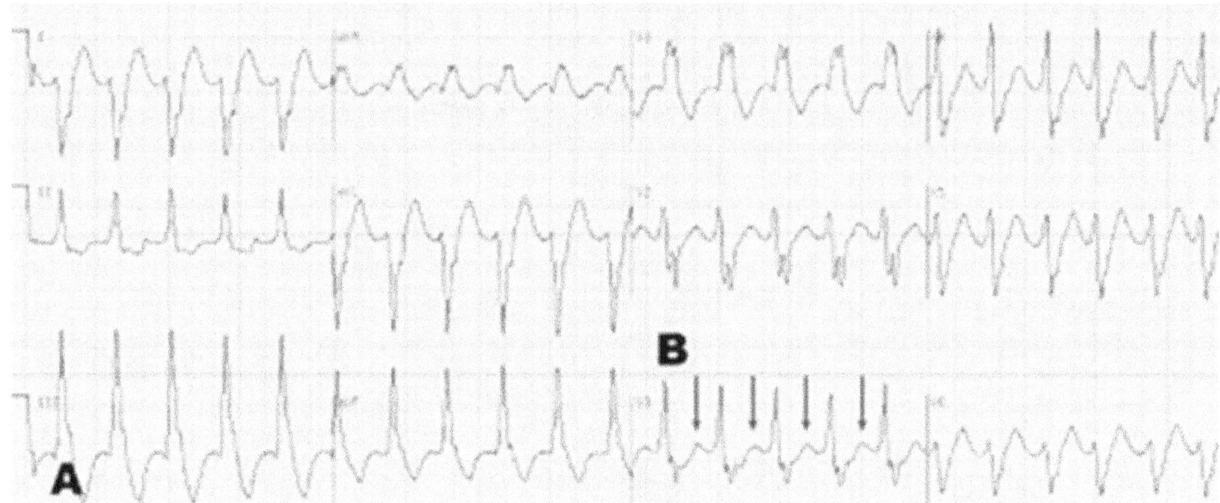

Figure 10-4

(Figure 10-4) Pay no attention to the letters and markings. Lead V1 manifests a QRS with an RBBB-like morphology which means the ventricular impulse originated in the *left* ventricle. All the QRS complexes in the inferior leads have tall R waves pointing up to the area of the ventricle where the origin of the impulse was located, in this case, the outflow tract. The *right* ventricle has an outflow tract (RVOT) and the *left* ventricle also has an outflow tract (LVOT). So, the impulse activating the left ventricle originated in the left ventricular outflow tract (LVOT). Tachycardias originating in either the right or left outflow tract have the *same characteristics and prognosis* and are *managed in the same way.*

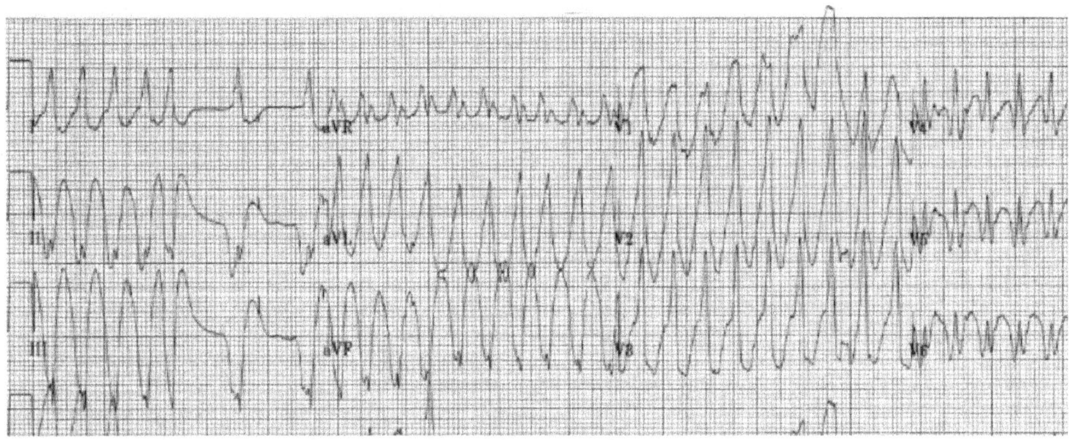

Figure 10-5

With Figure 10-5 the ECG has become more complex. However, a quick look at Lead V1 reveals an RBBB-like morphology (originating in the *left* ventricle) and QS waves in the inferior leads, indicating the origin of the impulse is in the apex of the left ventricle.

REMEMBER! | QRS complexes with tall R waves in the inferior leads indicate the impulse is coming from the *upper* part of the ventricle (outflow tract) and QRS complexes with deep S waves in the inferior leads mean the impulse is coming from the *lower* part of the ventricle (apex).

Let's see if you can maintain your speed as the ECGs get even more complicated.

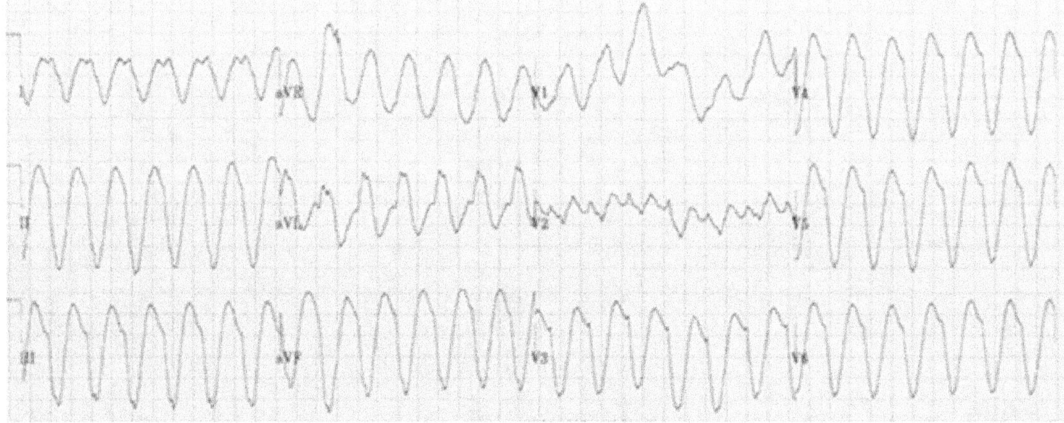

Figure 10-6

(Figure 10-6) Lead V1 manifests a monophasic upright QRS which indicates an RBBB-like morphology (and origin in the left ventricle) and all the inferior leads have QS complexes indicating an origin in the *apex* of the left ventricle.

OK... This next one (Figure 10-7) requires some thought. I'm going to bump up the complexity a bit...

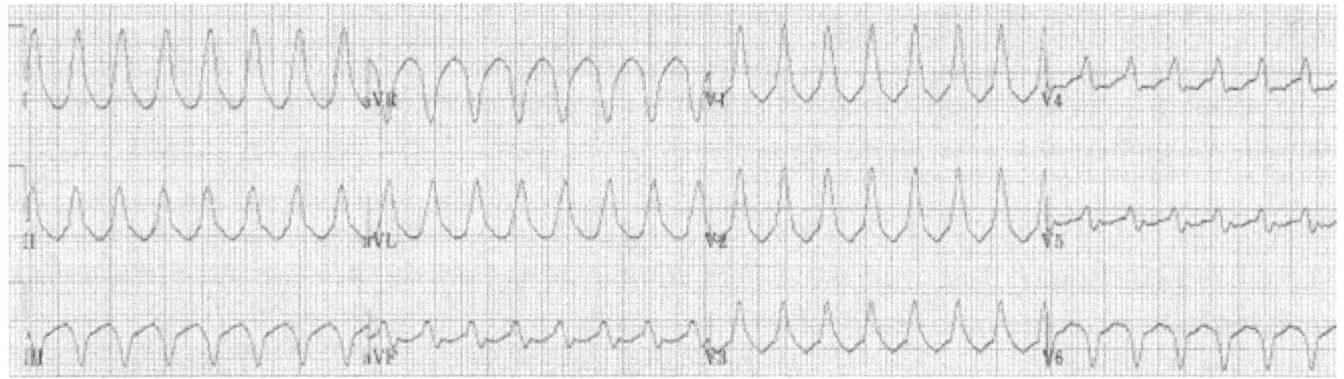

Figure 10-7

Did the QRS complexes in the inferior leads confuse you? Leads II and aVF have QRS complexes that are upright but Lead III has a QRS complex that is inverted.

In this ECG (Figure 10-7), you are presented with a situation in which not all the inferior leads are in agreement: two are upright and one is negative. The mean vector of all the inferior leads is not going to be pointing as straight down as before. Here's a tip for you:

> **TIP |** Lead aVF is the quintessential superior-inferior lead. It has no right or left vectors. When the inferior leads are not all concordant, base your decision on Lead aVF.

The bottom line is that not all the inferior leads need to point up to have an inferior axis (or *outflow* tract site of origin).

Step 3 – Precordial Transition

At this point, I check the precordial transition to validate my impression and more specifically localize the ectopic focus. This is quick and easy as long as you are familiar with interpreting the transition, so here it is – "in a nutshell:" left-sided ectopic foci will have early precordial transitions ranging from before Lead V1 to around Lead V3. The *earlier* the transition, the more leftward the location of the ectopic focus in the left ventricle. Right-sided ectopic foci will have late transitions, from around Lead V4 to beyond Lead V6. The *later* the transition, the more rightward the ectopic focus in the right ventricle.

What does it look like when a left-sided transition occurs *before* Lead V1? There is a dominant R wave in Lead V1 that continues throughout the precordial leads. A late transition beyond Lead V6 will manifest an rS complex in Lead V6. The closer the transition is to Lead V3 (either ventricle), the closer the focus is to the interventricular septum.

Step 4 – An Initial R Wave in Lead aVR or ÂQRS in the Right Upper Quadrant?

Next, inspect Lead aVR. If the initial deflection is a dominant R wave, then a diagnosis of ventricular tachycardia is strongly suggested.

Check Leads I and aVF to see if the mean QRS axis (ÂQRS) is in the *northwest quadrant* ("No Man's Land"), characterized by negative QRS complexes in both Leads I and aVF. If so, it is a good indicator of an ectopic ventricular rhythm (VT) – but... it's not 100% accurate. Class 1c anti-arrhythmic medications in toxic levels - especially flecainide - can cause this. Hyperkalemia can also result in mean QRS axes in the NW quadrant. If you know that the patient is not taking any Class 1c anti-arrhythmic agents and is not experiencing hyperkalemia, then you can certainly keep your impression of ventricular tachycardia.

Step 5 – Classic Bundle Branch Block in Leads V1 or V6?

Check Leads V1 and V6 to see if *either* one represents a classic RBBB morphology or a classic LBBB morphology. If *just one* of the two leads manifests a classic pattern, then a diagnosis of SVT with aberrancy is strongly favored. If *neither* Lead V1 *nor* Lead V6 manifest a classic bundle branch block pattern, then VT is very likely.

Summary of the "5 Step Start"

1. Look at Lead V1 and determine in *which ventricle* the rhythm is originating.

2. Look at Leads II, III, and aVF to determine if the impulse is originating in the *outflow* tract or *apex*.

3. Check the precordial transition to determine more exactly where the ventricular impulse is originating.

4. Is there a dominant R wave in Lead aVR? Look at Leads I and aVF to see if the impulse vector is directed toward the "northwest quadrant." If so (and there are no Class I anti-arrhythmic drugs or hyperkalemia), that would strongly suggest an origin of the impulse in the lower ventricle; thus, ventricular tachycardia is favored.

5. Check Leads V1 and V6 to see if *either* one manifests a classic bundle branch block pattern – right or left. If just one manifests a classic pattern, *supraventricular tachycardia with aberrancy* is favored.

Just So There Is No Misunderstanding | The "5 Step Start" is the approach that I use *before* starting an algorithm. It is NOT offered to be a tested or proven algorithm. It does not *replace* an algorithm. I still depend on one or more algorithms I have become proficient in using due to practice, practice, practice!

Recommended Reading:

Lam P, MD, Saba S, MD. Approach to the Evaluation and Management of Wide Complex Tachycardias. *Indian Pacing and Electrophysiology Journal.* 2(4): 120-126 (2002).

I have found the *Indian Pacing and Electrophysiology Journal* to be a great source of review articles often focusing on topics for the non-specialist.

Katritsis DG, and Brugada J. Differential Diagnosis of Wide QRS Tachycardias. *Arrhythmia & Electrophysiology Review.* 2020;9(3):155–60.

Kashou AH, MD, et al. Wide Complex Tachycardia Differentiation: A Reappraisal of the State-of-the-Art. *J Am Heart Assoc.* 2020;9:e016598. DOI: 10.1161/JAHA.120.016598.

Garner JB, Miller JM. Wide complex tachycardia—ventricular tachycardia or not ventricular tachycardia, that remains the question. *Arrhythm Electrophysiol Rev.* 2013;2:23–29.

Chapter 11

The Algorithms and Methods

Things To Watch for in Every Algorithm and Method

There are many algorithms, methods, and criteria for diagnosing wide complex tachycardias. And more are published every day! I have chosen to discuss and train you in depth using those that are more amenable to use in urgent and emergent situations. Many published algorithms are not feasible for use in stressful, emergent cases. Some require measuring up to seven criteria and then assigning weighted values to them while others are nothing more than unvalidated, "cherry-picked" criteria from other published algorithms and methods. Many have either no validation studies or validation studies that fail to substantiate the claims made about the derivation study. Here is some advice for evaluating algorithms and methods for their feasibility of use and reliability.

A few paragraphs are typically included pointing out how *other* algorithms and methods were not found to be as accurate in validation studies but somehow *theirs will* remain accurate and reliable... until, of course, the first independent validation study is published, in which *their* method is found to be every bit as *insensitive, nonspecific* and/or *inaccurate* as the others.

Why does this happen? There are several possible explanations: the original authors may simply be more adept and skillful at using their own method, or the patient population they studied may have produced *by chance* tachydysrhythmias that were more amenable to recognition by their algorithm or method. Or perhaps the selected omission of certain types of tachydysrhythmias increased the sensitivity and/or specificity of their method.

Now let's talk about some "validation studies." If you have read as many "validation" studies as I have, you will begin to notice that some actually alter the methods used in the derivation studies so that they are no longer the same algorithm or method as in the original article; or they interpret the methods in ways never intended by the original authors. Example: some authors critiquing the Brugada algorithm insist on stating that the First Step was created to decide if there were any concordance of the precordial leads – and *that* is what *they* are looking for in the First Step. That has got to be some of the most blatant and egregious misinformation I have ever seen! There is *absolutely no mention of concordance in the Brugada article* and the Brugadas *et al.* state very clearly and specifically how they came to include the First Step... and it had *nothing* to do with concordance!

1. Understand that EACH algorithm and method has failure *built-in!*

Please understand that you will *never* achieve 100% accuracy with any of the algorithms or methods because *failure is built-in.* Here's why I say that: none of the algorithms or methods take into consideration *all the types of wide complex tachycardias.* Antidromic AVRT is often not included in the studies; fascicular and bundle branch tachycardias are frequently not included, either. Such omissions will result in a given algorithm or method being insensitive to those tachydysrhythmias. Why are these different tachydysrhythmias omitted from the derivation study? Perhaps because they would make the method too difficult, cumbersome, or less specific. By their omissions, the algorithm or method will appear more sensitive and more specific. That always looks good while one is trying to promote one's own study. But the answer may actually lie in #2 (next)...

2. The patients in the derivation study are not like YOUR patients.

Let's face it... it's really difficult to acquire patients who are having episodes of wide complex tachycardias to study them, and it's especially difficult to locate and study the rarer types. Therefore, the majority of these patients had *scheduled electrophysiology studies*, and many of the tachydysrhythmias were *artificially induced in the EP lab.* Many of these patients may or may not have an increased amount of organic heart disease which could be different than your patients. In addition, the conditions of initiation of the dysrhythmias are different than in your patients.

3. Where to Find the Information Just Discussed

You can usually find information regarding which dysrhythmias were excluded and how the recordings of the dysrhythmias were obtained under two subtitles in any journal article: **METHODS** and **LIMITATIONS**. Always glance at these sections if you have questions about the accuracy and/or reliability of the algorithm or method they are promoting.

Remember This!

Always be aware that all the algorithms and methods allow for only *one* diagnosis – *ventricular tachycardia.* "But wait," you say. "If it's not ventricular tachycardia then it's SVT with aberrancy!"

SVT *is not a diagnosis*! It's just a general term for at least eight (possibly more) diagnoses. It's similar to telling a patient, "Your diagnosis is *illness*."

Is it sinus tachycardia, reentrant sinus tachycardia, atrial tachycardia, atrial flutter, atrial fibrillation, junctional tachycardia, multifocal atrial tachycardia, AVNRT, AVRT or permanent junctional reciprocating tachycardia? The prognosis and treatment of these various dysrhythmias is quite different – some are relatively benign while other have the potential for episodes with fatal outcomes. Some are very conducive to tachycardia-induced cardiomyopathy while others are not.

SVT is a *pseudo*-diagnosis! Granted, if you are managing the patient in an emergency room or urgent care center, you will likely not be able to arrive at a definitive diagnosis. But you *must* understand this and it is very important that a definitive diagnosis eventually be made. A diagnosis of an AVNRT is generally benign, but an AVRT means the patient has an accessory pathway *which could prove fatal in the event of an atrial fibrillation or atrial flutter!*

Recommended Reading:

Alzand BS, Crijns HJ. Diagnostic criteria of broad QRS complex tachycardia: decades of evolution. *Europace*. 2011;13:465–472.

Kashou AH, MD, et al. Wide Complex Tachycardia Differentiation: A Reappraisal of the State-of-the-Art. *J Am Heart Assoc*. 2020;9:e016598. DOI: 10.1161/JAHA.120.016598.

Sousa PA, Pereira S, Candeias R, de Jesus I. The value of electrocardiography for differential diagnosis in wide QRS complex tachycardia. *Rev Port Cardiol*. 2014;33(3):165-173.

Wellens HJJ. Ventricular tachycardia: diagnosis of broad QRS complex tachycardia. *Heart*. 2001;86:579±585.

Chapter 12

The Brugada Algorithm

The Brugada algorithm consists of four steps. Two are easy, two will require some practice, and a few may require the use of calipers and/or a magnifying lens (if you are not using digital calipers). The third step (identifying AV dissociation) requires practice and experience. The fourth step (morphological criteria) has always been viewed as the most problematic because people try to memorize the morphological criteria and it's just too darn difficult to remember – especially while under stress! I am going to teach you all four steps and there will be no memory issues. Here's how the Brugada algorithm works: the first three steps are worded so that any "Yes!" answer indicates ventricular tachycardia. You stop with the first "Yes!" answer because you have your diagnosis at that point; there's no need to go any further. This is *important* because *the steps with better specificity and accuracy are placed first*. Otherwise, you may find yourself in a paradoxical situation in which a "Yes" answer in Step 2 indicating a diagnosis of VT could be followed by a Step 4 result that suggests the (incorrect) diagnosis of SVT with aberrancy. Avoid this by stopping at the first "Yes" answer.

In Step 4 a "YES!" answer will still diagnose ventricular tachycardia using the "Jones Modification" of Step 4, but the question will be asked differently. This is the same as the third step of the Vereckei Algorithm #1 (2007).

Step 1: Is there an absence of an RS complex in all precordial leads?

This pertains to rS, RS, or Rs complexes, though you will usually see an rS complex if any are present. Some people interpret this to mean that the absence of RS complexes indicates that the Brugadas are looking for *concordance*.

> **STOP RIGHT THERE! |** Precordial concordance means that the QRS complexes in all precordial leads are strictly monophasic – either monophasic R waves or monophasic QS waves and all have the same polarity.

Saying that Step 1 is a search for precordial concordance is *total misinformation!* One could still have a QR wave or rSR'. When concordance was first described, it was defined as all positive <u>monophasic</u> QRS complexes (meaning monophasic R waves) or all negative <u>monophasic</u> QRS complexes (meaning monophasic QS complexes). Of late, some people are now defining it as "mostly" positive QRS complexes or "mostly" negative QRS complexes in "most" precordial leads. **That is not correct!** What's more, the people who depend on the "mostly" definitions do not suggest how much "mostly" refers to. In their original paper in which they presented these criteria, the Brugadas *et al. never mentioned or even alluded to the word concordance.* **Concordance is not part of the Brugada criteria or algorithm.**

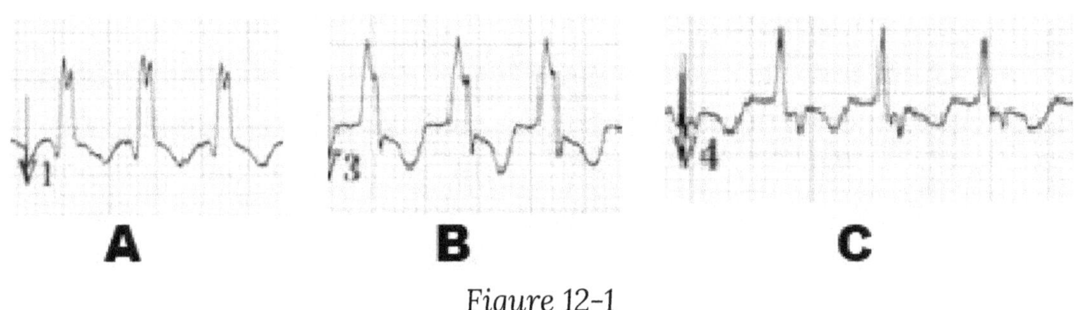

Figure 12-1

As a refresher (Figure 12-1)...

A is a qR complex. It automatically disqualifies the precordial leads from consideration of concordance since it is not monophasic. It also establishes the lack of a classic, complete RBBB in Lead V1. But it can still be present and not counted as an RS complex.

B is an Rs complex. It leads to a "NO!" answer in Step 1 of the Brugada algorithm and it also disqualifies the precordial leads from consideration of concordance. Do you notice something else unusual in this lead*?

C is also an Rs complex with the same disqualifications. It also has the same unusual finding.*

> ***PEARL |** When you see an inverted T wave immediately following an S wave, always consider the presence of *ischemia – whether there is a tachycardia or not.* This is called a *primary* repolarization abnormality and it is very abnormal. Ischemia is a known cause of ventricular tachycardia.

Here is an example of an ECG without any RS complexes in the precordial leads but also without either form of concordance (Figure 12-2):

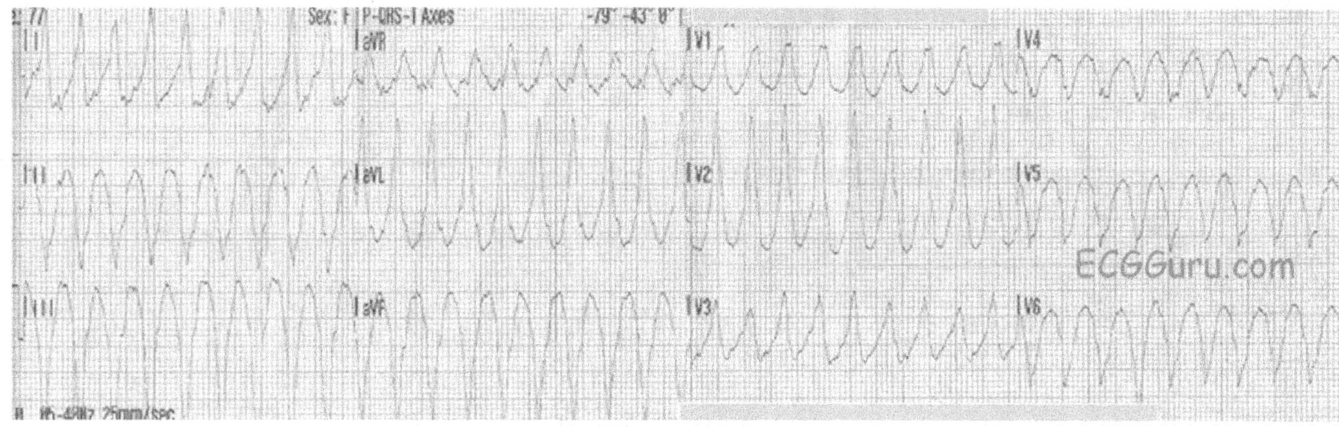

Figure 12-2

Returning to **Step 1**: If the answer is "Yes!" we have a diagnosis of ventricular tachycardia and we STOP; otherwise, we proceed to...

Step 2: If one or more RS complexes are present, do any of them have an onset R to S nadir > 100 msec?

Please note that the Brugadas were very specific about the use of the words *greater than* **(>)** and *not* **"equal to or greater than"** **(≥)**. This measurement is made from the *beginning* of the R wave where it leaves the baseline (not the peak) to the *nadir* (the lowest peak) of the S wave. Don't worry about what to do if there is a q wave because this step applies *only* to **biphasic RS complexes**. The reasoning behind this measurement is that in ventricular tachycardia, the depolarization wave originates in the myocardium and travels through the myocardium by cell-to-cell propagation. This is going to cause a slower initial inscription on the ECG paper. Conversely, a depolarization wave originating in the atria and entering the ventricles through the His-Purkinje system will have an initial inscription on the ECG that is more rapid due to conduction through the normal conducting pathways up to the point that a block or delay is encountered.

At this point there is a problem in their reasoning: this concept – which is indeed reasonable and valid – pertains *only* to ventricular ectopy originating in the working myocardium. But three ventricular tachycardias can develop within the His-Purkinje system (HPS) itself: *fascicular tachycardia* which is *benign* and *bundle branch tachycardia* and *interfascicular tachycardia* which *are highly* dangerous. All these tachydysrhythmias can have R-to-S nadir measurements less than 100 msec (and often less than 80 msec). It is still possible for them to be detected by the Brugada algorithm and correctly diagnosed as ventricular tachycardia, but there is also a significant chance they will be missed.

The Brugada algorithm is also not sensitive to impulses entering the ventricles via an antegrade accessory pathway. The Brugadas did not distinguish between an antegrade impulse entering the ventricles through an accessory pathway and ventricular tachycardia since both impulses originated in the ventricular myocardium so an antidromic AVRT will be counted as ventricular tachycardia.

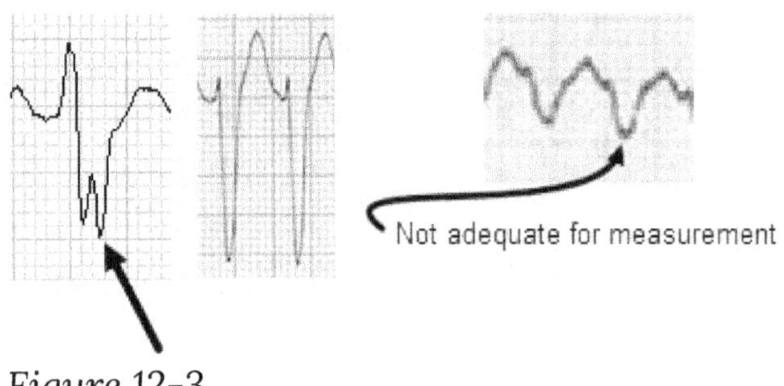

Figure 12-3

Please note in Figure 12-3 that if there is more than one nadir in the S wave, you measure to the *second* nadir because you are measuring duration. Also, the nadir must come to a sufficient point that an exact measurement can be made; a rounded nadir cannot be used.

The Brugadas also make it very clear that an R-to-S nadir that equals 100 msec cannot be considered a "YES!" answer. They had several supraventricular tachycardias with aberrant conduction that were *exactly* 100 msec. All ventricular tachycardias were *greater than* 100 msec. So, exactly 100 msec gets a "NO!" answer.

The two snippets in Figure 12-4 (below) are from Lead V1 (different patients) recorded during documented ventricular tachycardias. In **A**, there is no need for caliper measurements. You can easily see that the R-to-S nadir will be greater than 100 msec (that's 2.5 small squares). The rS complex in **B** is very close to 100 msec. Here's the difference you should learn – the wide QRS developed in *ventricular myocardium* and is wide – likely – for two reasons: 1) slow cell-to-cell conduction and 2) most probably structural heart disease rendering conduction even more problematic. This VT is very dangerous! The narrower rS (**B**) is from the *right ventricular outflow tract*, most likely on or very near the interventricular septum. There are pathways nearby that can facilitate the conduction of an impulse, so it tends to be narrower and better formed. Compare the two r waves and the two S wave descents. Note the subtle difference in slopes. This ventricular tachycardia is considered *benign* (if it doesn't occur too frequently). **More on this beginning in Chapter 19...**

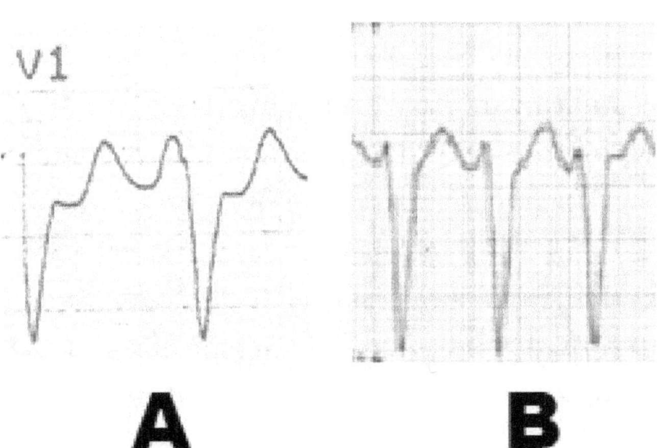

Figure 12-4

If the answer is "Yes!" we have a diagnosis of ventricular tachycardia and we STOP; otherwise, we proceed to...

Step 3: Is there evidence of AV dissociation?

The recognition of AV dissociation and VA dissociation requires *study*, *practice*, and *experience*. Bear in mind that evidence of AV or VA dissociation is visible in only about 20% of wide complex tachycardias. If signs are present – and you are *experienced* and *skilled* at recognizing these signs – it should take you no more than about 20 seconds to locate them. Therefore, if you are not as experienced at recognizing the signs of AV or VA dissociation, don't spend more than 20 seconds looking for it if you are in the process of managing a patient with a wide complex tachycardia. This workbook has given you the tools you will need to accomplish this task (Chapters 9 and 24), so search online for wide complex tachycardias and practice, practice, practice! We have already discussed AV dissociation at length, so if the answer is "Yes!" we have a diagnosis of ventricular tachycardia and we STOP; otherwise, we proceed to...

Step 4: Are the morphological criteria for ventricular tachycardia present in *both* Lead V1 *and* Lead V6?

This is the step that gives the Brugada algorithm its bad reputation as a "difficult-to-remember" algorithm. There's a tremendous difference between rote memorization and understanding the concepts and reasons behind something.

> **PEARL |** If you *understand* something, you won't have to memorize it. When was the last time you forgot that fire will burn you?

If I gave you 100 pieces of paper numbered 1 to 100, then randomly put 96 of them in Box A and 4 in Box B, then told you to memorize the contents of each box, would you seriously try to memorize the 96 numbers in Box A? Yet so many people try to memorize the "96 numbers in Box A" when it comes to learning the fourth step of the Brugada algorithm by trying to memorize *all the exceptions* to a classic bundle branch block pattern. However, let's not blame them; that is somewhat the way it is presented in the Brugadas' original article. Let's learn how to use the morphological criteria in the Fourth Step.

Learning the Fourth Step of the Brugada Algorithm

The first thing to do is decide on the QRS morphology in Lead V1. You've already learned how to do that. After deciding which morphology is present, you have only two leads to consider: V1 and V6. We do not evaluate the limb leads in the Brugada Algorithm except during Step 3 – the search for AV dissociation.

RBBB-like Morphology

Anything *other than* this pattern in V1 with these two patterns in V6 points to ventricular tachycardia (Figure 12-5):

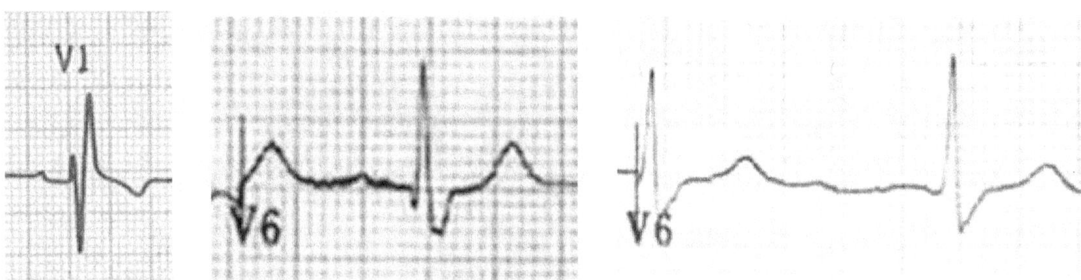

Figure 12-5

So, with an RBBB-like morphology, if the QRS complex in Lead V1 is anything *other than* the classic triphasic rSR′ of complete RBBB, VT is favored.

Let me point out a few things about the classic, complete RBBB (cRBBB) pattern in Lead V1:

1. It is produced by impulses traveling through the His bundle followed by the Purkinje system (bundle branches, fascicles). Only two other dysrhythmias can produce that exact morphology and both are rare: *bundle branch tachycardia* and *fascicular tachycardia*. Thankfully, the lethal one is the rarer of the two.

2. The pattern of a classic, complete RBBB does *not* include a tall r wave. It includes a tall R′ wave.

3. An ectopic impulse originating in the ventricular working myocardium *cannot produce that same pattern*. It just cannot do it! However, ventricular tachycardia originating in or near a conducting fiber can! The closest resemblance is simply a deflection on the same side of the baseline (RBBB-*like*) which has *very little to do with the origin of the impulse* – it just tells us which ventricle was activated first! An ectopic impulse can originate in either ventricle and a supraventricular impulse can *activate* either ventricle first. *Identifying which ventricle was activated first does not give us a diagnosis – it just gives us a starting point in our analysis of the dysrhythmia.*

Moving to Lead V6, the same criteria hold except for an RS complex. If there is an RS complex the R/S ratio must be greater than 1.0 (R wave height greater than S wave depth) to indicate a classic, complete RBBB pattern in Lead V6. Remember: **to diagnose ventricular tachycardia, the criteria for classic, complete RBBB must be ABSENT in <u>both</u> leads, not just one!**

TIP | The morphological criteria have less specificity than the first, second, or third steps. For a more detailed discussion, see: "Read This! – The Problem No One Mentions..." at the end of this chapter.

To summarize:

Lead V1: Anything other than some variation of rSR' suggests ventricular tachycardia. An rSR', however, does not rule out ventricular tachycardia.

Lead V6: Anything other than some variation of qRs suggests ventricular tachycardia *unless it is an RS complex*, in which case the R wave must be taller than the S wave depth to clinch the diagnosis of supraventricular tachycardia. This stipulation always raises a question...

What if there is an rS complex in Lead V6 with a classic RBBB pattern in Lead I and an anterior fascicular block pattern noted in the limb leads? Does that create a problem when using the Brugada algorithm? After all, the Vereckei algorithm (discussed later) takes anterior fascicular block into consideration.

The answer is "No, it does not create a problem." First, *the presence of a classic RBBB pattern in Lead V1 during Step 4 will automatically result in the diagnosis of SVT with aberrancy.* Remember: a *classic bundle branch morphology* in just *one* of the two leads – V1 or V6 – is all that is necessary to RULE OUT ventricular tachycardia. A potential problem here would be *posterior fascicular tachycardia* - a ventricular tachycardia arising in or very close to the posterior fascicle of the left ventricle.

> **PEARL |** A complete RBBB with rS complexes in Leads II, III, and aVF indicates an anterior fascicular block *only* when there is normal conduction from above the division of the His bundle into the right and left bundle branches). During an ectopic rhythm, such as ventricular tachycardia, such a pattern does *not* indicate block – it indicates the *origin of the ectopic rhythm from the posterior fascicle or very near to it.*

LBBB-like Morphology

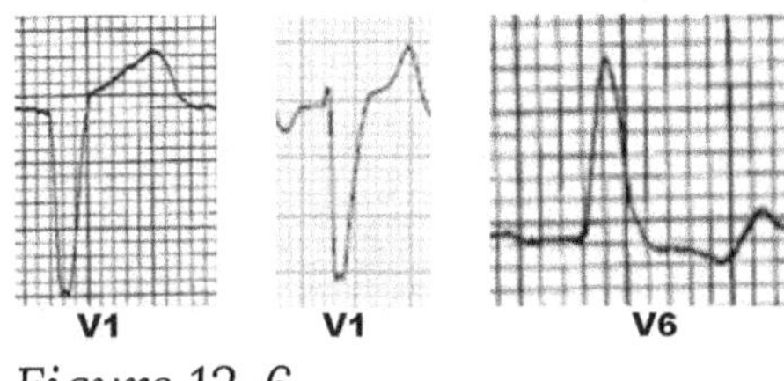

Figure 12-6

With LBBB-like morphology, when we analyze Lead V1 we must do a little more measuring and also understand that we are now going to do the same measurement of the **onset R to S nadir** as in Step 2. At this point, since we still have not made a diagnosis of ventricular tachycardia (or we would not be doing this step), the Brugadas are going to let us lower our standards and will now allow a measurement of **greater than (>) 60 msec** to make a diagnosis instead of greater than 100 msec. (This is in accordance with the original Kindwall criteria which established the morphological criteria for LBBB in 1988.) Even if that doesn't qualify, an r wave greater than 30 msec in duration in Lead V1 is suggestive of ventricular tachycardia. If that doesn't work, any notching in the S wave will qualify. Remember: since *this is only Lead V1 being considered* at this point, we can't diagnose ventricular tachycardia unless Lead V6 *also* fails to manifest any sign of classic LBBB morphology. To diagnose ventricular tachycardia, BOTH Leads V1 and V6 must not have any deflections indicating a *classic* LBBB. If needed, refer to Figure 12-6 (middle snippet) to refresh your memory of a *classic* LBBB morphology.

In Lead V6, the main thing to remember is that a Q or q or QS is highly suggestive of ventricular tachycardia. The Brugadas also included the presence of a monophasic R wave in Lead V6 as an indication of SVT-A (a classic, complete LBBB pattern) rather than VT, but don't rely on this finding too much: true, it was present in 31/31 (100%) patients with SVT-A, but it was also present in 29/35 (83%) patients with VT – not very discriminating at all.

> **TIP |** Why is a notch on the downslope of the S wave so important, other than as a sign of a previous myocardial infarction? In the presence of a complete LBBB, the S wave represents late activation of the left ventricle. The location of the notch on the downslope of the S wave specifically localizes the old MI to the left ventricle – the most common site for MIs. Without a LBBB you would not be able to see it.

The Brugadas did not specify where on the S wave the notch needed to be, but Cabrera's sign (indicative of a previous MI in LBBB) is a notch on the *upslope* of the S wave and Josephson's sign is a notch on the *downslope* of the S wave near the nadir. So it appears the Brugadas are relying on statistics.

Cabrera's sign: notch on *the upslope* of the S wave in Lead V1 but *only in the presence of complete* LBBB

Josephson's sign: notch on the *downslope* of the S wave "near" the nadir (also *only during* complete LBBB)

> **PEARL |** A memory aid here: Josephson has two O's at the beginning and end and "downslope" also has two O's at the beginning and end.

TIP | The issue of notching as a diagnostic aid pertains *only* to the notching seen with a left bundle branch block-like morphology. The fact that the notches are either on the *downslope near the nadir* or on the *upslope* of the S wave indicates the portion of the QRS representative of left ventricular activation. The first 40 msec or so would represent activation of the right ventricle.

To summarize:

Lead V1: Signs of initial slow propagation due to origination in the peripheral myocardium – R to S nadir > 60 msec, R wave duration > 30 msec in an rS complex or a notch in the S wave

Lead V6: The presence of any Q or q wave (including QS)

The Jones Modification of Step 4

The question remains, "Do BOTH Leads V1 and V6 FAIL to demonstrate a *classic* bundle branch block morphology?"

If "YES!", then the diagnosis is ventricular tachycardia. If "NO!", then the diagnosis is supraventricular tachycardia with aberrancy. This maintains the original pattern of "YES!" = VT and "NO!" = SVT-A.

While it helps to know all the possible presentations of the QRS complexes of the morphological criteria, *it is not necessary.* Just learn – *thoroughly* – what the classic criteria for RBBB and LBBB look like in BOTH Leads V1 *and* V6 and know that *anything different supports ventricular tachycardia.* The Jones Method of Step 4 is not about learning all the *exceptions* – it's about learning the RULE!

In my years of teaching, I have found that while most of my students are quite familiar with the classic patterns in Lead V1, they often have no idea what the classic pattern should look like in Lead V6 – for either bundle branch block morphology. Learn it *now* so you won't have to be concerned about it when a *real* WCT patient arrives.

More thoughts on the Brugada algorithm

The further you get into the algorithm, the less discriminatory the criteria. The first three steps are very good at distinguishing between supraventricular tachycardia with aberrant conduction (SVT-A) and VT. However, by the time you get to the morphological criteria, the difference between the two dysrhythmias becomes less and less distinctive. For example, in LBBB-like morphology, a monophasic R in Lead V6 is supposed to favor SVT-A over VT because 100% of patients (31 out of 31) with SVT-A had this finding; however, 83% of patients with VT (29 out of 35) also had a monophasic R wave. This means you have only a 1 in 5 chance of making an assured, correct diagnosis of SVT-A based on this criterion.

What exactly IS the Jones Modification of Step 4? The Jones Modification simply states that instead of looking for all the different exceptions to a classic bundle branch block in Leads V1 and V6, just remember exactly what a classic bundle branch block should look like in both leads. Anything different means it is NOT a classic bundle branch block. In other words, why learn the classic patterns PLUS all conceivable exceptions when you only have to know the classic patterns?

All numbers involved in comparative measurements are greater than (>), <u>not</u> equal to or greater than (≥). This includes

> 1. **R-to-S nadir in any precordial lead >** 100 msec (RBBB-like pattern, Step 2),
>
> 2. **R-to-S nadir in Lead V1 >** 60 msec (LBBB-like pattern, morphological criteria: Step 4) and
>
> 3. **R wave in Lead V1 >** 30 msec (LBBB-like pattern, morphological criteria: Step 4).

Despite all the different morphological patterns involved, you only need to remember six complexes (and you already know all or most of them):

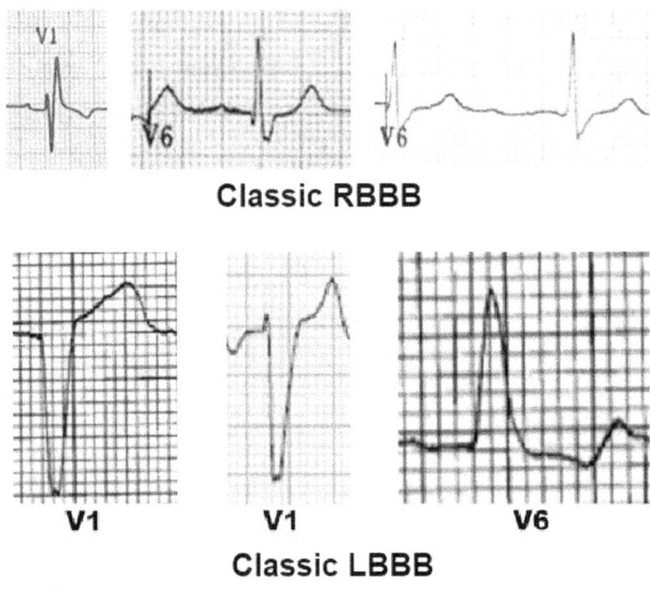

12-7

The **classic triphasic (rSR')** in Lead V1 and the **qRs** or **Rs** in Lead V6 for classic RBBB morphology and the **rS** or **QS** in Lead V1 and the **monophasic R** wave in Lead V6 for classic LBBB morphology. If these patterns are missing in BOTH Leads V1 and V6 then the diagnosis is ventricular tachycardia.

You need to remember just three numbers: 100, 60, and 30 (which are all msec)

The R to S nadir measurement appears <u>twice</u>:

The first time it appears in **Step 2** where the cut-off is > 100 msec (our standards are still high at that point). The measurement in Step 2 applies to *any precordial lead (and <u>only</u> precordial leads).*

The second time it appears is in **Step 4** (morphological criteria, Lead V1) for LBBB-like morphology where the cut-off is lowered to 60 msec. The measurement in Step 4 applies *only to Lead V1 and the LBBB-like morphology.*

Read This! – The Problem No One Mentions...

According to the fourth Step of the Brugada Algorithm, if either Lead V1 or Lead V6 manifests a classic RBBB pattern, then the diagnosis is SVT with aberrant conduction. But there is a problem that I never see mentioned regarding the Brugada Criteria:

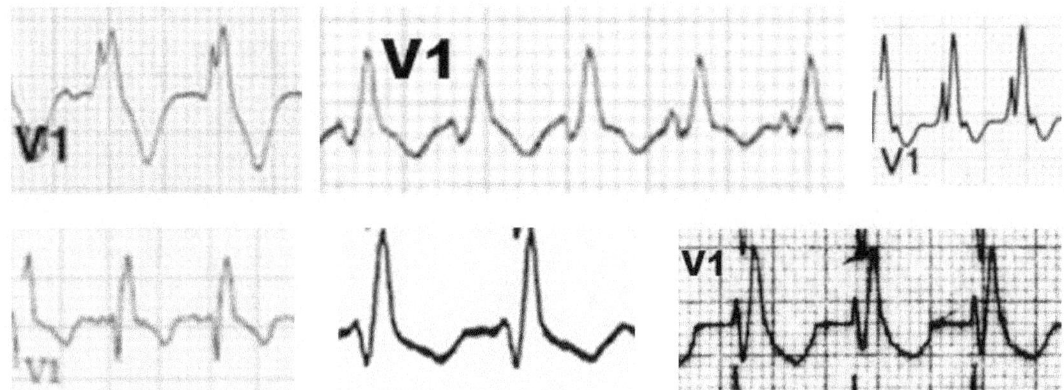

Figure 12-8 | All snippets are from documented ventricular tachycardias!

Ventricular tachycardia – under certain circumstances and depending on the type of tachycardia – can also present with a classic RBBB pattern in Lead V1 (Figure 12-8). If you are basing your diagnosis on the fourth step and specifically on the fact that there is a classic RBBB morphology in Lead V1 – you could be diagnosing a ventricular tachycardia as an SVT. **This is a very dangerous mistake!** It can also occur when using the Lead II Peak Time Method.

Misdiagnosing an SVT as a VT will not present any immediate dangers to the patient. If you misdiagnose an SVT and treat it as a VT – what have you done? You just treated an SVT, because the treatment is very similar – or the same!

However, if you misdiagnose a VT as an SVT, what could happen? Let's say you give several doses of adenosine and it doesn't work. Many would then try verapamil – which could prove disastrous!

If you are depending on the fourth step of the Brugada Algorithm to make your diagnosis – and there is a classic RBBB morphology in Lead V1 – be very, very careful. Validate your impression with other criteria or algorithms. If you still question your diagnosis, perform a D/C cardioversion.

NEVER give verapamil to a patient with a wide complex tachycardia if...

    1. you are not convinced of the diagnosis of a fascicular tachycardia or even an outflow

tract tachycardia, and

2. you have little experience in managing a patient with profound cardiovascular collapse.

Recommended Reading:

Brugada P, Brugada J, Mont L, Smeets J, Andries EW. A new approach to the differential diagnosis of a regular tachycardia with a wide QRS complex. *Circulation.* 1991;83:1649–1659.

Classic! This is the first method for differentiating wide complex tachycardias with a step-by-step approach.

Jastrzebski M, Kukla P, Czarnecka D, and Kawecka-Jaszcz K. Comparison of five electrocardiographic methods for differentiation of wide QRS-complex tachycardias. *Europace.* (2012) 14, 1165–1171 doi:10.1093/europace/eus015.

Kindwall KE, MD, Brown J, RN, Josephson ME, MD. Electrocardiographic Criteria for Ventricular Tachycardia in Wide Complex Left Bundle Branch Block Morphology Tachycardias. *Am J Cardiol.* 1988;61:1279-1283.

Practicing With the Brugada Algorithm

Brugada Algorithm

1. Is there a lack of RS complexes (rS, RS, Rs) in *all* precordial leads?
2. If one or more RS complexes are present, do any have an R-to-S nadir > 100 msec?
3. Is there any evidence of AV dissociation in any of the twelve leads on the ECG?
4. Are the morphological criteria for VT met in *both* Leads V1 and V6?

Criteria for RBBB-like Morphology

1. Is there anything other than a classic triphasic (rSR′) pattern in Lead V1?
2. Is there anything other than a classic triphasic (qRs) pattern in Lead V6?
    a. If so, is it an RS complex?
    b. If an RS complex is present, is the R/S ratio < 1.0 (i.e., is the depth of the S wave greater than the height of the R wave)?

Criteria for LBBB-like Morphology

1. Is the R-to-S nadir > 60 msec in Lead V1?
    a. If not, is the r wave duration in Lead V1 > 30 msec?
    b. If not, is there any notching of the downslope of the S wave in Lead V1?
2. Is there a Q or QS in Lead V6?

Practice ECG #1

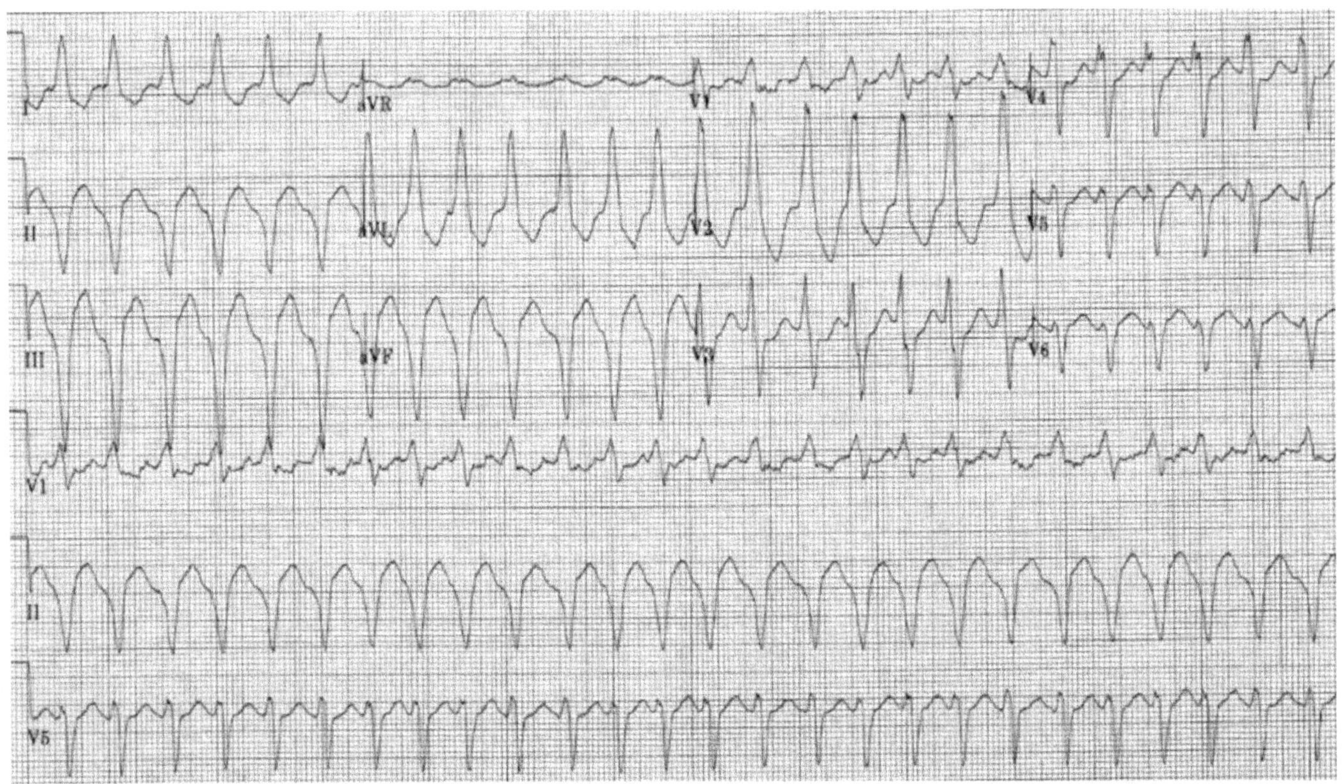

Figure 12-9

Brugada Algorithm

1. Is there a lack of RS complexes (rS, RS, Rs) in *all* precordial leads?
2. If one or more RS complexes are present, do any have an R-to-S nadir > 100 msec?
3. Is there any evidence of AV dissociation in any of the twelve leads on the ECG?
4. Are the morphological criteria for VT met in *both* Leads V1 and V6?

Criteria for RBBB-like Morphology

1. Is there anything other than a classic triphasic (rSR′) pattern in Lead V1?
2. Is there anything other than a classic triphasic (qRs) pattern in Lead V6?
    a. If so, is it an RS complex?
    b. If an RS complex is present, is the R/S ratio < 1.0 (i.e., is the depth of the S wave greater than the height of the R wave)?

Criteria for LBBB-like Morphology

1. Is the R-to-S nadir > 60 msec in Lead V1?
    a. If not, is the r wave duration in Lead V1 > 30 msec?
    b. If not, is there any notching of the downslope of the S wave in Lead V1?
2. Is there a Q or QS in Lead V6?

Practice ECG #2

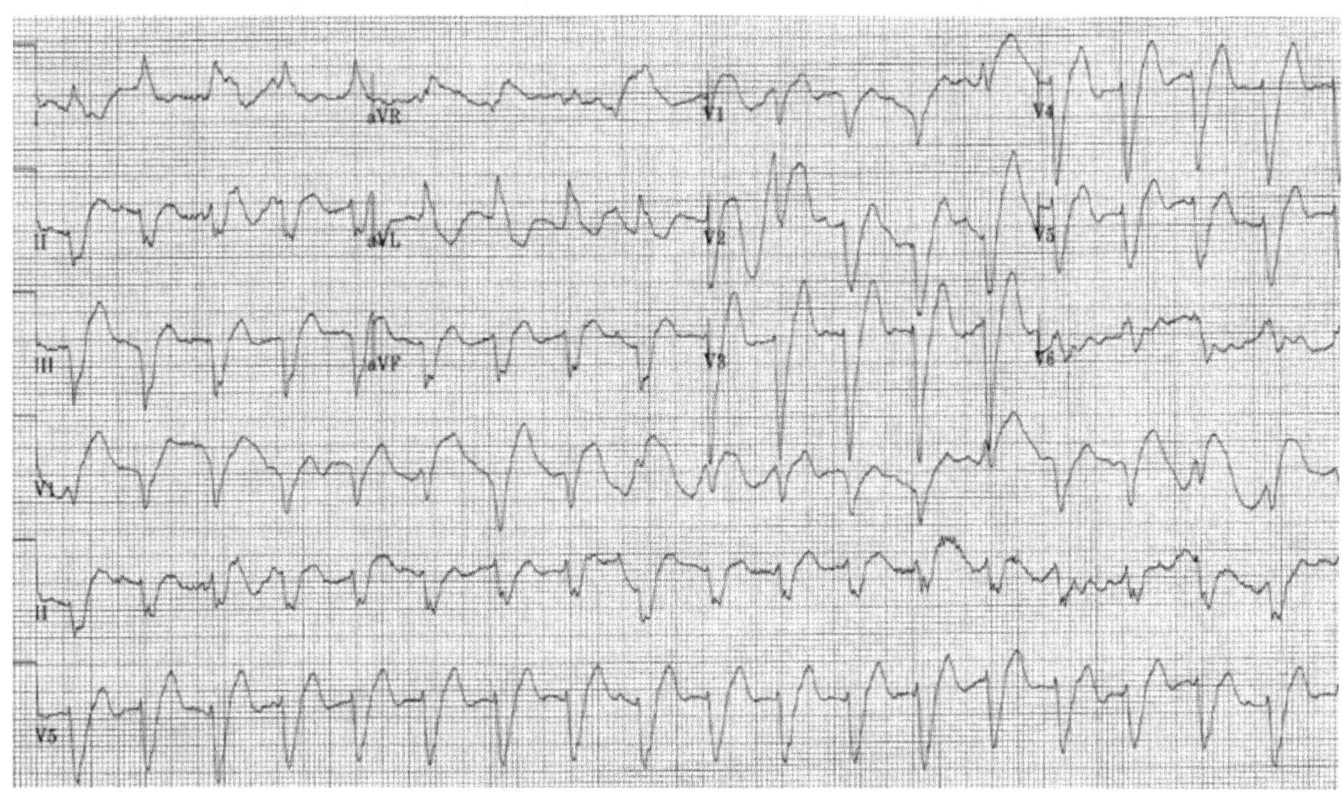

Figure 12–10

Brugada Algorithm

1. Is there a lack of RS complexes (rS, RS, Rs) in *all* precordial leads?
2. If one or more RS complexes are present, do any have an R-to-S nadir > 100 msec?
3. Is there any evidence of AV dissociation in any of the twelve leads on the ECG?
4. Are the morphological criteria for VT met in *both* Leads V1 and V6?

Criteria for RBBB-like Morphology

1. Is there anything other than a classic triphasic (rSR′) pattern in Lead V1?
2. Is there anything other than a classic triphasic (qRs) pattern in Lead V6?
   a. If so, is it an RS complex?
   b. If an RS complex is present, is the R/S ratio < 1.0 (i.e., is the depth of the S wave greater than the height of the R wave)?

Criteria for LBBB-like Morphology

1. Is the R-to-S nadir > 60 msec in Lead V1?
   a. If not, is the r wave duration in Lead V1 > 30 msec?
   b. If not, is there any notching of the downslope of the S wave in Lead V1?
2. Is there a Q or QS in Lead V6?

Practice ECG #3

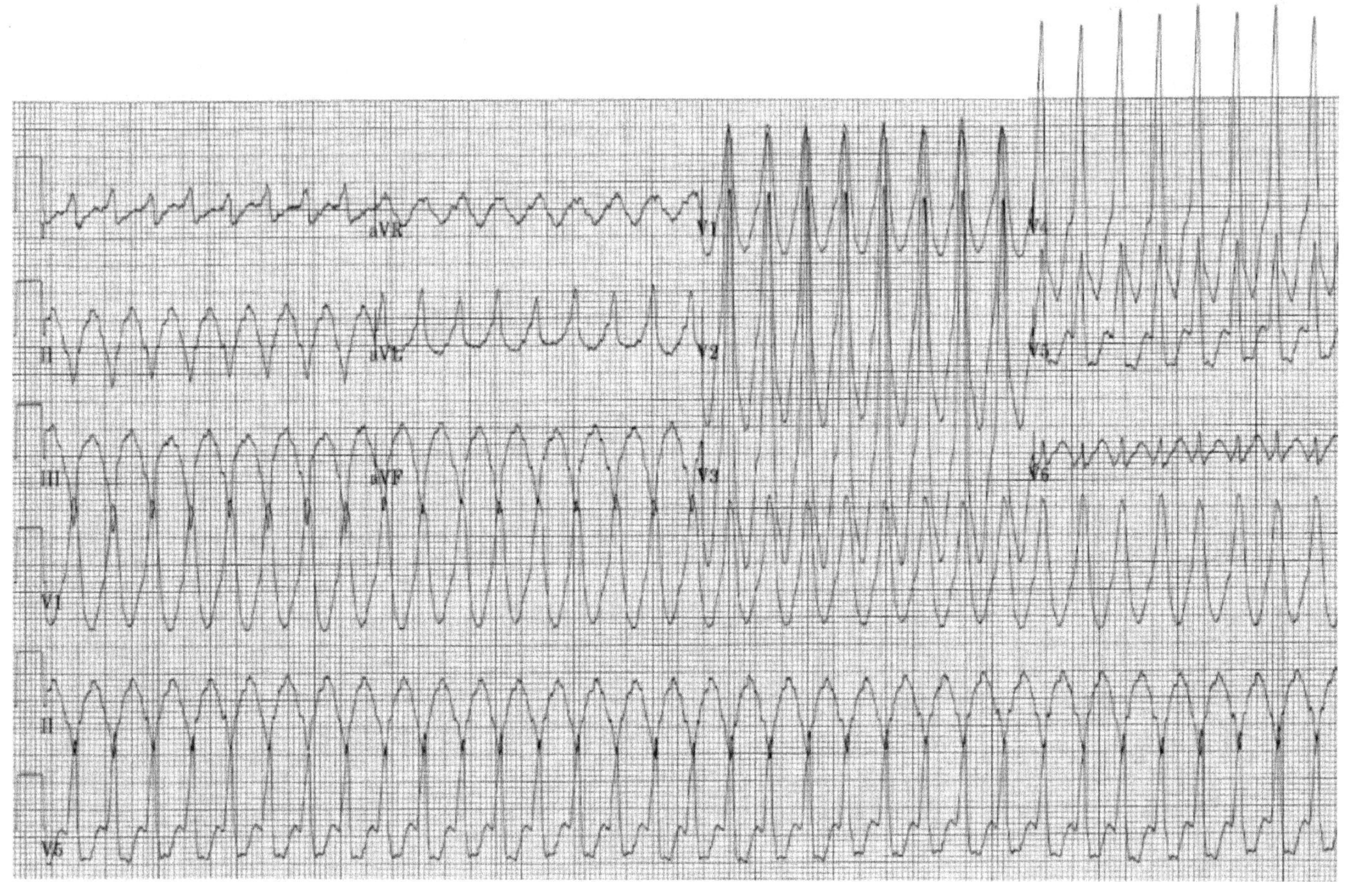

Figure 12-11

Brugada Algorithm

1. Is there a lack of RS complexes (rS, RS, Rs) in *all* precordial leads?
2. If one or more RS complexes are present, do any have an R-to-S nadir > 100 msec?
3. Is there any evidence of AV dissociation in any of the twelve leads on the ECG?
4. Are the morphological criteria for VT met in *both* Leads V1 and V6?

Criteria for RBBB-like Morphology

1. Is there anything other than a classic triphasic (rSR′) pattern in Lead V1?
2. Is there anything other than a classic triphasic (qRs) pattern in Lead V6?
    a. If so, is it an RS complex?
    b. If an RS complex is present, is the R/S ratio < 1.0 (i.e., is the depth of the S wave greater than the height of the R wave)?

Criteria for LBBB-like Morphology

1. Is the R-to-S nadir > 60 msec in Lead V1?
    a. If not, is the r wave duration in Lead V1 > 30 msec?
    b. If not, is there any notching of the downslope of the S wave in Lead V1?
2. Is there a Q or QS in Lead V6?

Practice ECG #4

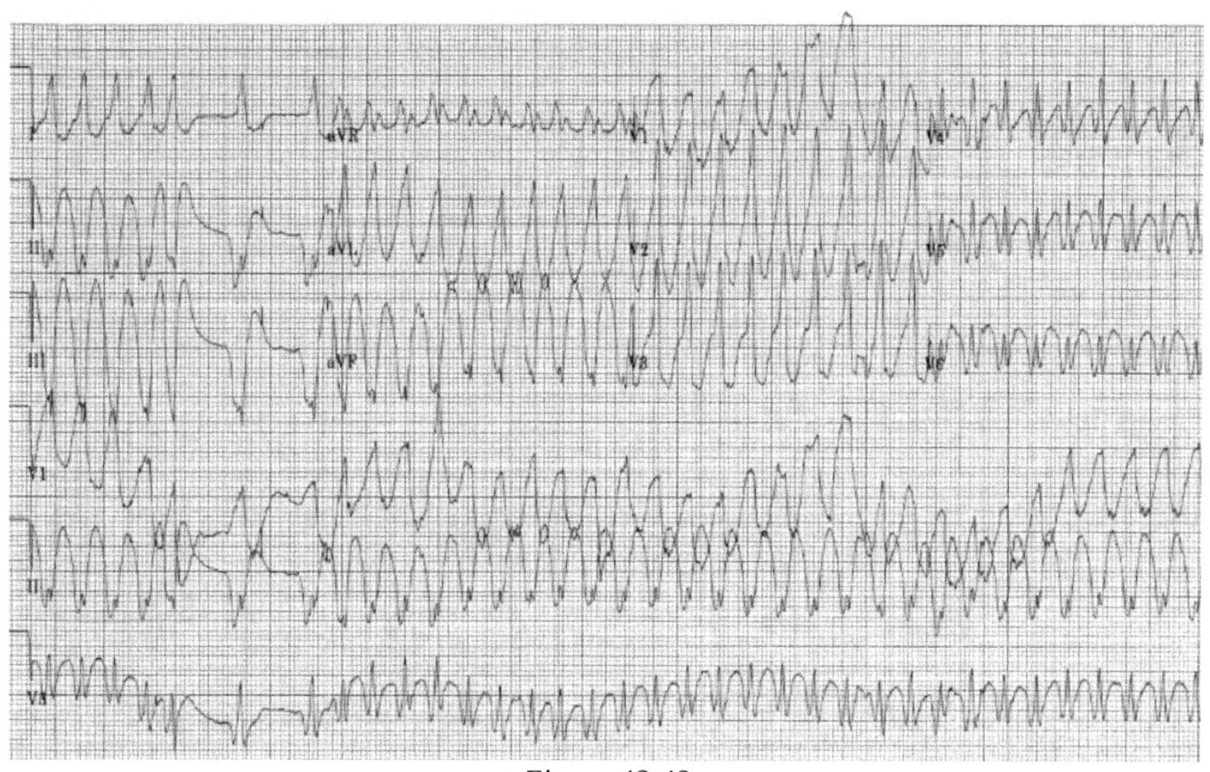

Figure 12-12

Brugada Algorithm

1. Is there a lack of RS complexes (rS, RS, Rs) in *all* precordial leads?
2. If one or more RS complexes are present, do any have an R-to-S nadir > 100 msec?
3. Is there any evidence of AV dissociation in any of the twelve leads on the ECG?
4. Are the morphological criteria for VT met in *both* Leads V1 and V6?

Criteria for RBBB-like Morphology

1. Is there anything other than a classic triphasic (rSR′) pattern in Lead V1?
2. Is there anything other than a classic triphasic (qRs) pattern in Lead V6?
   a. If so, is it an RS complex?
   b. If an RS complex is present, is the R/S ratio < 1.0 (i.e., is the depth of the S wave greater than the height of the R wave)?

Criteria for LBBB-like Morphology

1. Is the R-to-S nadir > 60 msec in Lead V1?
   a. If not, is the r wave duration in Lead V1 > 30 msec?
   b. If not, is there any notching of the downslope of the S wave in Lead V1?
2. Is there a Q or QS in Lead V6?

Practice ECG #5

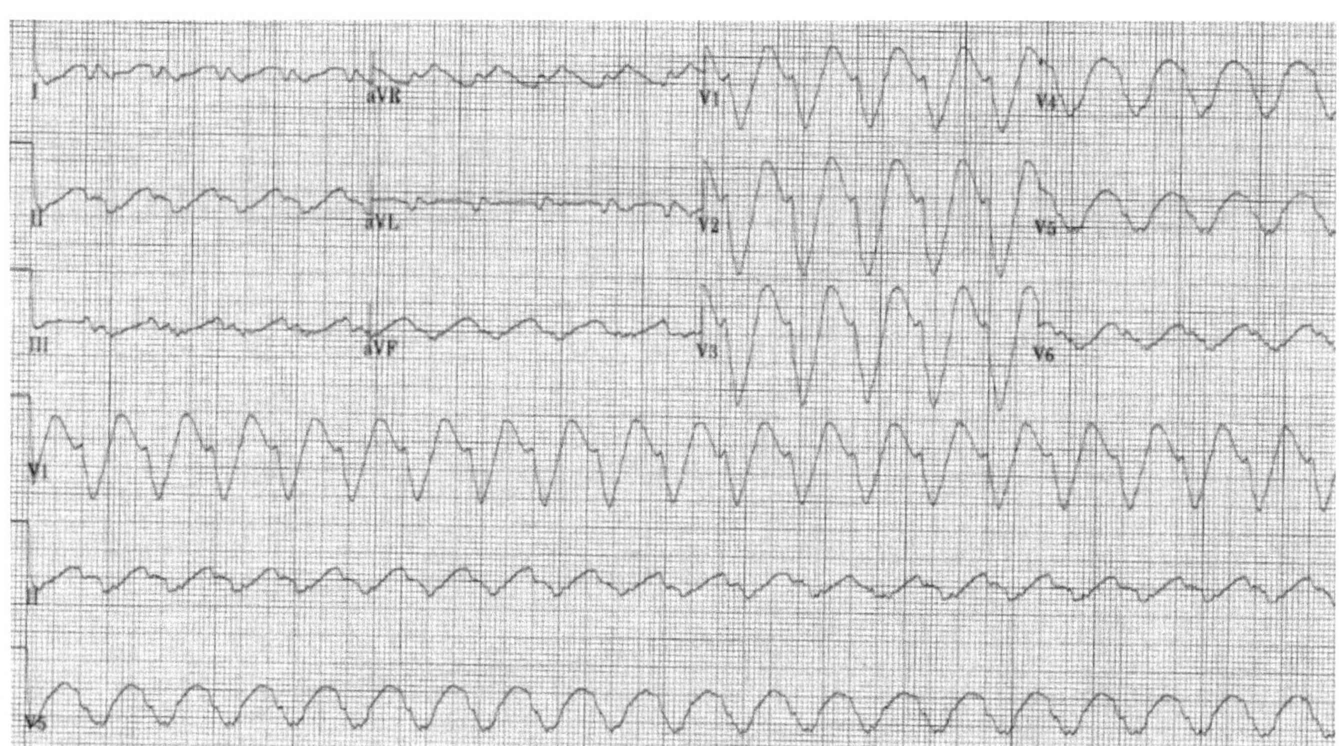

Figure 12-13

Brugada Algorithm

1. Is there a lack of RS complexes (rS, RS, Rs) in *all* precordial leads?
2. If one or more RS complexes are present, do any have an R-to-S nadir > 100 msec?
3. Is there any evidence of AV dissociation in any of the twelve leads on the ECG?
4. Are the morphological criteria for VT met in *both* Leads V1 and V6?

Criteria for RBBB-like Morphology

1. Is there anything other than a classic triphasic (rSR′) pattern in Lead V1?
2. Is there anything other than a classic triphasic (qRs) pattern in Lead V6?
    a. If so, is it an RS complex?
    b. If an RS complex is present, is the R/S ratio < 1.0 (i.e., is the depth of the S wave greater than the height of the R wave)?

Criteria for LBBB-like Morphology

1. Is the R-to-S nadir > 60 msec in Lead V1?
    a. If not, is the r wave duration in Lead V1 > 30 msec?
    b. If not, is there any notching of the downslope of the S wave in Lead V1?
2. Is there a Q or QS in Lead V6?

Practice ECG #6

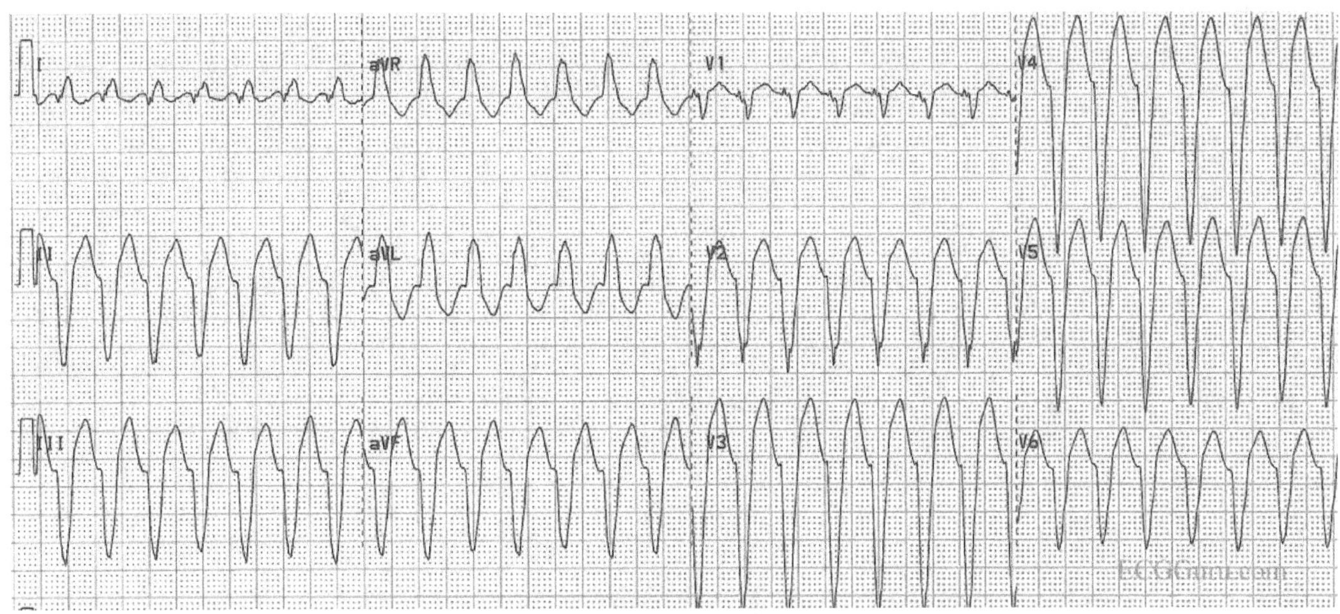

Figure 12-14

Brugada Algorithm

1. Is there a lack of RS complexes (rS, RS, Rs) in *all* precordial leads?
2. If one or more RS complexes are present, do any have an R-to-S nadir > 100 msec?
3. Is there any evidence of AV dissociation in any of the twelve leads on the ECG?
4. Are the morphological criteria for VT met in *both* Leads V1 and V6?

Criteria for RBBB-like Morphology

1. Is there anything other than a classic triphasic (rSR′) pattern in Lead V1?
2. Is there anything other than a classic triphasic (qRs) pattern in Lead V6?
    a. If so, is it an RS complex?
    b. If an RS complex is present, is the R/S ratio < 1.0 (i.e., is the depth of the S wave greater than the height of the R wave)?

Criteria for LBBB-like Morphology

1. Is the R-to-S nadir > 60 msec in Lead V1?
    a. If not, is the r wave duration in Lead V1 > 30 msec?
    b. If not, is there any notching of the downslope of the S wave in Lead V1?
2. Is there a Q or QS in Lead V6?

Practice ECG #7

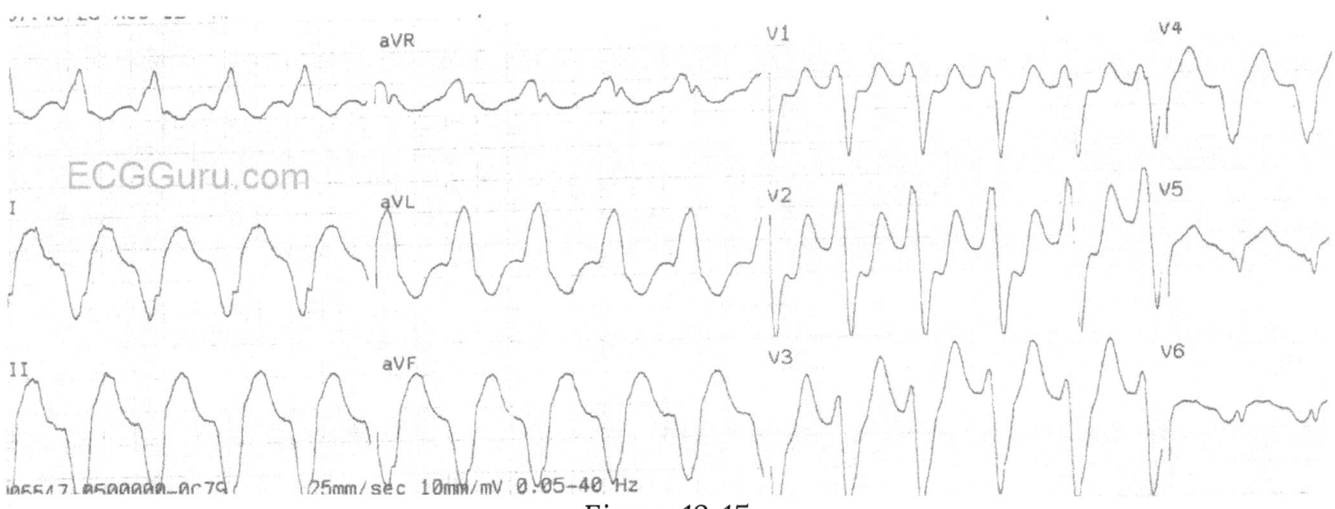

Figure 12-15

Brugada Algorithm

1. Is there a lack of RS complexes (rS, RS, Rs) in *all* precordial leads?
2. If one or more RS complexes are present, do any have an R-to-S nadir > 100 msec?
3. Is there any evidence of AV dissociation in any of the twelve leads on the ECG?
4. Are the morphological criteria for VT met in *both* Leads V1 and V6?

Criteria for RBBB-like Morphology

1. Is there anything other than a classic triphasic (rSR′) pattern in Lead V1?
2. Is there anything other than a classic triphasic (qRs) pattern in Lead V6?
   a. If so, is it an RS complex?
   b. If an RS complex is present, is the R/S ratio < 1.0 (i.e., is the depth of the S wave greater than the height of the R wave)?

Criteria for LBBB-like Morphology

1. Is the R-to-S nadir > 60 msec in Lead V1?
   a. If not, is the r wave duration in Lead V1 > 30 msec?
   b. If not, is there any notching of the downslope of the S wave in Lead V1?
2. Is there a Q or QS in Lead V6?

Practice ECG #8

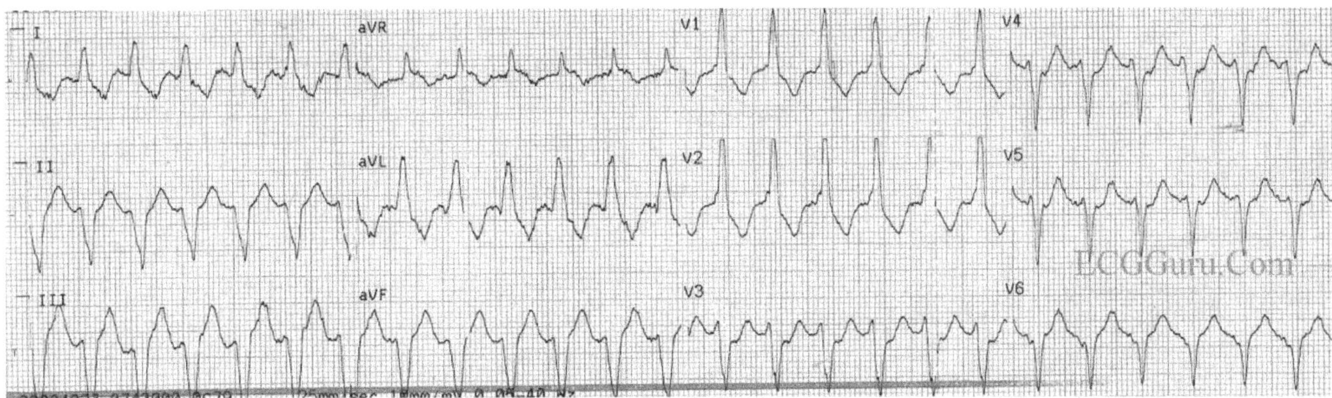

Figure 12-16

Brugada Algorithm

1. Is there a lack of RS complexes (rS, RS, Rs) in *all* precordial leads?
2. If one or more RS complexes are present, do any have an R-to-S nadir > 100 msec?
3. Is there any evidence of AV dissociation in any of the twelve leads on the ECG?
4. Are the morphological criteria for VT met in *both* Leads V1 and V6?

Criteria for RBBB-like Morphology

1. Is there anything other than a classic triphasic (rSR′) pattern in Lead V1?
2. Is there anything other than a classic triphasic (qRs) pattern in Lead V6?
   a. If so, is it an RS complex?
   b. If an RS complex is present, is the R/S ratio < 1.0 (i.e., is the depth of the S wave greater than the height of the R wave)?

Criteria for LBBB-like Morphology

1. Is the R-to-S nadir > 60 msec in Lead V1?
   a. If not, is the r wave duration in Lead V1 > 30 msec?
   b. If not, is there any notching of the downslope of the S wave in Lead V1?
2. Is there a Q or QS in Lead V6?

Practice ECG #9

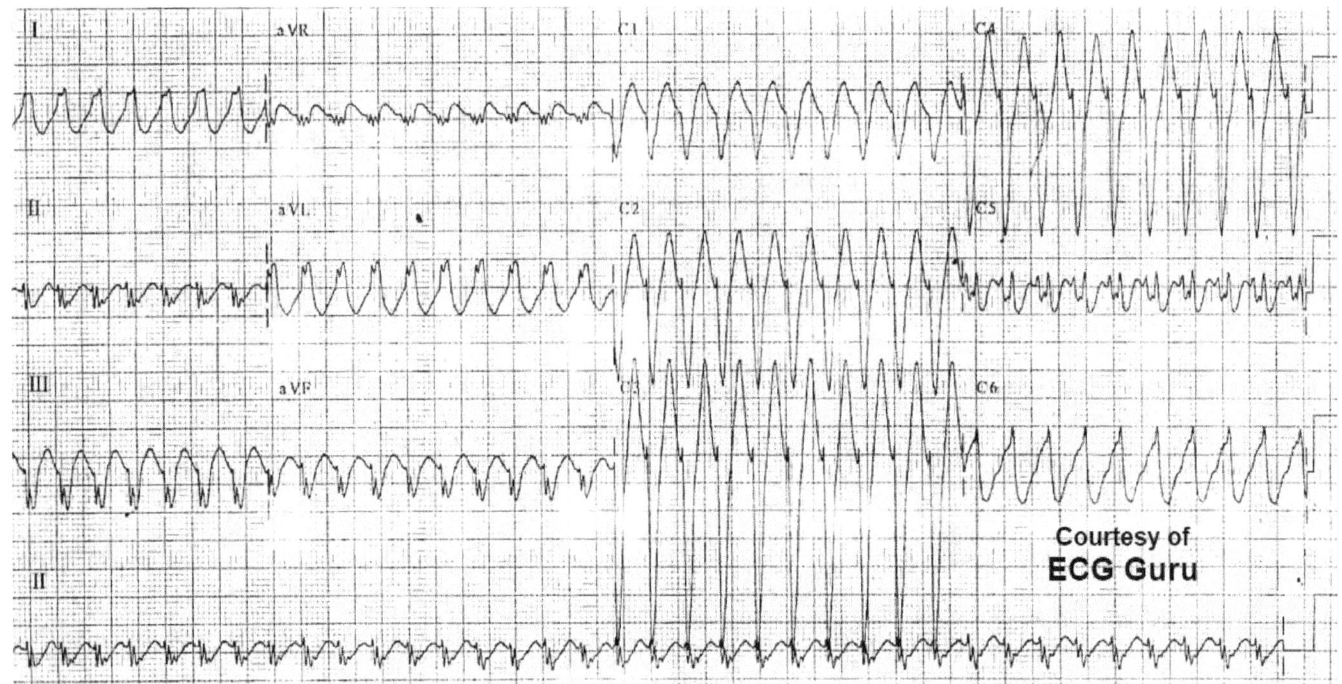

Figure 12-17

Brugada Algorithm

1. Is there a lack of RS complexes (rS, RS, Rs) in *all* precordial leads?
2. If one or more RS complexes are present, do any have an R-to-S nadir > 100 msec?
3. Is there any evidence of AV dissociation in any of the twelve leads on the ECG?
4. Are the morphological criteria for VT met in *both* Leads V1 and V6?

Criteria for RBBB-like Morphology

1. Is there anything other than a classic triphasic (rSR′) pattern in Lead V1?
2. Is there anything other than a classic triphasic (qRs) pattern in Lead V6?
   a. If so, is it an RS complex?
   b. If an RS complex is present, is the R/S ratio < 1.0 (i.e., is the depth of the S wave greater than the height of the R wave)?

Criteria for LBBB-like Morphology

1. Is the R-to-S nadir > 60 msec in Lead V1?
   a. If not, is the r wave duration in Lead V1 > 30 msec?
   b. If not, is there any notching of the downslope of the S wave in Lead V1?
2. Is there a Q or QS in Lead V6?

Practice ECG #10

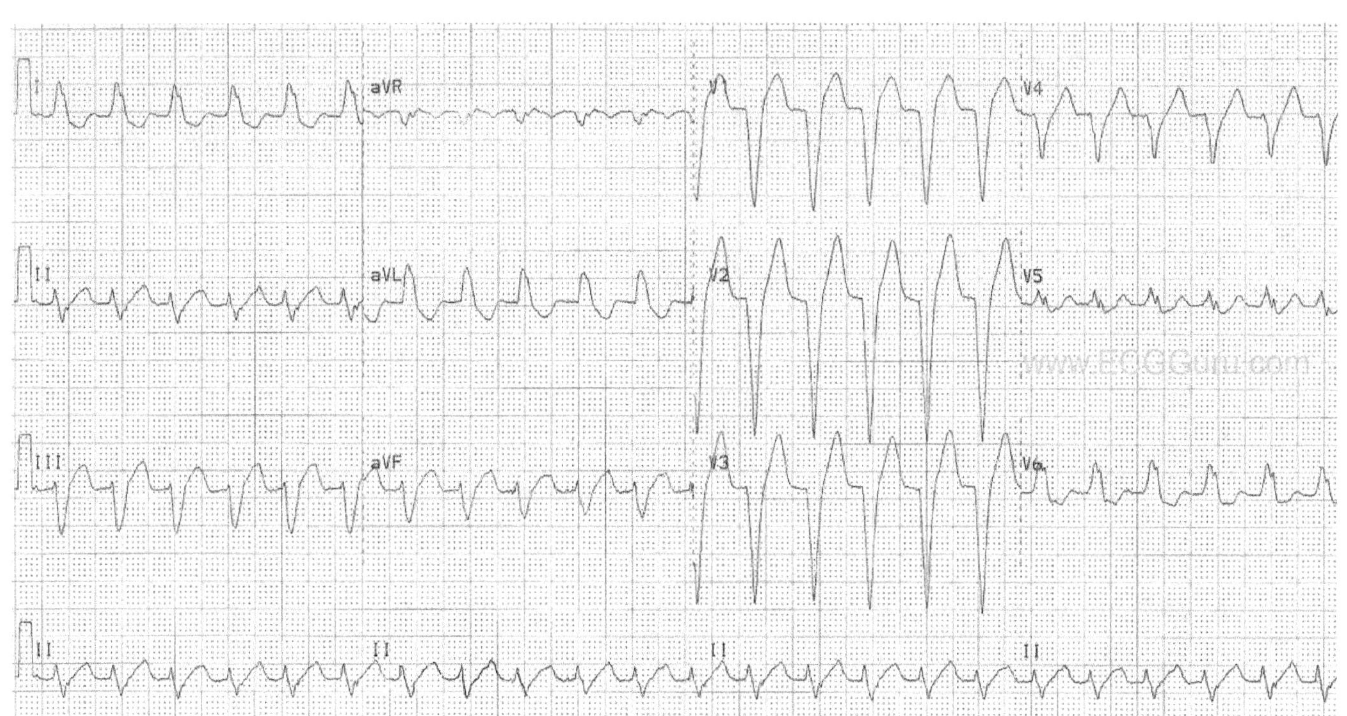

Figure 12-18

Chapter 13

The Vereckei Algorithms

Vereckei Algorithm #1 (2007, Not Limited to Lead aVR)

In 2007, Dr. Andras Vereckei introduced the first of two algorithms for the differential diagnosis of wide complex tachycardias. Like the Brugada algorithm, it consists of four steps in a stepwise decision-tree format. Vereckei felt that the use of the morphological criteria in the Brugada algorithm made it difficult to use in practical clinical situations and possibly contributed to less accuracy. His goal was to create an algorithm that did not depend on the morphological criteria... and he (almost) did!

Step 1: Is there evidence of AV dissociation present?

This step is the same as Step 3 of the Brugada Algorithm and it suffers from the same issues. AV dissociation is diagnosed only in about 20% of wide complex tachycardias. It is seen *almost* exclusively in ventricular tachycardias. Either it is simply not present, or it is present but often difficult to detect except by the most experienced and skillful electrocardiographer (that means YOU!). Although it is not 100% proof that ventricular tachycardia is the cause, conditions other than ventricular tachycardia causing AV dissociation during a wide complex tachycardia are so rare that their likelihood is negligible.

Be careful that you don't confuse VA *association* with AV *dissociation*.

> **PEARL |** The presence of P or P′ waves in a wide complex tachycardia doesn't necessarily prove anything. Therefore, you must know *how to interpret them* when you find them!

With VA association, a retrograde P′ wave appears *at the same R-P′ interval following each QRS complex*. Those P′ waves are being produced by an impulse traveling up the His bundle, crossing through the AV node retrograde, and then exciting the atria. *"But wait a minute!"* you exclaim. *"Isn't that* evidence of ventricular tachycardia?" Unfortunately, no. An antidromic

AVRT presenting as a wide complex tachycardia can do *the same thing!* Even an orthodromic tachycardia with either a fixed or rate-related bundle branch block could present that way.

However, if there are P′ waves appearing at a fixed R-P′ interval, and suddenly one fails to appear – look very closely! If there is no change in the ventricular rhythm then you are seeing a *ventriculoatrial block* and evidence of VA *dissociation!* A VA block is definite evidence of an ectopic ventricular rhythm – *even more so than AV dissociation!*

> **FYI |** If AV dissociation is not 100% assurance of ventricular tachycardia, then what other dysrhythmias could cause it? **1)** AVNRT **PLUS** a block of the upper common pathway **PLUS** aberrant conduction and **2)** junctional tachycardia (very rare!) **PLUS** aberrant conduction WITH a retrograde block into the atria.

As I have recommended before, if you are very experienced and skillful at recognizing AV dissociation, you will likely find it within about 20 seconds. If not, and you are in the process of managing a patient currently experiencing a wide complex tachycardia, don't spend more than about 20 seconds looking for it before continuing with the management of your patient (which includes completing the rest of the algorithm or moving on to DC cardioversion).

Just as with the Brugada Algorithm, if your answer to Step 1 is "YES!" then **STOP**. You've just diagnosed *ventricular tachycardia.*

Step 2: Is there an initial R wave present in Lead aVR?

Again, be very careful here! This seems like a very simple question – but it's NOT! What most discussions of this step of the First Vereckei algorithm fail to mention is that Vereckei is NOT referring to ALL R waves – just *monophasic R waves* and RS *waves where the R wave is large and at least similar in amplitude to the S wave.* He specifically excludes rS complexes! The reason for the exclusion of rS complexes is because they can occur:

1. as a normal variant

2. during an SVT with an initial superiorly directed vector,

3. due to a previous inferior myocardial infarction, and

4. due to activation of the ventricle by an accessory bypass tract (*atriofascicular* and *nodofascicular* tracts).

What do YOU think of these QRS complexes from Lead aVR (Figure 13-1)? Do the R waves qualify for use in the First Vereckei algorithm? Choose "Y" (YES!) or "N" (NO!).

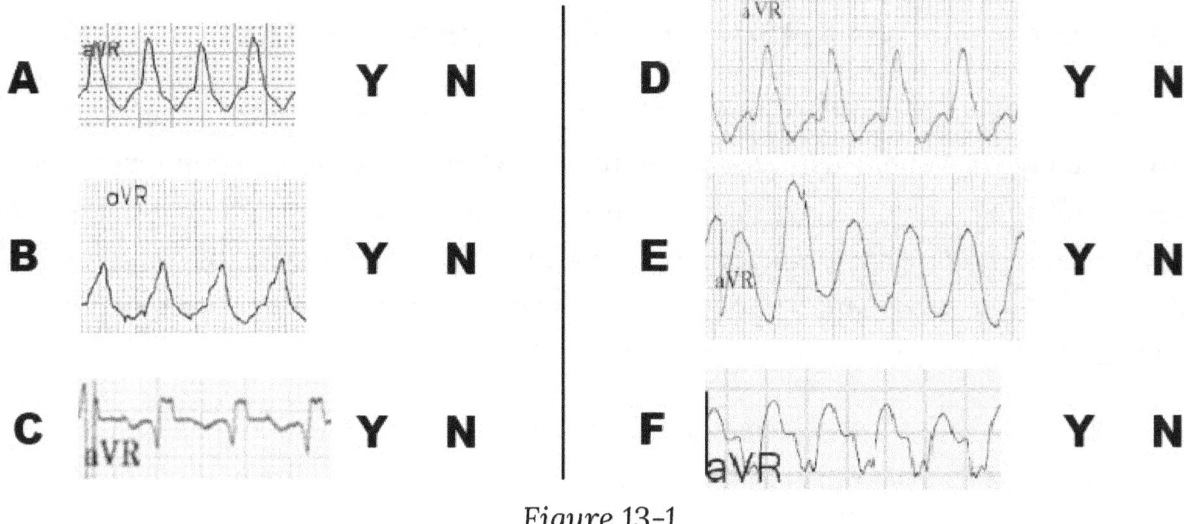

Figure 13-1

Answers to Figure 13-1:

(**A**): Y

(**B**): Y

(**C**): No, there is an initial Q wave.

(**D**): No, there is an initial q wave.

(**E**): Y

(**F**): No, there is an rS complex.

If your answer to Step 2 is "YES!" then **STOP**. You've just diagnosed ventricular tachycardia.

Step 3: Is the QRS morphology unlike classic bundle branch block or classic anterior or posterior fascicular block?

So, what have we here? It's nothing more than the morphological criteria – but Vereckei is approaching it "through the back door" (so to speak) – just as I did with the *Jones Modification* in Step 4 of the Brugada Algorithm. Instead of asking you to check for every possible QRS morphology *other* than the classic morphology, he is going straight to the heart of the matter and simply asking you if the classic bundle branch block morphology is present or not. He also includes the classic morphology of anterior and posterior fascicular blocks which are not mentioned in the Brugada Algorithm (or in the original article, for that matter). Note that he doesn't mention any *specific* leads – particularly Lead V1.

If your answer to Step 3 is "YES!" then **STOP**. You've just diagnosed ventricular tachycardia.

Step 4: The Ventricular Activation Velocity Ratio (V_i / V_t)

OK... Vereckei complained about the complexity of the fourth step of the Brugada Algorithm (though certainly with some justification) so here is where most people complain about the complexity of the Vereckei Algorithms #1 and #2. The chances are – when you use either of these algorithms – you will end up here in Step 4 about 50 – 60% of the time and have to deal with this step! There will be many times that you simply *cannot complete this step* due to the type or quality of the QRS morphologies on the WCT tracing.

"Well," you say. "I will just find a good example of a monophasic R wave, measure 0.04 seconds (one small square) from the onset and one small square back from the end of the QRS. If the onset measurement (V_i) is taller, then the WCT is a supraventricular tachycardia. If the onset (V_i) is the same height or shorter than the termination measurement (V_t), then it is ventricular tachycardia. Simple... no?

NO! Here's the problem... at no point in the derivation study of the First Vereckei Algorithm (2007) did Vereckei et al use a *monophasic* R to calculate (V_i / V_t). All computations using the ventricular activation velocity ratio (V_i / V_t) used only *biphasic* or *multiphasic* QRS complexes. And they were very clear about this!

Why? They never stated precisely, but *in my opinion*, a monophasic R wave in Lead aVR would have diagnosed ventricular tachycardia in Step 2; a monophasic R in any *other* lead would strongly suggest an impulse traveling *away* from the positive pole of Lead aVR (right shoulder) which would be more suggestive of an SVT with aberrancy.

> **Remember! |** Vereckei et al. are trying to *prove* that the WCT is ventricular tachy-cardia. SVT with aberrancy will be a *diagnosis of exclusion.*

The instructions in this – the First Vereckei Algorithm are to *find the QRS with the most visible and most rapid onset*. And you can use *any* lead – not just Lead aVR! The QRS diagram in Figure 13-2 is very similar to the one used in the original 2007 article. See the next section, "Vereckei Algorithm #2 (2008, The aVR Algorithm) for a discussion of the QRS morphology chosen in *that* version of the algorithm.

> **TIP |** At no point in either of the Vereckei algorithms is the ventricular activation velocity ratio (Vi/Vt) calculated using a monophasic R wave. I know it would be easier, but it just can't happen!

Calculating the Vi/Vt Ratio

1. Measure from the baseline to Point A.

2. Measure from Point A to Point B.

3. Add the two lengths together using their absolute values (no minus signs). The sum = Vi.

4. Measure from Point C to Point D.

5. Measure from Point D down to the baseline at Point E.

6. Add the two lengths together using their absolute values (no minus signs). The sum = Vt.

7. Now divide Vi / Vt.

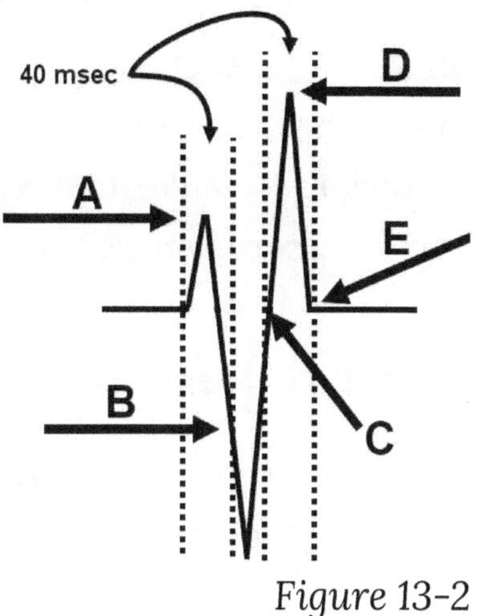

Figure 13-2

If equal to or less than 1.0 – ventricular tachycardia
If greater than 1.0 – SVT with aberrancy

If your answer to Step 4 is ≤ 1.0 then you've just diagnosed *ventricular tachycardia*. Otherwise, the diagnosis is *supraventricular tachycardia* by exclusion.

More Thoughts on the Vereckei Algorithm #1

While the Brugada algorithm used only the precordial leads except for Step 3 (the search for AV dissociation) the Vereckei Algorithm #1 is *not limited to the precordial or limb leads* – except for Step 2 which deals only with Lead aVR.

Vereckei Algorithm #2 (2008, The aVR Algorithm)

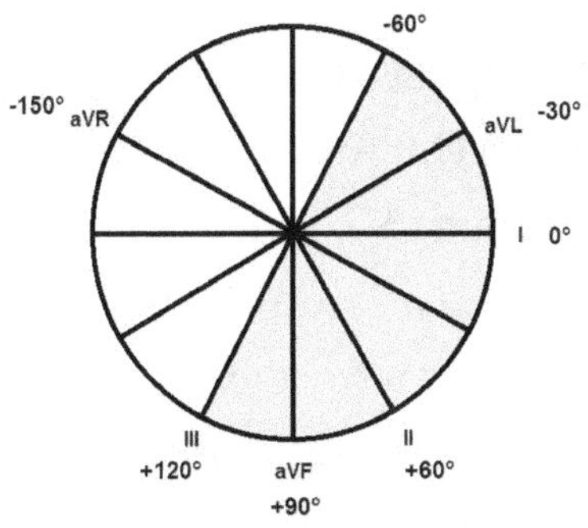

Figure 13-3

In 2008, Vereckei et al produced a *second* version of their algorithm. What was unique about this algorithm (at the time) was that it was limited to examining just one lead – Lead aVR. They focused on Lead aVR because, during normal *sinus rhythm* and most *supraventricular tachycardias*, the activation of the ventricles traveled *away* from the right arm electrode (aVR positive pole) producing a QS wave in that lead (Figure 13-3). Therefore, they reasoned that a ventricular ectopic impulse would be traveling in the opposite direction.

A vector traveling up and to the right, vertically up, or up and to the left (white area on the HRG, Figure 13-3), would still register as an initial R wave in Lead aVR as long as the vector was between +120° and -60° on the hexaxial reference grid (Figure 13-3, shaded area) and on the same side as the positive pole for Lead aVR. And they were right. The only problem: dysrhythmias other than ventricular tachycardia can result in the same vectors, such as *posterior fascicular tachycardia, bundle branch tachycardia, previous myocardial infarctions,* and *accessory bypass tracts.*

Step 1: Is there an initial R wave?

Again, this refers only to a monophasic R or an RS but not an rS – until Step 2. The R wave must be at least as large or larger than the S wave (R ≥ S).

If your answer to Step 1 is "YES!" then **STOP**. You've just diagnosed ventricular tachycardia.

Step 2: Is there an initial r or q wave > 40 msec?

In some criteria, you may see a value such as > 30 msec while another article will list the same value as > 40 msec. This is not too unusual, and the reason is practical – measuring 40 msec on a printed 12-lead ECG is easier and more reliable than trying to measure 30 msec without the use of digital calipers. The width > 40 msec indicates a slow onset of the depolarization which suggests that its origin is in the working ventricular myocardium. This concept was taken from the 1988 Kindwall et al criteria. These were four criteria that were developed to diagnose wide complex tachycardias with an LBBB-like morphology. They were *not* arranged in a *stepwise algorithm* – just a list of four criteria.

If your answer to Step 2 is "YES!" then **STOP**. You've just diagnosed ventricular tachycardia.

Step 3: Is there a notch on the descending limb of a *negative onset* and *predominantly negative* QRS?

The identification of a notch on the downslope of the S wave as a sign suggestive of ventricular tachycardia was initially introduced by Mark Josephson, MD in 1988 with the Kindwall criteria (Josephson was also one of the authors). However, it was reserved for Leads V1 and V2 in wide complex tachycardias *with a left bundle branch block-like morphology.* It was significant as a sign of a previous anterior myocardial infarction of the left ventricle. Infarctions leave scars in the myocardium which may become a focus of reentrant tachycardia. When not serving as a focus of reentry, it can act as a cause for slowing of conduction and, therefore, the appearance of a notch in the downslope of the S wave.

Vereckei applies the concept of a notched downslope of the S wave to Lead aVR using it as a general sign of slowed conduction.

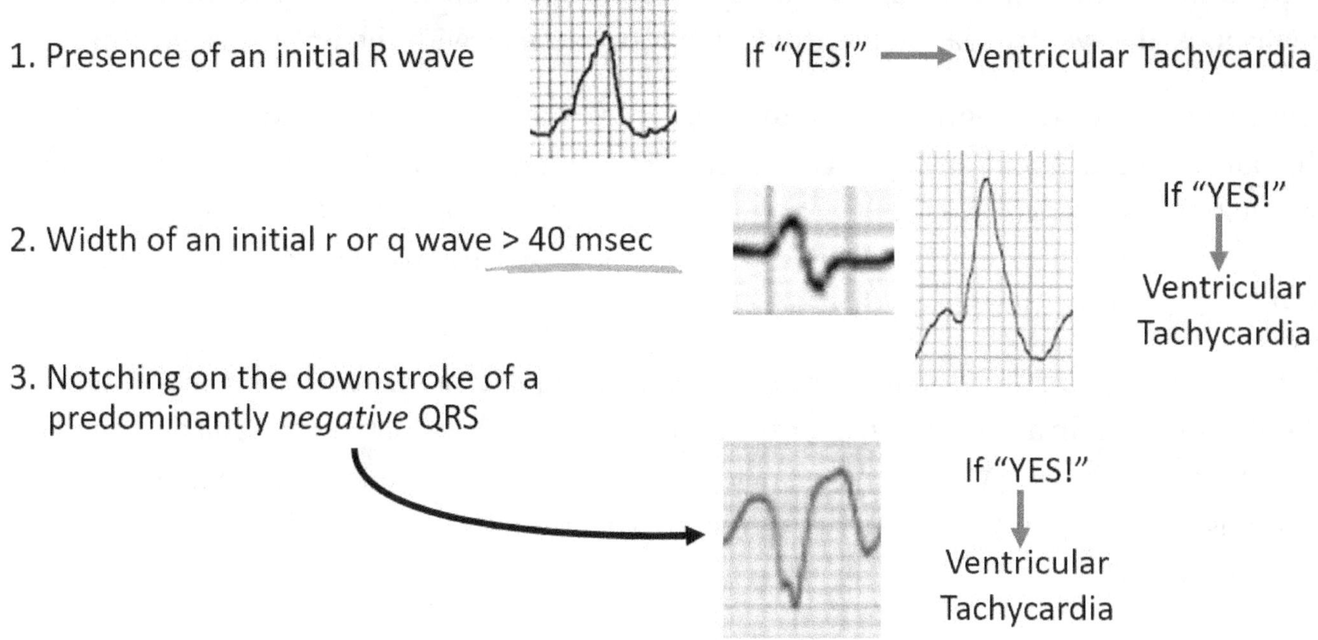

Figure 13-4 The First Three Steps

If your answer to any part of Step 3 is "YES!" then **STOP**. You've just diagnosed ventricular tachycardia.

Step 4: The Ventricular Activation Velocity Ratio

This remains the same as in the Vereckei Algorithm #1 except only the QRS in Lead aVR – and only Lead aVR – can be used (refer back to Figure 13-2). It is assumed the QRS will be *biphasic* or *multiphasic* because if it is monophasic the diagnosis of ventricular tachycardia would already have been made in Step 1.

If your answer to Step 4 is ≤ 1.0 then you've just diagnosed ventricular tachycardia. Otherwise, the diagnosis is supraventricular tachycardia.

More Thoughts on the Vereckei Algorithm #2

The issue with the fourth step of the Vereckei Algorithm #2 is the same as with the Vereckei Algorithm #1.

Two algorithms limit use to just one lead: the **Vereckei Algorithm #2** using Lead aVR and the **Lead II R Wave Peak Time – Pava Method** (which will be discussed next). The use of either method depends on the ability to view the deflections in the leads accurately. And remember, when using Step 4 of the Vereckei Algorithms you must use a *biphasic* or *multiphasic* QRS. You should not be making measurements of the Vi/Vt ratio on monophasic R waves in Lead aVR while using this algorithm. If you are, then *you missed the diagnosis two steps earlier!*

Using either of the Vereckei Algorithms, antidromic supraventricular tachycardia will likely be diagnosed as ventricular tachycardia. That also happens with the Brugada algorithm.

The Second Vereckei algorithm (aVR) divides ventricular tachycardias into two groups for the purpose of diagnosis using this algorithm. The *first* group are those tachydysrhythmias originating in the apical area and characterized by an initial dominant R wave in Lead aVR. The *second* group are those tachydysrhythmias arising elsewhere in the working myocardium that present with initial slowing on the QRS complex.

Although we all want to be as accurate as possible in our diagnoses, mistaking an SVT for a VT should not result in a bad outcome for the patient. The patient will typically still do quite well. Mistaking a VT for an SVT, however, can lead to a very bad outcome for the patient. Be very cautious of any algorithm, method, or criteria in which a mistake will likely involve diagnosing a VT as an SVT!

Recommended Reading:

Dendi R, Josephson ME. A new algorithm in the differential diagnosis of wide complex tachycardia – Editorial. *European Heart Journal.* (2007) 28, 525–526.

Kindwall KE, MD, Brown J, RN, Josephson ME, MD. Electrocardiographic Criteria for Ventricular Tachycardia in Wide Complex Left Bundle Branch Block Morphology Tachycardias. *Am J Cardiol.* 1988;61:1279-1283.

Vereckei A, Duray G, Szenasi G, Altemose GT, Miller JM. Application of a new algorithm in the differential diagnosis of wide QRS complex tachycardia. *Eur Heart J.* 2007;28:589–600.

Vereckei A, Duray G, Szenasi G, Altemose GT, Miller JM. New algorithm using only lead aVR for differential diagnosis of wide QRS complex tachycardia. *Heart Rhythm.* 2008;5:89–98.

Vereckei A, MD, et al. The Application of a New, Modified Algorithm for the Differentiation of Regular Ventricular and Pre-Excited Tachycardias. *Heart, Lung and Circulation.* (2023) 32, 719–725.

Practicing with the Vereckei Algorithms (#1 and #2)

Vereckei Algorithm #1

Step 1: Is AV dissociation present?

Step 2: Is there an initial R wave in Lead aVR? (Cannot be rS)

Step 3: Is the QRS morphology unlike classic BBB or fascicular block?

Step 4: Ventricular Activation Velocity Ratio (Vi / Vt)

Vereckei Algorithm #2 (Lead aVR *only*)

Step 1: Is there an initial R wave? (Cannot be rS)

Step 2: Is there an initial r or q wave > 40 msec?

Step 3: Is there a notch on the descending limb of a negative onset and predominantly negative QRS?

Step 4: Ventricular Activation Velocity Ratio (Vi / Vt)

ECG #1

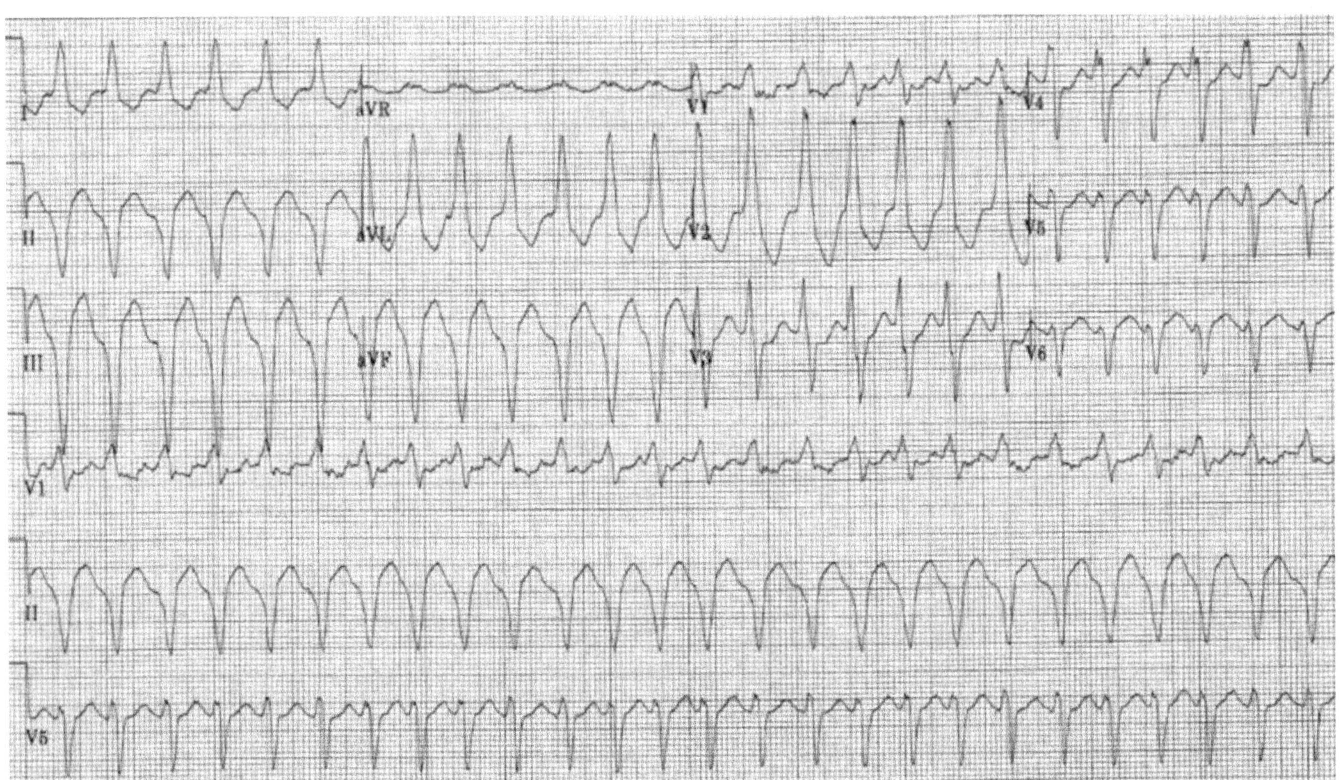

Figure 13-5

Vereckei Algorithm #1

Step 1: Is AV dissociation present?

Step 2: Is there an initial R wave in Lead aVR? (Cannot be rS)

Step 3: Is the QRS morphology unlike classic BBB or fascicular block?

Step 4: Ventricular Activation Velocity Ratio (Vi / Vt)

Vereckei Algorithm #2 (Lead aVR *only*)

Step 1: Is there an initial R wave? (Cannot be rS)

Step 2: Is there an initial r or q wave > 40 msec?

Step 3: Is there a notch on the descending limb of a negative onset and predominantly negative QRS?

Step 4: Ventricular Activation Velocity Ratio (Vi / Vt)

ECG #2

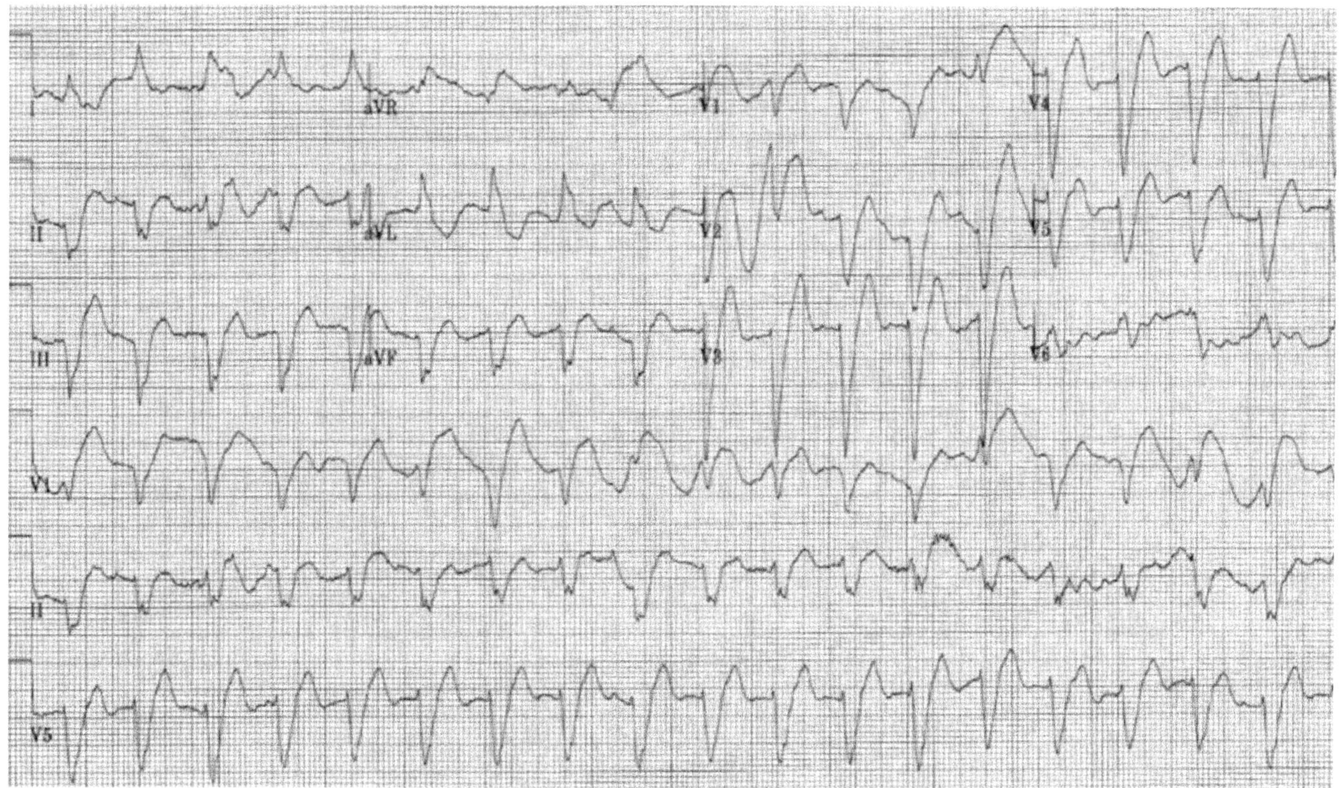

Figure 13-6

Vereckei Algorithm #1

Step 1: Is AV dissociation present?

Step 2: Is there an initial R wave in Lead aVR? (Cannot be rS)

Step 3: Is the QRS morphology unlike classic BBB or fascicular block?

Step 4: Ventricular Activation Velocity Ratio (Vi / Vt)

Vereckei Algorithm #2 (Lead aVR *only*)

Step 1: Is there an initial R wave? (Cannot be rS)

Step 2: Is there an initial r or q wave > 40 msec?

Step 3: Is there a notch on the descending limb of a negative onset and
predominantly negative QRS?

Step 4: Ventricular Activation Velocity Ratio (Vi / Vt)

ECG #3

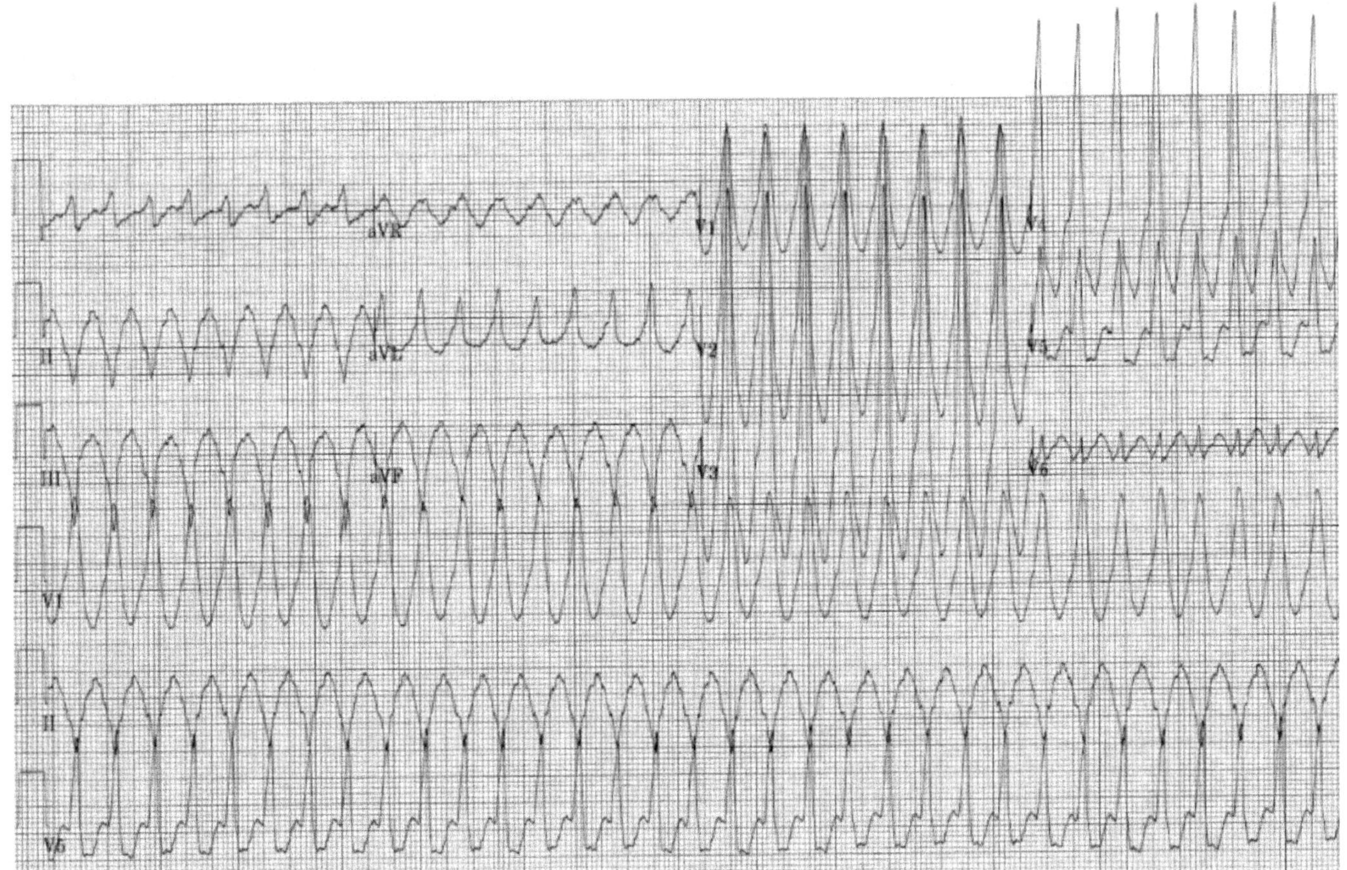

Figure 13-7

Vereckei Algorithm #1

Step 1: Is AV dissociation present?

Step 2: Is there an initial R wave in Lead aVR? (Cannot be rS)

Step 3: Is the QRS morphology unlike classic BBB or fascicular block?

Step 4: Ventricular Activation Velocity Ratio (Vi / Vt)

Vereckei Algorithm #2 (Lead aVR *only*)

Step 1: Is there an initial R wave? (Cannot be rS)

Step 2: Is there an initial r or q wave > 40 msec?

Step 3: Is there a notch on the descending limb of a negative onset and predominantly negative QRS?

Step 4: Ventricular Activation Velocity Ratio (Vi / Vt)

ECG #4

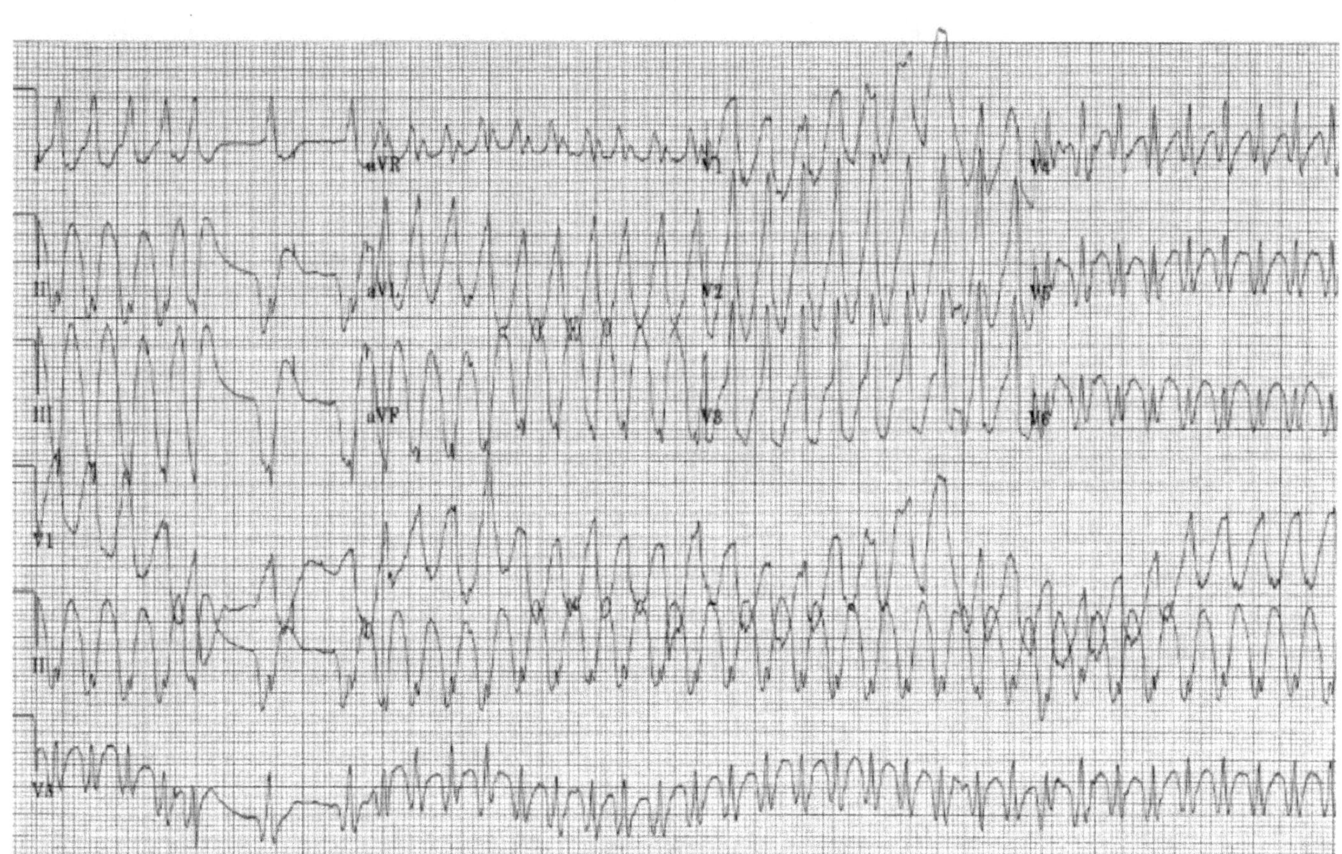

Figure 13-8

Vereckei Algorithm #1

Step 1: Is AV dissociation present?

Step 2: Is there an initial R wave in Lead aVR? (Cannot be rS)

Step 3: Is the QRS morphology unlike classic BBB or fascicular block?

Step 4: Ventricular Activation Velocity Ratio (Vi / Vt)

Vereckei Algorithm #2 (Lead aVR *only*)

Step 1: Is there an initial R wave? (Cannot be rS)

Step 2: Is there an initial r or q wave > 40 msec?

Step 3: Is there a notch on the descending limb of a negative onset and predominantly negative QRS?

Step 4: Ventricular Activation Velocity Ratio (Vi / Vt)

ECG #5

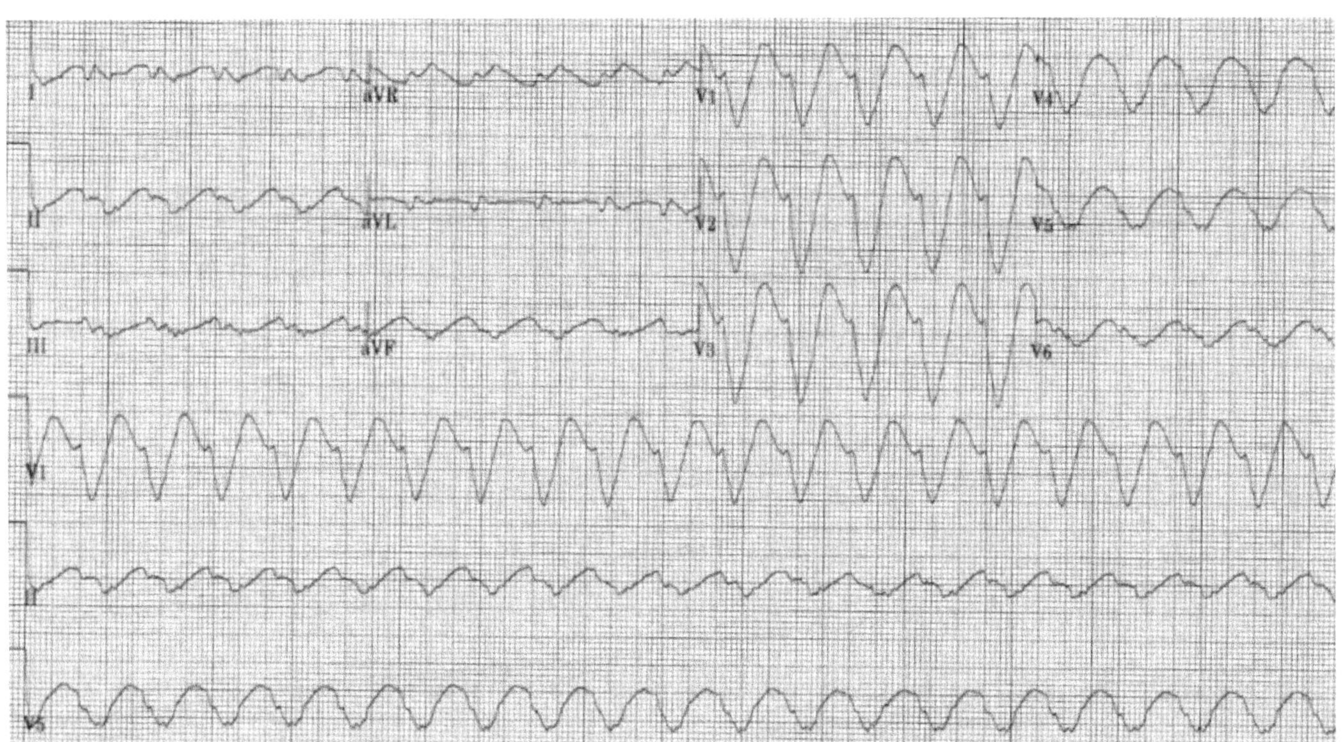

Figure 13-9

Vereckei Algorithm #1

Step 1: Is AV dissociation present?

Step 2: Is there an initial R wave in Lead aVR? (Cannot be rS)

Step 3: Is the QRS morphology unlike classic BBB or fascicular block?

Step 4: Ventricular Activation Velocity Ratio (Vi / Vt)

Vereckei Algorithm #2 (Lead aVR *only*)

Step 1: Is there an initial R wave? (Cannot be rS)

Step 2: Is there an initial r or q wave > 40 msec?

Step 3: Is there a notch on the descending limb of a negative onset and
predominantly negative QRS?

Step 4: Ventricular Activation Velocity Ratio (Vi / Vt)

ECG #6

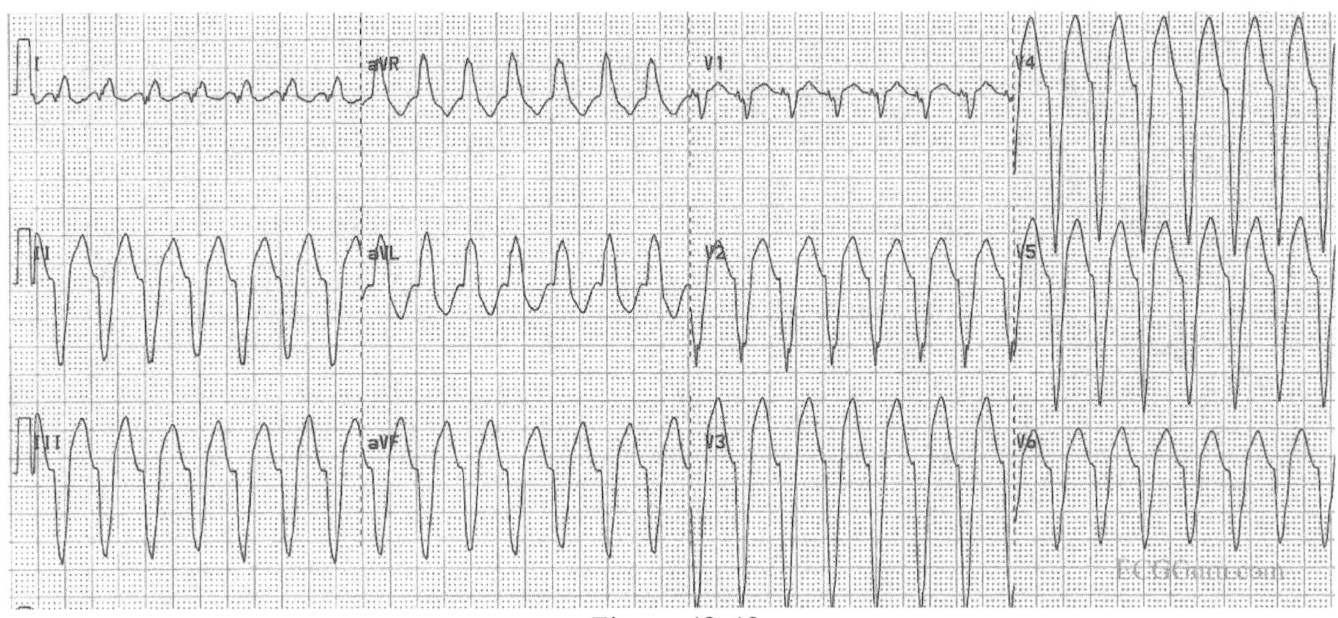

Figure 13-10

Vereckei Algorithm #1

Step 1: Is AV dissociation present?

Step 2: Is there an initial R wave in Lead aVR? (Cannot be rS)

Step 3: Is the QRS morphology unlike classic BBB or fascicular block?

Step 4: Ventricular Activation Velocity Ratio (Vi / Vt)

Vereckei Algorithm #2 (Lead aVR *only*)

Step 1: Is there an initial R wave? (Cannot be rS)

Step 2: Is there an initial r or q wave > 40 msec?

Step 3: Is there a notch on the descending limb of a negative onset and predominantly negative QRS?

Step 4: Ventricular Activation Velocity Ratio (Vi / Vt)

ECG #7

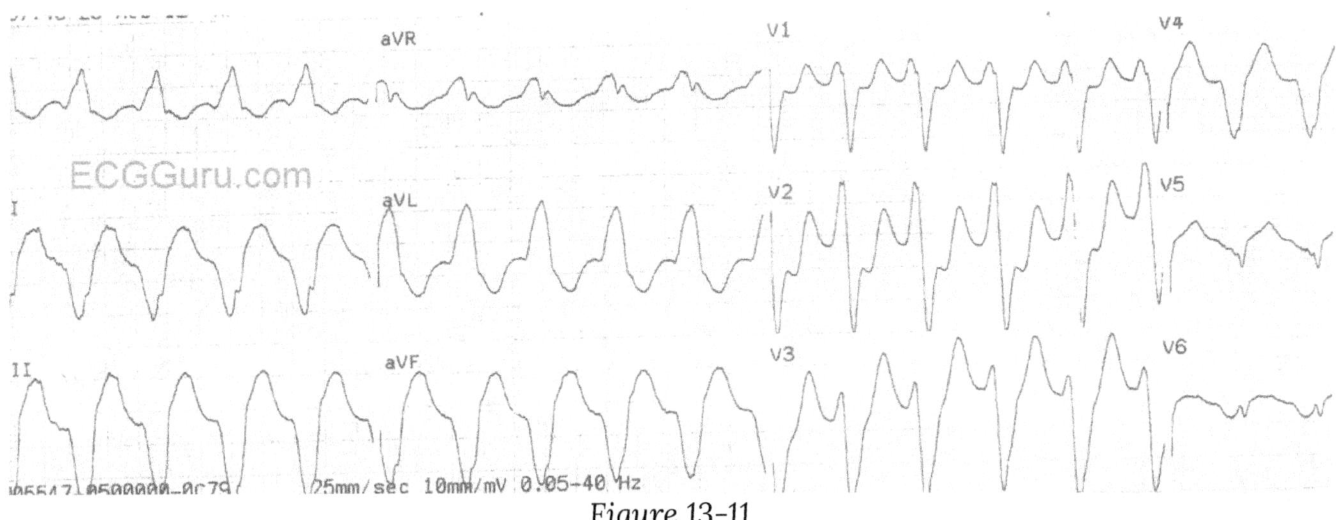

Figure 13-11

Vereckei Algorithm #1

Step 1: Is AV dissociation present?

Step 2: Is there an initial R wave in Lead aVR? (Cannot be rS)

Step 3: Is the QRS morphology unlike classic BBB or fascicular block?

Step 4: Ventricular Activation Velocity Ratio (Vi / Vt)

Vereckei Algorithm #2 (Lead aVR *only*)

Step 1: Is there an initial R wave? (Cannot be rS)

Step 2: Is there an initial r or q wave > 40 msec?

Step 3: Is there a notch on the descending limb of a negative onset and predominantly negative QRS?

Step 4: Ventricular Activation Velocity Ratio (Vi / Vt)

ECG #8

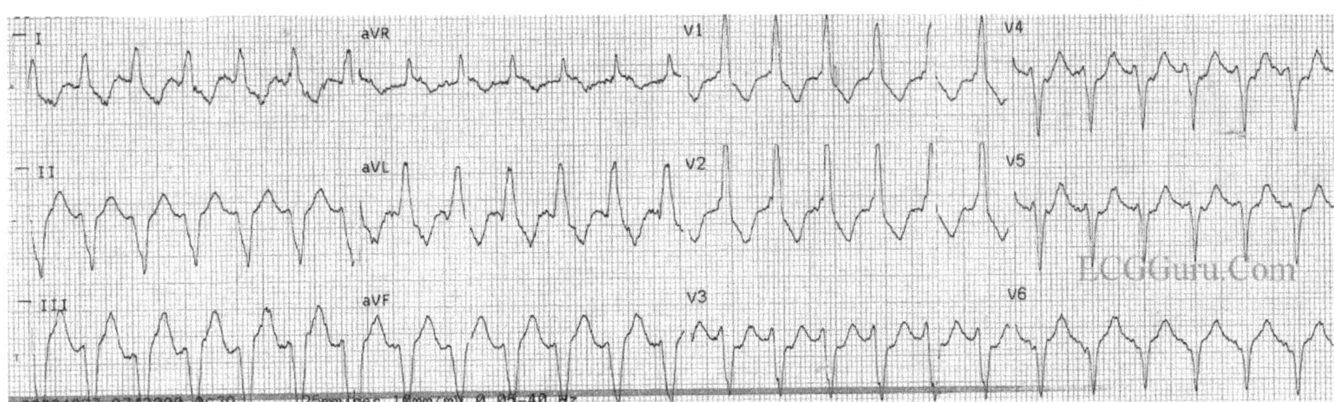

Figure 13-12

Vereckei Algorithm #1

Step 1: Is AV dissociation present?

Step 2: Is there an initial R wave in Lead aVR? (Cannot be rS)

Step 3: Is the QRS morphology unlike classic BBB or fascicular block?

Step 4: Ventricular Activation Velocity Ratio (Vi / Vt)

Vereckei Algorithm #2 (Lead aVR *only*)

Step 1: Is there an initial R wave? (Cannot be rS)

Step 2: Is there an initial r or q wave > 40 msec?

Step 3: Is there a notch on the descending limb of a negative onset and predominantly negative QRS?

Step 4: Ventricular Activation Velocity Ratio (Vi / Vt)

ECG #9

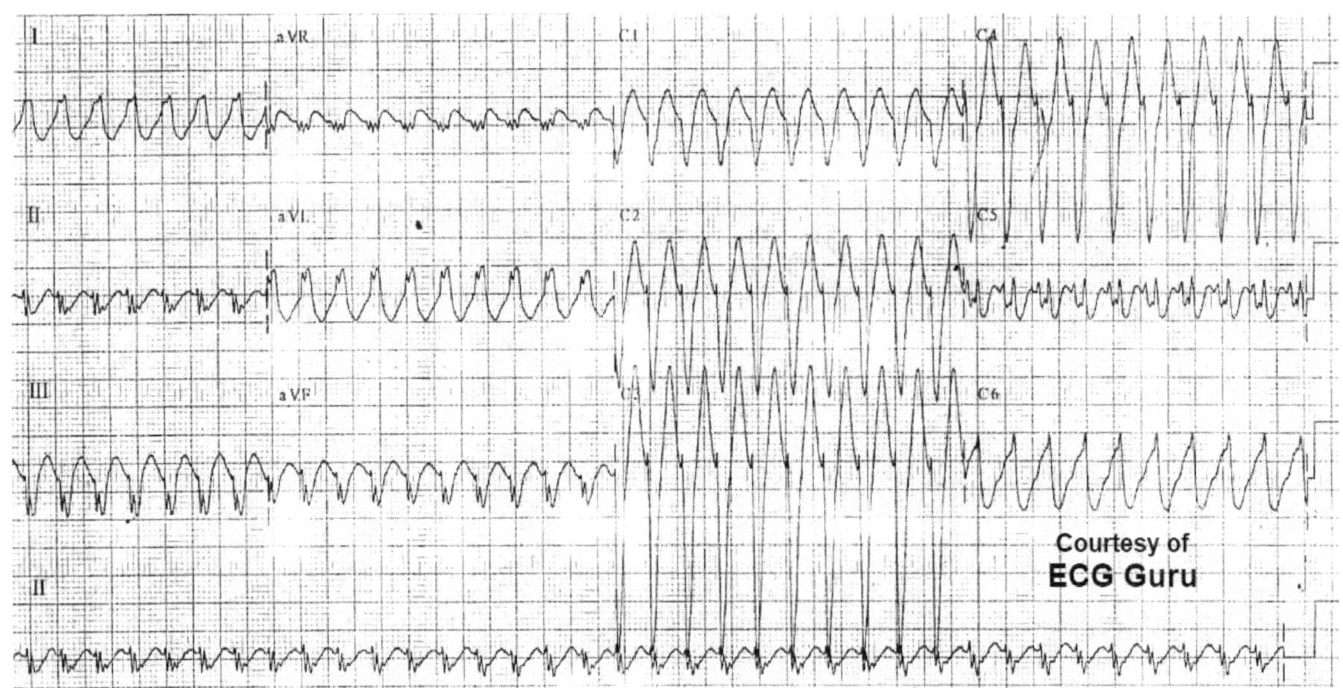

Figure 13-13

Vereckei Algorithm #1

Step 1: Is AV dissociation present?

Step 2: Is there an initial R wave in Lead aVR? (Cannot be rS)

Step 3: Is the QRS morphology unlike classic BBB or fascicular block?

Step 4: Ventricular Activation Velocity Ratio (Vi / Vt)

Vereckei Algorithm #2 (Lead aVR *only*)

Step 1: Is there an initial R wave? (Cannot be rS)

Step 2: Is there an initial r or q wave > 40 msec?

Step 3: Is there a notch on the descending limb of a negative onset and predominantly negative QRS?

Step 4: Ventricular Activation Velocity Ratio (Vi / Vt)

ECG #10

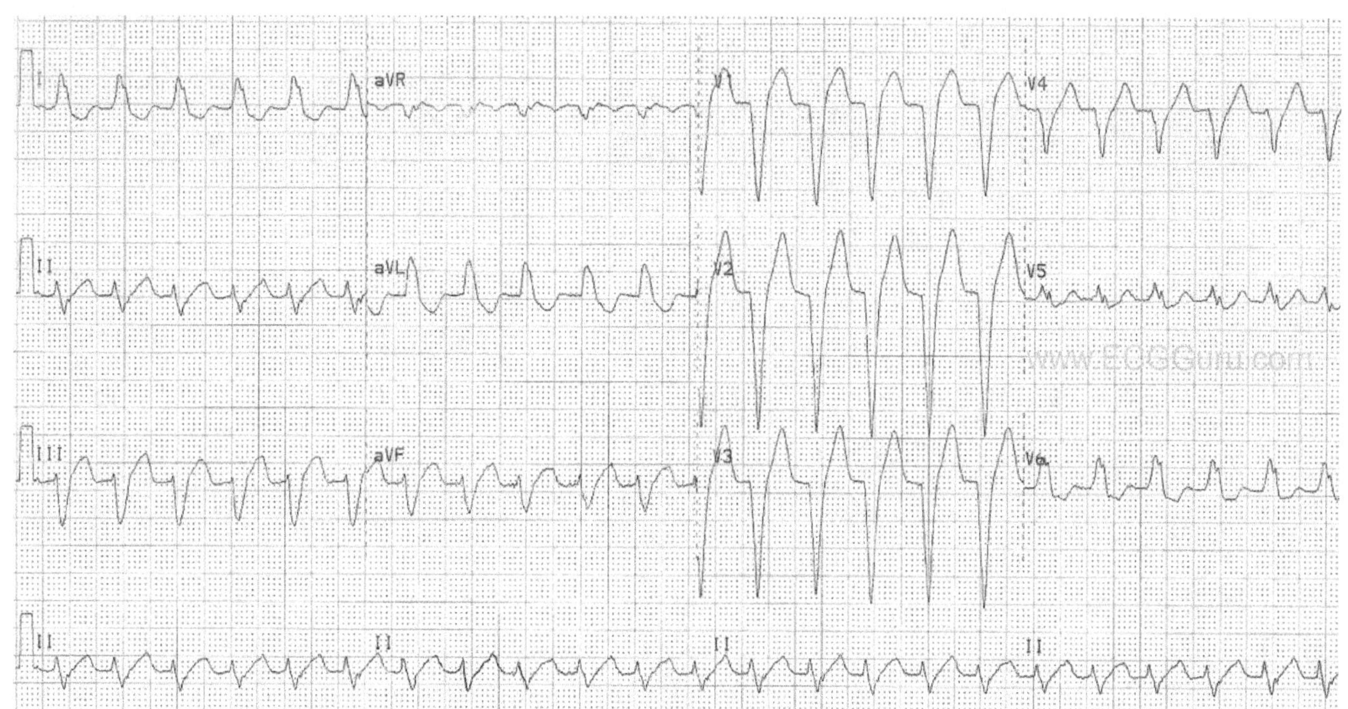

Figure 13-14

Chapter 14

The R Wave Peak Time

Pava Method

How to Measure the R Wave Peak Time (Pava Method)

The R Wave Peak Time (RWPT), or "Pava Method," was introduced in 2010. In addition to the *Vereckei Algorithm #2*, it is based on the findings in just one lead: Lead II. The basis of this value is very similar to the ventricular activation velocity ratio – ectopic ventricular rhythms will be slow from the beginning of the deflection because the impulse is being conducted from cell to cell. R wave peak time replaces the old terminology: *intrinsicoid deflection.*

There is a little "quirk" regarding the RWPT... despite its name, *it does not require the presence of an R wave.* As Pava et al defined it as: "[the] QRS duration from initiation of depolarization until the first change of the polarity, independent of whether the QRS deflection was positive or negative." And, unlike the ventricular activation velocity ratio, there is no restriction on the QRS morphology to be used.

How to measure the RWPT (Figure 14-1):

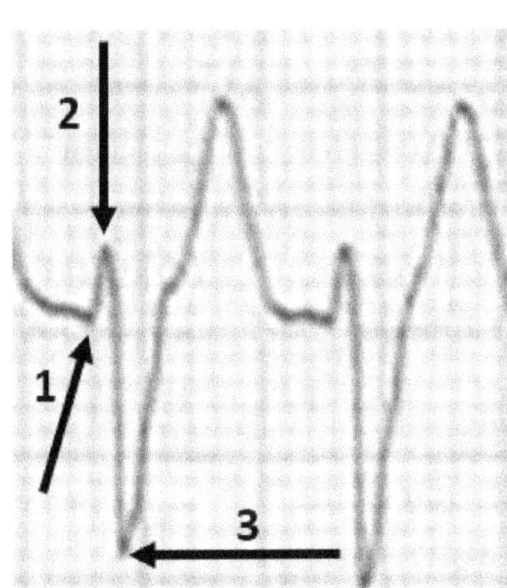

Measure from the onset of the *first* deflection of the QRS, whether it's a Q, an R, or an S (arrow labeled "1"). Then identify the first change in polarity (arrow labelled "2"). Note that in this case, the first change in polarity is where the upslope of the R wave reaches its peak and then begins a downward slope. It is *not* at the nadir of the S wave (arrow labeled "3"). Can you determine how many msec are between the first arrow (1) and the second arrow (2)? Is it ≥ 50 msec? Are you sure – even with the Lead II enlarged many times?

Figure 14-1

Here is a negative Lead II (Figure 14-2). First, you must identify the onset of the QRS. *It needs to be as exact as possible because we are measuring in milliseconds!* We measure from the onset of the QS deflection to its nadir which represents the first change in polarity.

Be very careful of your measurements. Here are two things you CANNOT do:

1. you CANNOT move to a different lead because measuring it will be easier. You must use Lead II and Lead II ONLY!

2. you CANNOT "overlook" a polarity change because it is small and/or early in the deflection!

Here is an example (Figure 14-2):

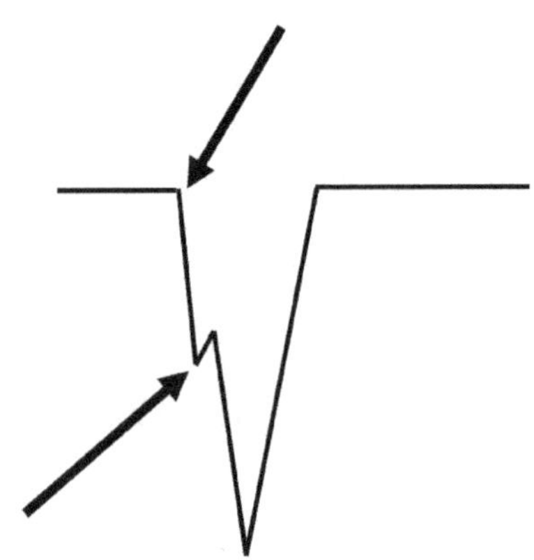

Do NOT be tempted to measure from the onset of the QRS to the nadir of the S wave. Similarly, if the QRS begins with a Q wave, the onset of the QRS is the onset of the Q wave and the first change in polarity will be the nadir of the Q wave.

Figure 14-2

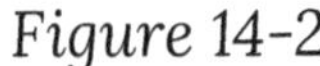

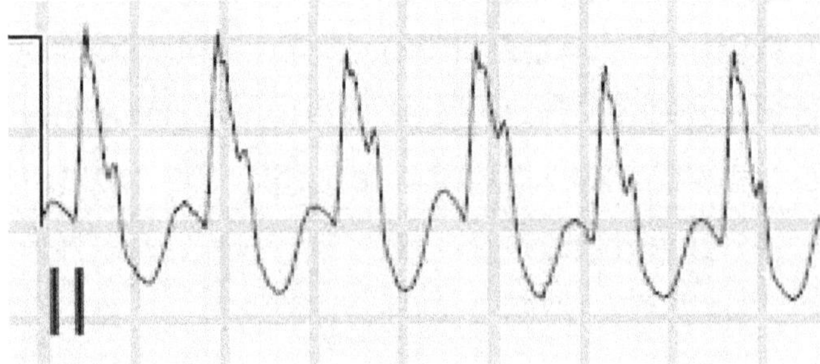

Figure 14-3

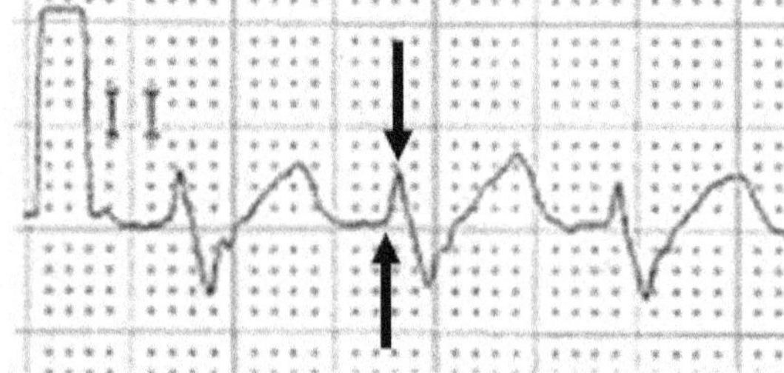

Figure 14-4

Let's look at Figure 14-3. This morphology is a qR with a notched R wave. Here's a question for you: where does the q wave begin? The first change in polarity would be the nadir of the q wave, but where do we measure from? You will not be able to use this Lead II, so you had better have another acceptable algorithm that you can use instead. Figure 14-4 is much easier.

TIP | Just because only a single lead is involved, don't assume that using the algorithm or method is going to be easy! You had better be proficient at using a second (different) algorithm if needed.

Recommended Reading:

Jastrzebski M, Kukla P, Czarnecka D, and Kawecka-Jaszcz K. Comparison of five electrocardiographic methods for differentiation of wide QRS-complex tachycardias. *Europace*. (2012) 14, 1165–1171 doi:10.1093/europace/eus015.

Pava LF, Perafan P, Badiel M, et al. R-Wave peak time at DII: a new criterion for differentiating between wide complex QRS tachycardias. *Heart Rhythm*. 2010;7:922–926.

Szelényi ZDG, Katona G, Fritúz G, et al. Comparison of the "real-life" diagnostic value of two recently published electrocardiogram methods for the differential diagnosis of wide QRS complex tachycardias. *Acad Emerg Med*. 20(11); November 2013; pp. 1121-1130.

Practicing the R Wave Peak Time (Pava) Method

Measure from the onset of the first deflection of the QRS to the first change in polarity, whether positive or negative. If the duration is ≥ 50 msec then the diagnosis is **ventricular tachycardia**; otherwise, it is **supraventricular tachycardia**. I'm making it easy for you – I've enlarged these snippets, but I also placed a more realistic size next to the first one (if your ECGs are printed on paper)! Remember: the **R wave peak time** must be at least 50 msec; 49 msec doesn't qualify!

ECG Snippet #1

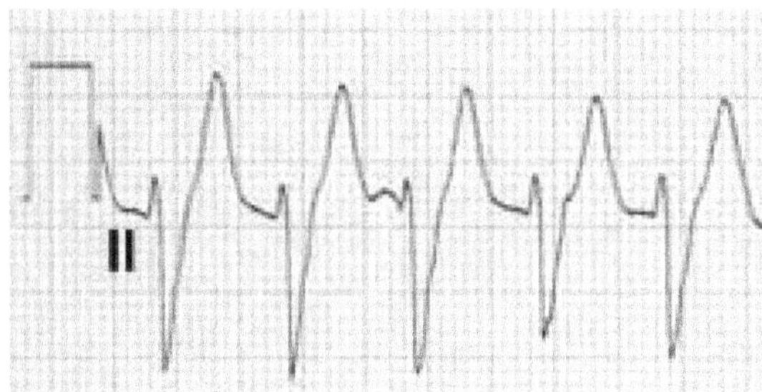

Figure 14-5

ECG Snippet #2

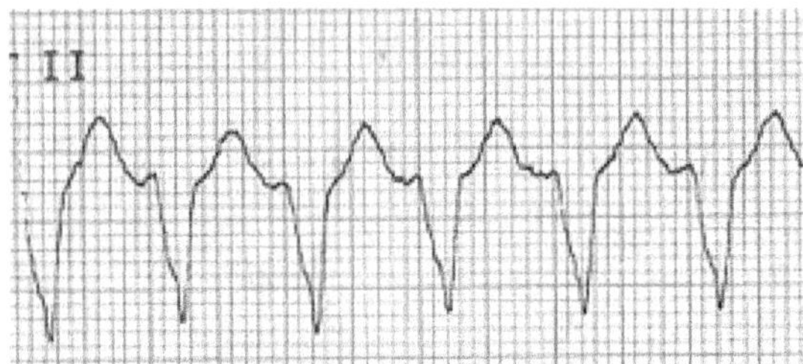

Figure 14-6

ECG Snippet #3

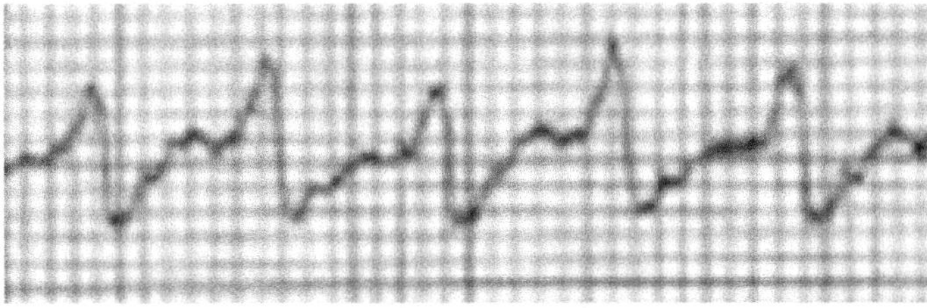

Figure 14-7

ECG Snippet #4

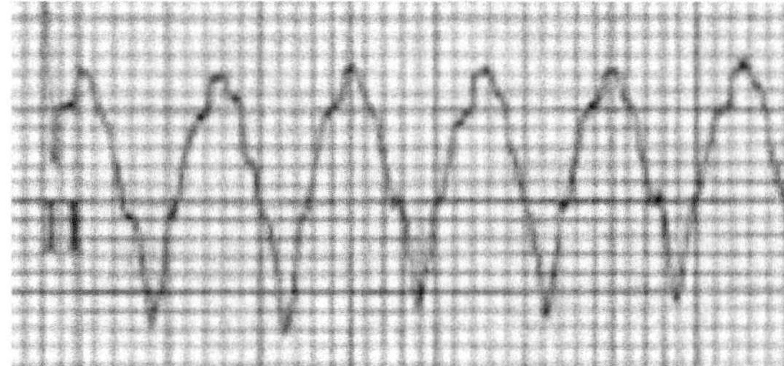

Figure 14-8

ECG Snippet #5

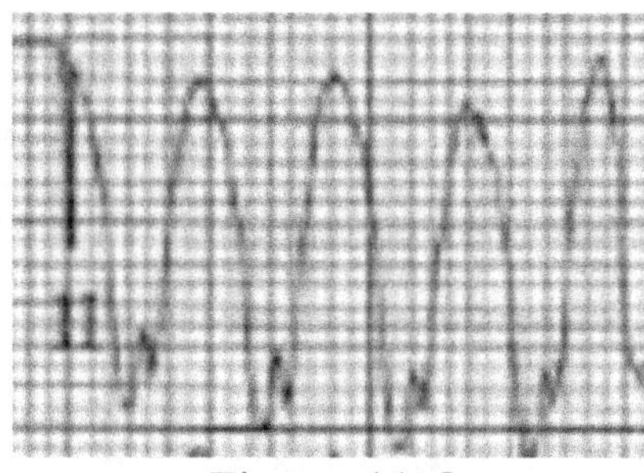

Figure 14-9

ECG Snippet #6

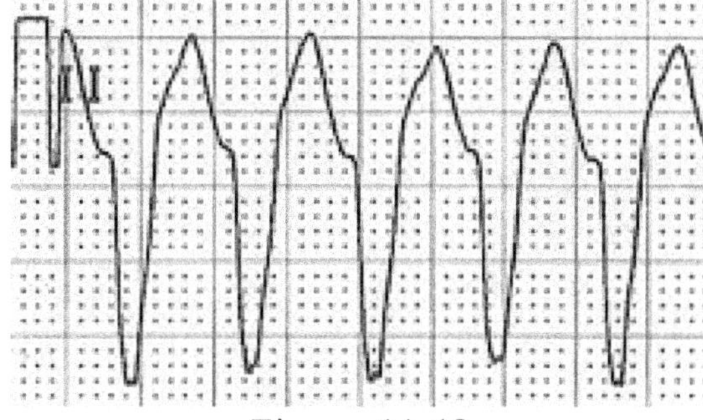

Figure 14-10

ECG Snippet #7

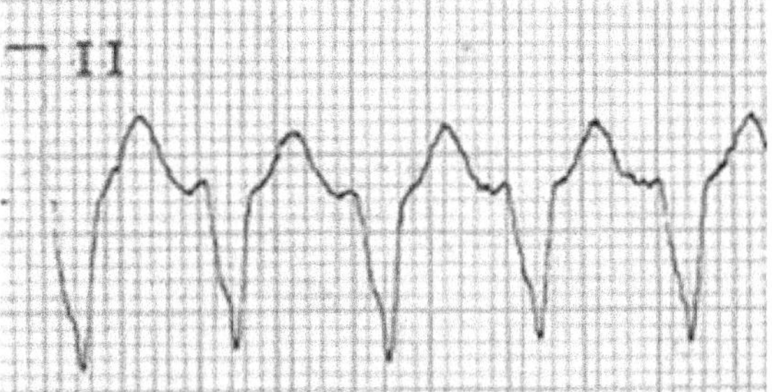

Figure 14-11

ECG Snippet #8

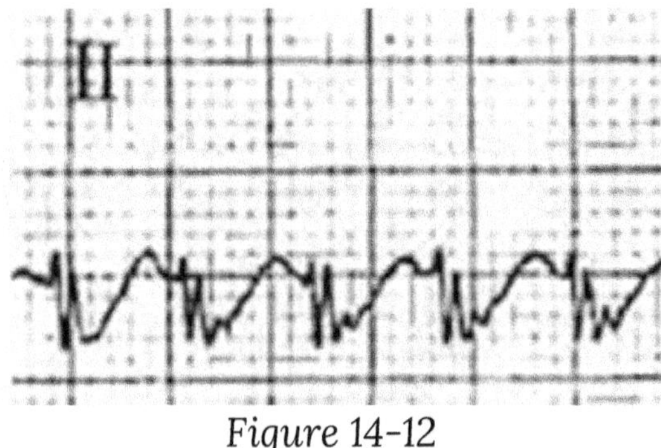

Figure 14-12

ECG Snippet #9

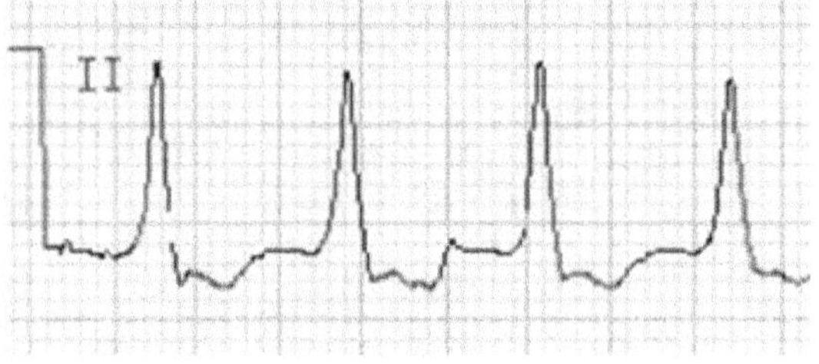

Figure 14-13

ECG Snippet #10

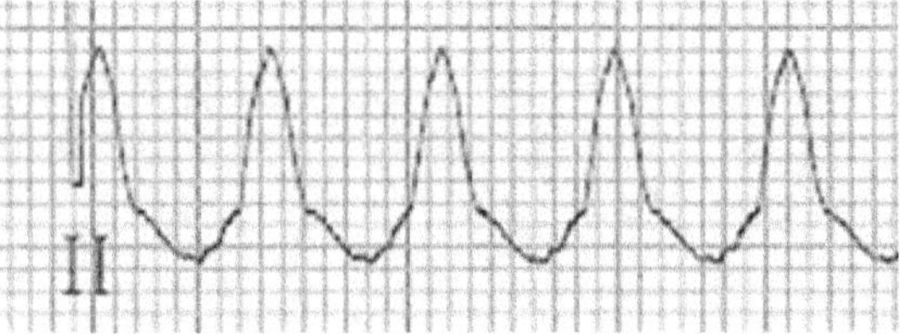

Figure 14-14

Chapter 15

The Limb Lead Method

2019 saw the appearance of a new algorithm for distinguishing between ventricular tachycardia (VT) and supraventricular tachycardia with aberrant conduction (SVT-A). It was published in the journal of the prestigious Heart Rhythm Society, "Heart Rhythm." Seventeen authors were listed – a very international group. The premise seems plausible and it is certainly usable in tense, emergent situations. Its only weakness appears to be several exceptions not covered by the algorithm and a lack of independent validation studies.

Limb Lead Algorithm Criteria

The Limb Lead Algorithm consists of three (3) criteria. If any ONE criterion is met, then the diagnosis is VT. The criteria are:

Step 1: Presence of a monophasic R wave in Lead aVR

Vereckei et al. presented a similar criterion in 2007 (they also allowed for an Rs wave). This represents an ectopic ventricular impulse traveling directly toward the positive pole of Lead aVR – something a supraventricular impulse entering the ventricles via the AV node and bundle branches would be most unlikely to do.

Step 2: Predominantly NEGATIVE QRS complexes in standard Leads I, II, and III

The exact morphology of the QRS complexes in those leads is not important as long as the QRS complexes are *predominantly* (net) NEGATIVE. They *do not have to be monophasic QS complexes*. This is much like the $S_1S_2S_3$ syndrome and indicates a far rightward mean QRS axis.

Step 3: Opposing QRS Complexes in the Limb Leads (OQL)

Monophasic concordant QRS complexes in all the INFERIOR leads (Leads II, III, and aVF), either monophasic R or monophasic QS.

Monophasic concordant QRS complexes involving two or more of the remaining limb leads (I, aVR, and aVL) of OPPOSITE POLARITY to the inferior leads.

> **TIP |** Look at the hexaxial reference grid (HRG): the only area on the grid where all three of the opposing limb leads (I, aVR, aVL) will be positive is between -60° and -90°.

Here is an ECG (limb leads only) that demonstrates "opposing QRS complexes in the limb leads (OQL)" (Figure 15-1):

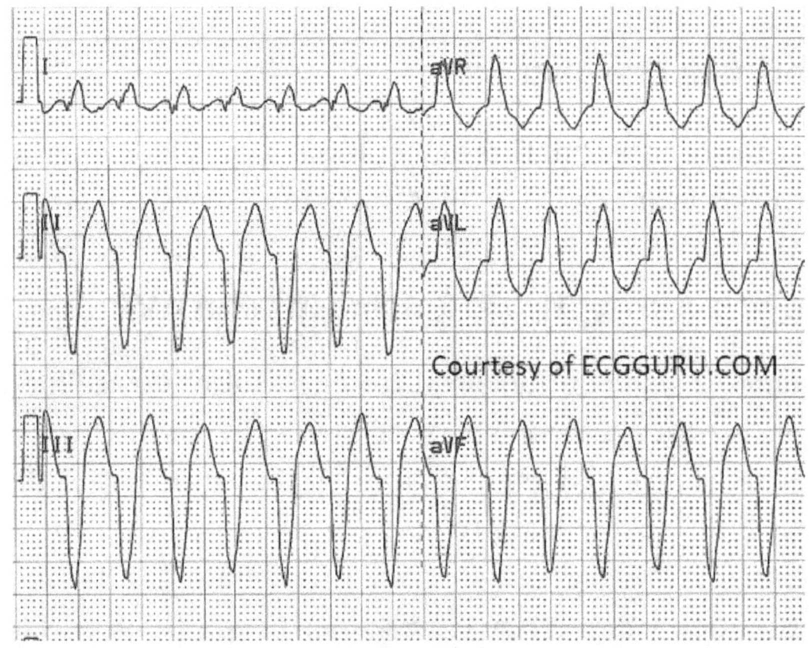

Figure 15-1

The OQL step is based on the different directions of depolarizations taken by SVTs entering the ventricles through the AV node and His-Purkinje system and VTs which tend to originate in either the superior ventricle (outflow tract) or inferior ventricle (apex). While the specificity was high, sensitivity was low. Step 1 ("monophasic R in Lead aVR") and Step 2 ("predominantly negative QRS complexes in Leads I, II, and III") were added to increase sensitivity. Step 1 is based on the Vereckei algorithm which suggests that an ectopically generated ventricular impulse will point to the positive pole of Lead aVR. Step 2 is based on the same assumption ("mean QRS axis in northwest quadrant").

Let's think about this...

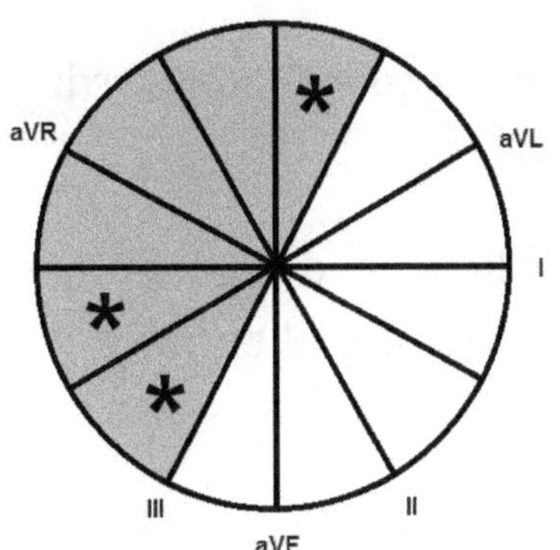

Figure 15-2

Step 1 is looking for a mean vector that will be located between +120° and -60°. That will include the shaded area on this Hexaxial Reference Grid (Figure 15-3):

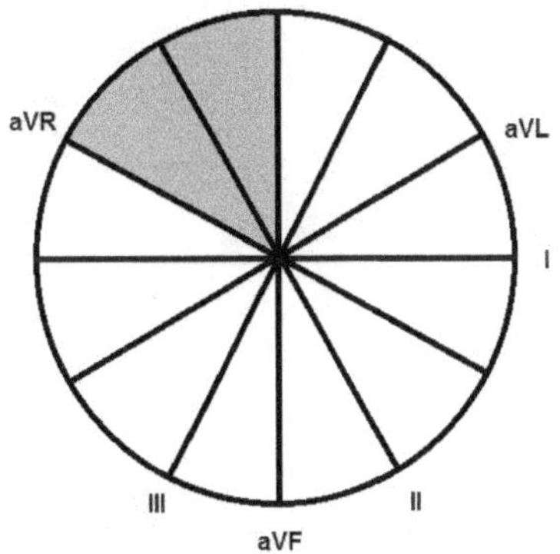

Figure 15-3

Step 2 is looking for a mean vector that will be located between -150° and -90°:

The shaded area is more restrictive and represents the only area on the Hexaxial Reference Grid that would result in net negative QRS complexes in *all* the standard limb leads (Leads I, II, and III).

A dominant R wave in Lead aVR would include vectors outside the right upper ("northwest") quadrant (note asterisks in Figure 15-2). Step 2 would obviously be a lot more specific for vectors in the right upper quadrant.

PEARL | Figure 15-3 is a diagram you should remember if you are serious about learning more electrocardiography. You will eventually encounter the $S_1S_2S_3$ finding which is usually mentioned in regard to severe right heart strain – often in association with acute cor pulmonale and as a sign of pulmonary emobilism. When there are deep S waves in all three standard leads (Leads I, II, and III), that indicates that the right ventricle is depolarizing late because it is under a lot of strain! That will send the mean QRS vector (ÂQRS) rightward into that portion of the right upper quadrant of the Hexaxial Reference Grid.

Recommended Reading:

Chen Q, Xu J, Gianni C, et al. [published online September 20, 2019]. Heart Rhythm. doi: 10.1016/j.hrthm.2019.09.021

Sison CP, MD. ECG Limb Lead Algorithm: Sensitive, Specific for Wide Complex Tachycardia Diagnosis.

https://www.thecardiologyadvisor.com//home/topics/arrhythmia/limb-lead-algorithm-sensitive-specific-for-wide-qrs-complex-tachycardia-diagnosis-on-electrocardiogram/

Practicing the Limb Lead (OQL) Algorithm

Limb Leads (OQL) Algorithm

Step 1: Presence of a monophasic R wave in Lead aVR

Step 2: Predominantly NEGATIVE QRS complexes in standard Leads I, II and III

Step 3: Opposing QRS Complexes in the Limb Leads (OQL)

Monophasic concordant QRS complexes in all the INFERIOR leads (Leads II, III and aVF), either monophasic R or monophasic QS.

Monophasic concordant QRS complexes involving two or more of the remaining limb leads (I, aVR and aVL) of OPPOSITE POLARITY to the inferior leads

ECG #1

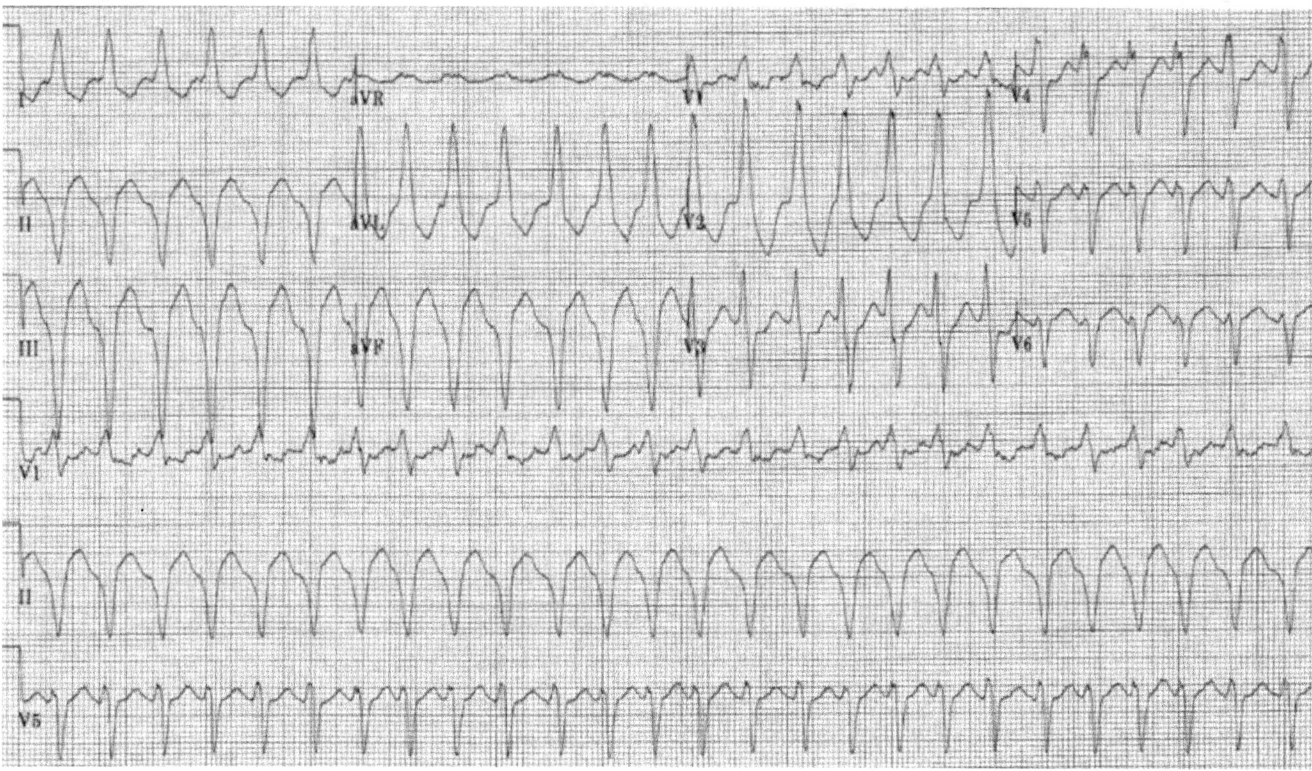

Figure 15-4

Limb Leads (OQL) Algorithm

Step 1: Presence of a monophasic R wave in Lead aVR

Step 2: Predominantly NEGATIVE QRS complexes in standard Leads I, II and III

Step 3: Opposing QRS Complexes in the Limb Leads (OQL)

Monophasic concordant QRS complexes in all the INFERIOR leads (Leads II, III and aVF), either monophasic R or monophasic QS.

Monophasic concordant QRS complexes involving two or more of the remaining limb leads (I, aVR and aVL) of OPPOSITE POLARITY to the inferior leads

ECG #2

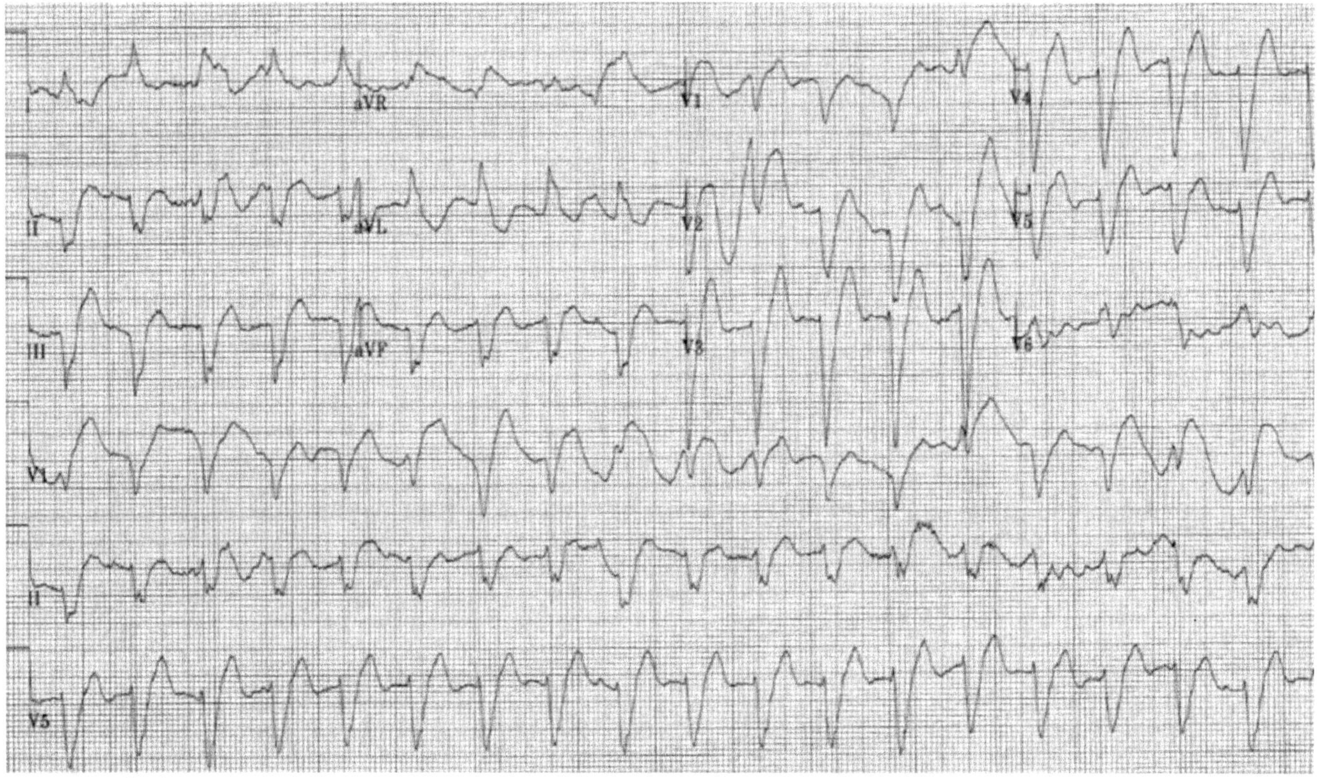

Figure 15-5

Limb Leads (OQL) Algorithm

Step 1: Presence of a monophasic R wave in Lead aVR

Step 2: Predominantly NEGATIVE QRS complexes in standard Leads I, II and III

Step 3: Opposing QRS Complexes in the Limb Leads (OQL)

> Monophasic concordant QRS complexes in all the INFERIOR leads (Leads II, III and aVF), either monophasic R or monophasic QS.

> Monophasic concordant QRS complexes involving two or more of the remaining limb leads (I, aVR and aVL) of OPPOSITE POLARITY to the inferior leads

ECG #3

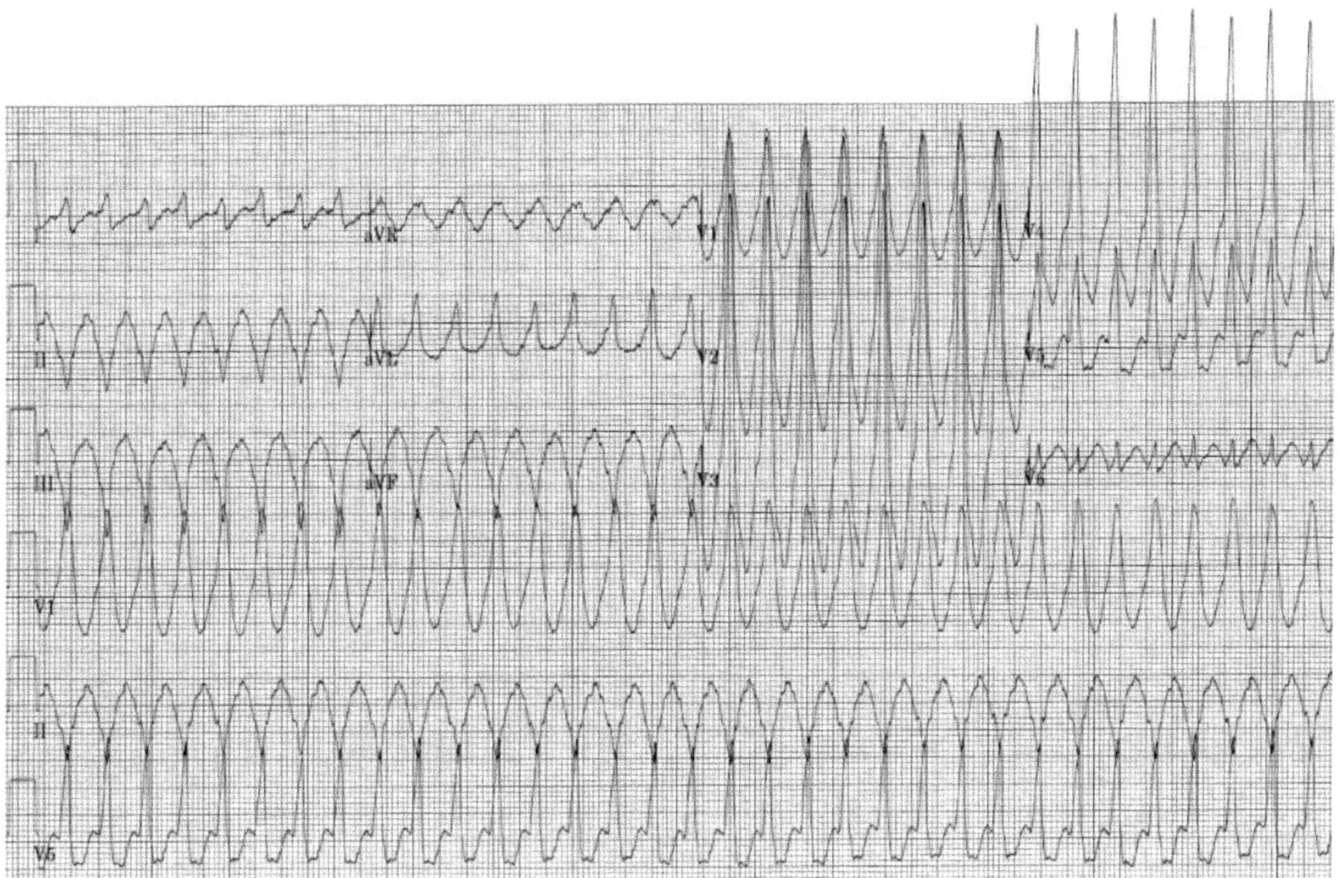

Figure 15-6

Limb Leads (OQL) Algorithm

Step 1: Presence of a monophasic R wave in Lead aVR

Step 2: Predominantly NEGATIVE QRS complexes in standard Leads I, II and III

Step 3: Opposing QRS Complexes in the Limb Leads (OQL)

Monophasic concordant QRS complexes in all the INFERIOR leads (Leads II, III and aVF), either monophasic R or monophasic QS.

Monophasic concordant QRS complexes involving two or more of the remaining limb leads (I, aVR and aVL) of OPPOSITE POLARITY to the inferior leads

ECG #4

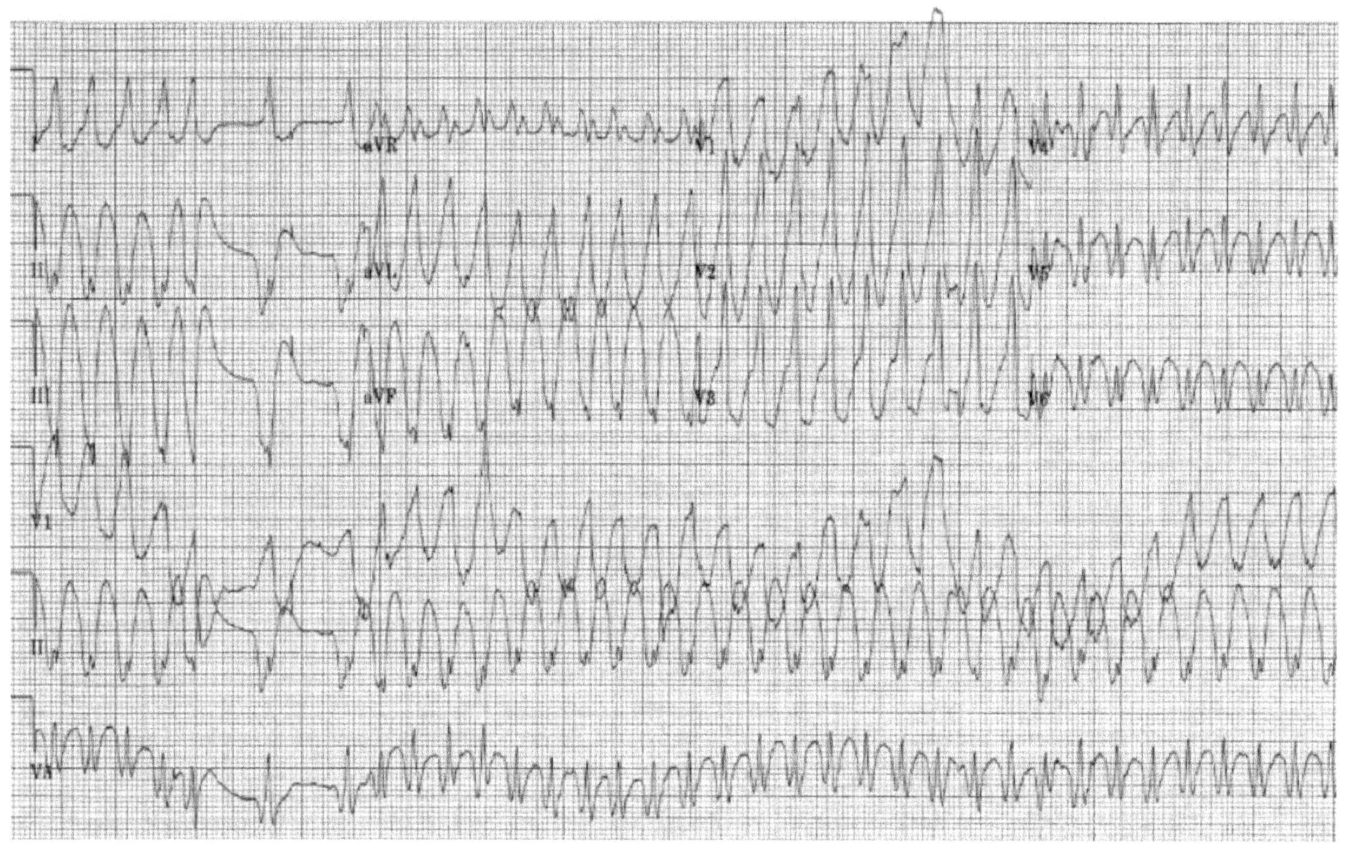

Figure 15-7

Limb Leads (OQL) Algorithm

Step 1: Presence of a monophasic R wave in Lead aVR

Step 2: Predominantly NEGATIVE QRS complexes in standard Leads I, II and III

Step 3: Opposing QRS Complexes in the Limb Leads (OQL)

Monophasic concordant QRS complexes in all the INFERIOR leads (Leads II, III and aVF), either monophasic R or monophasic QS.

Monophasic concordant QRS complexes involving two or more of the remaining limb leads (I, aVR and aVL) of OPPOSITE POLARITY to the inferior leads

ECG #5

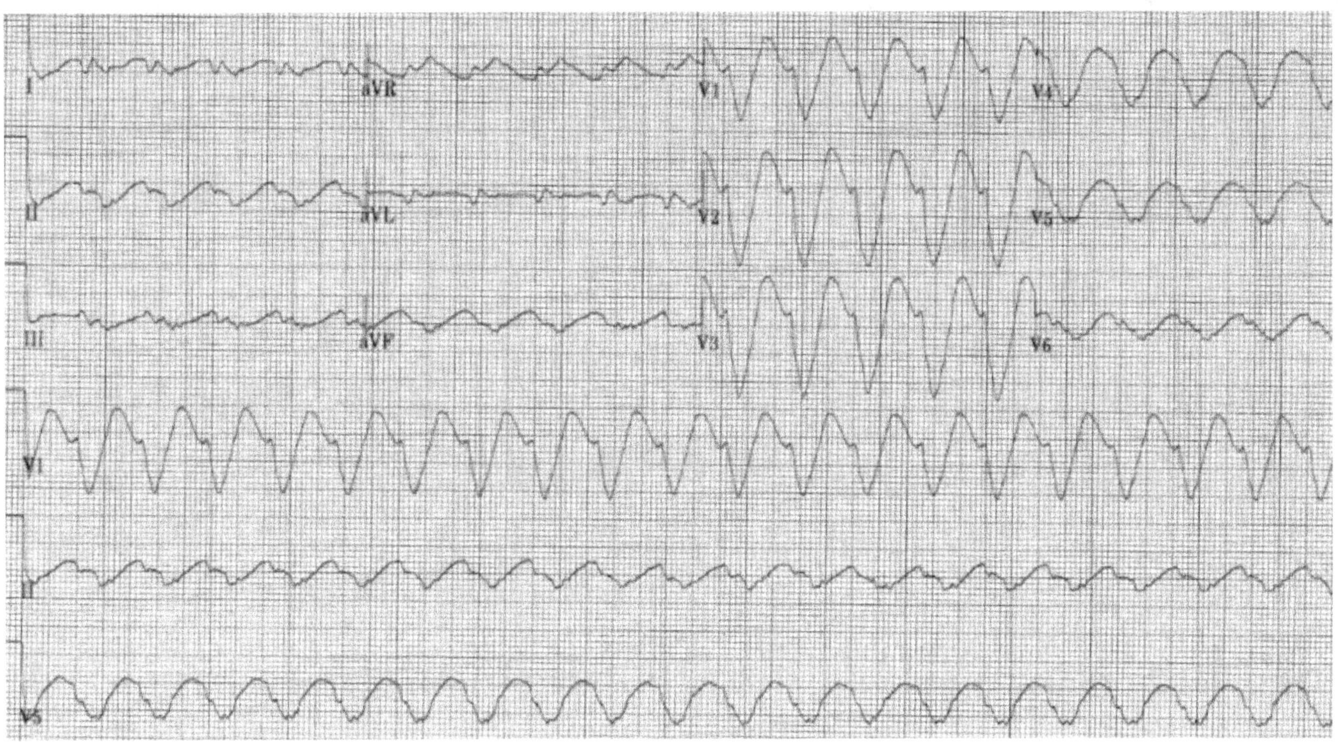

Figure 15-8

Limb Leads (OQL) Algorithm

Step 1: Presence of a monophasic R wave in Lead aVR

Step 2: Predominantly NEGATIVE QRS complexes in standard Leads I, II and III

Step 3: Opposing QRS Complexes in the Limb Leads (OQL)

> Monophasic concordant QRS complexes in all the INFERIOR leads (Leads II, III and aVF), either monophasic R or monophasic QS.

> Monophasic concordant QRS complexes involving two or more of the remaining limb leads (I, aVR and aVL) of OPPOSITE POLARITY to the inferior leads

ECG #6

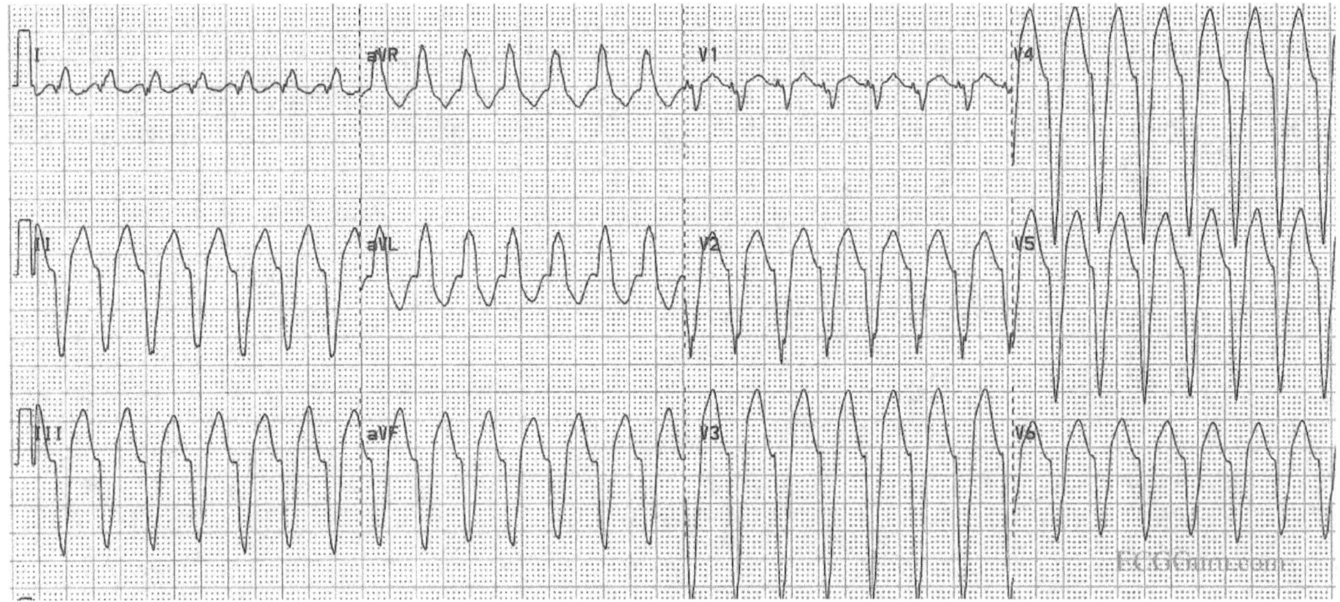

Figure 15-9

Limb Leads (OQL) Algorithm

Step 1: Presence of a monophasic R wave in Lead aVR

Step 2: Predominantly NEGATIVE QRS complexes in standard Leads I, II and III

Step 3: Opposing QRS Complexes in the Limb Leads (OQL)

Monophasic concordant QRS complexes in all the INFERIOR leads (Leads II, III and aVF), either monophasic R or monophasic QS.

Monophasic concordant QRS complexes involving two or more of the remaining limb leads (I, aVR and aVL) of OPPOSITE POLARITY to the inferior leads

ECG #7

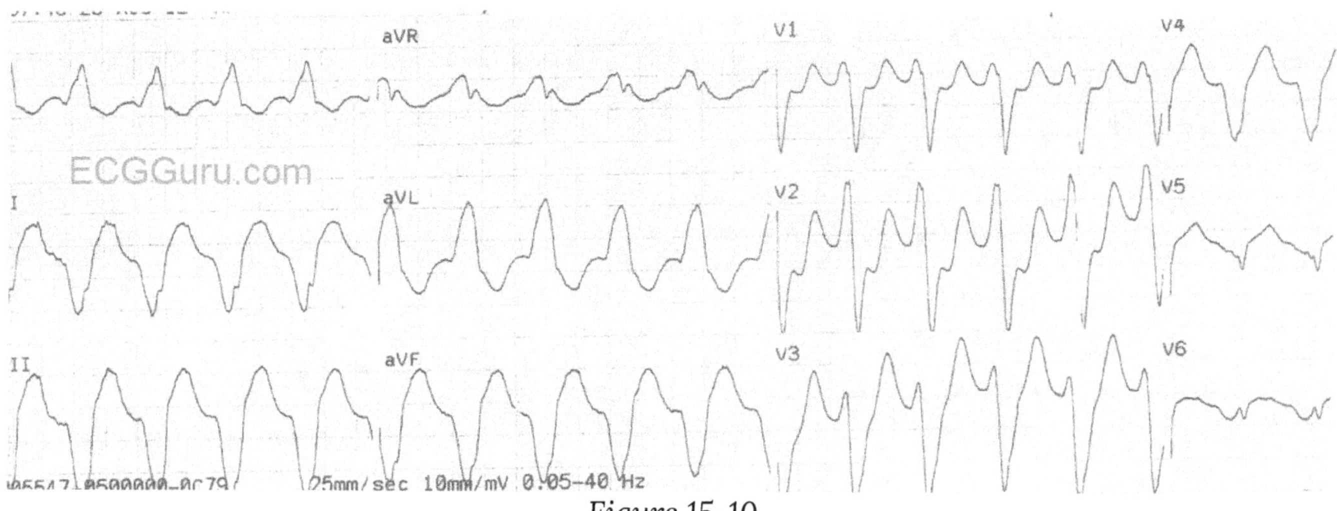

Figure 15-10

Limb Leads (OQL) Algorithm

Step 1: Presence of a monophasic R wave in Lead aVR

Step 2: Predominantly NEGATIVE QRS complexes in standard Leads I, II and III

Step 3: Opposing QRS Complexes in the Limb Leads (OQL)

> Monophasic concordant QRS complexes in all the INFERIOR leads (Leads II, III and aVF), either monophasic R or monophasic QS.

> Monophasic concordant QRS complexes involving two or more of the remaining limb leads (I, aVR and aVL) of OPPOSITE POLARITY to the inferior leads

ECG #8

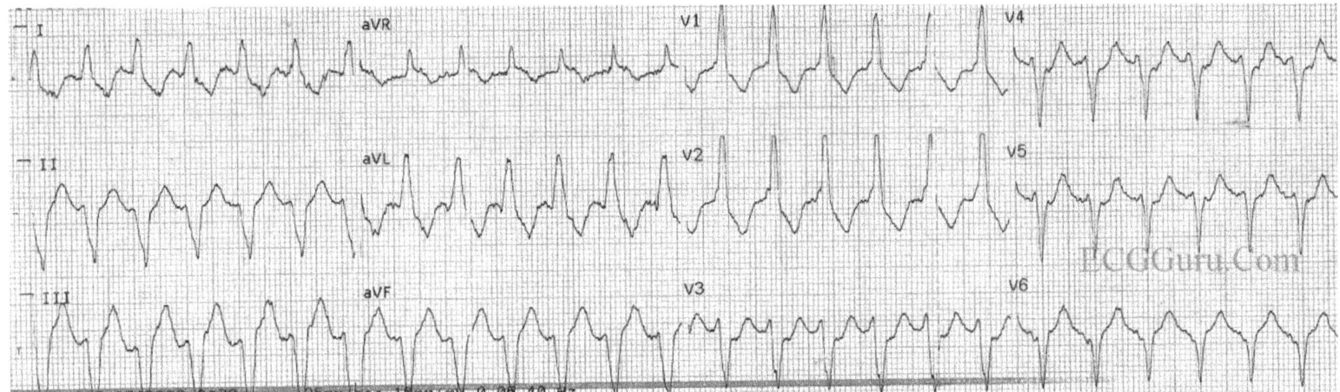

Figure 15-11

Limb Leads (OQL) Algorithm

Step 1: Presence of a monophasic R wave in Lead aVR

Step 2: Predominantly NEGATIVE QRS complexes in standard Leads I, II and III

Step 3: Opposing QRS Complexes in the Limb Leads (OQL)

Monophasic concordant QRS complexes in all the INFERIOR leads (Leads II, III and aVF), either monophasic R or monophasic QS.

Monophasic concordant QRS complexes involving two or more of the remaining limb leads (I, aVR and aVL) of OPPOSITE POLARITY to the inferior leads

ECG #9

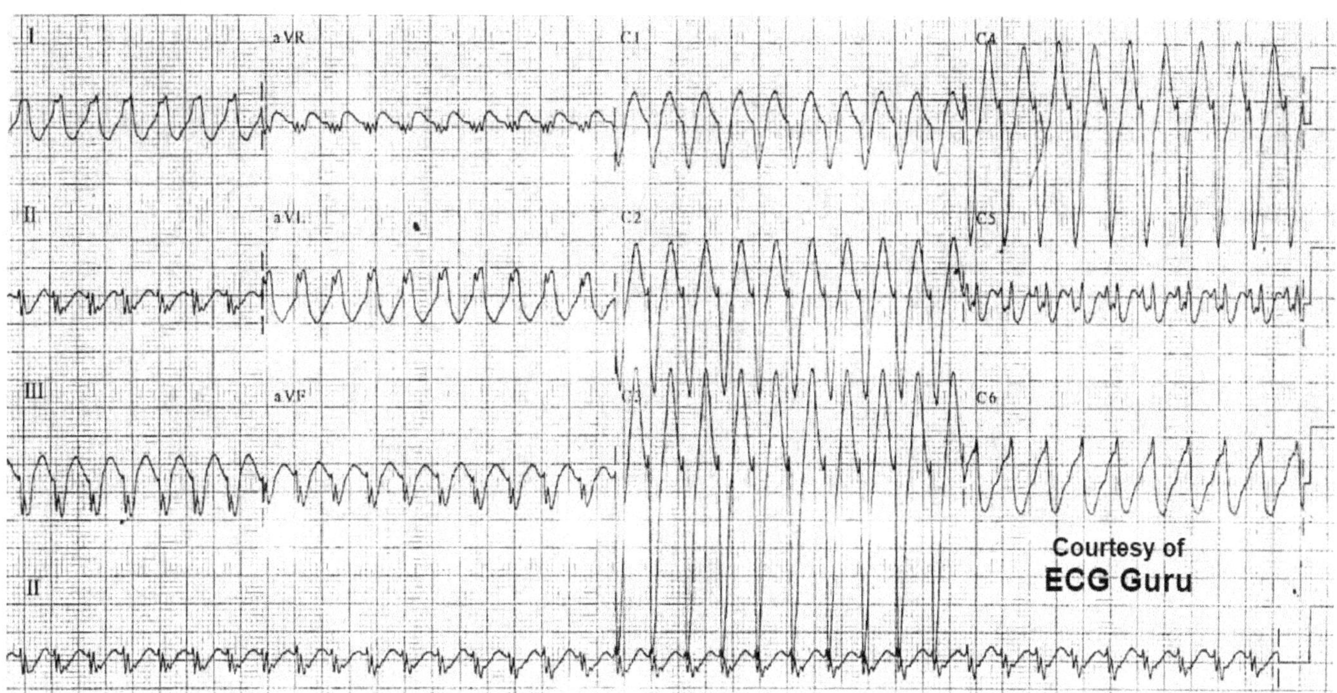

Figure 15-12

Limb Leads (OQL) Algorithm

Step 1: Presence of a monophasic R wave in Lead aVR

Step 2: Predominantly NEGATIVE QRS complexes in standard Leads I, II and III

Step 3: Opposing QRS Complexes in the Limb Leads (OQL)

Monophasic concordant QRS complexes in all the INFERIOR leads (Leads II, III and aVF), either monophasic R or monophasic QS.

Monophasic concordant QRS complexes involving two or more of the remaining limb leads (I, aVR and aVL) of OPPOSITE POLARITY to the inferior leads

ECG #10

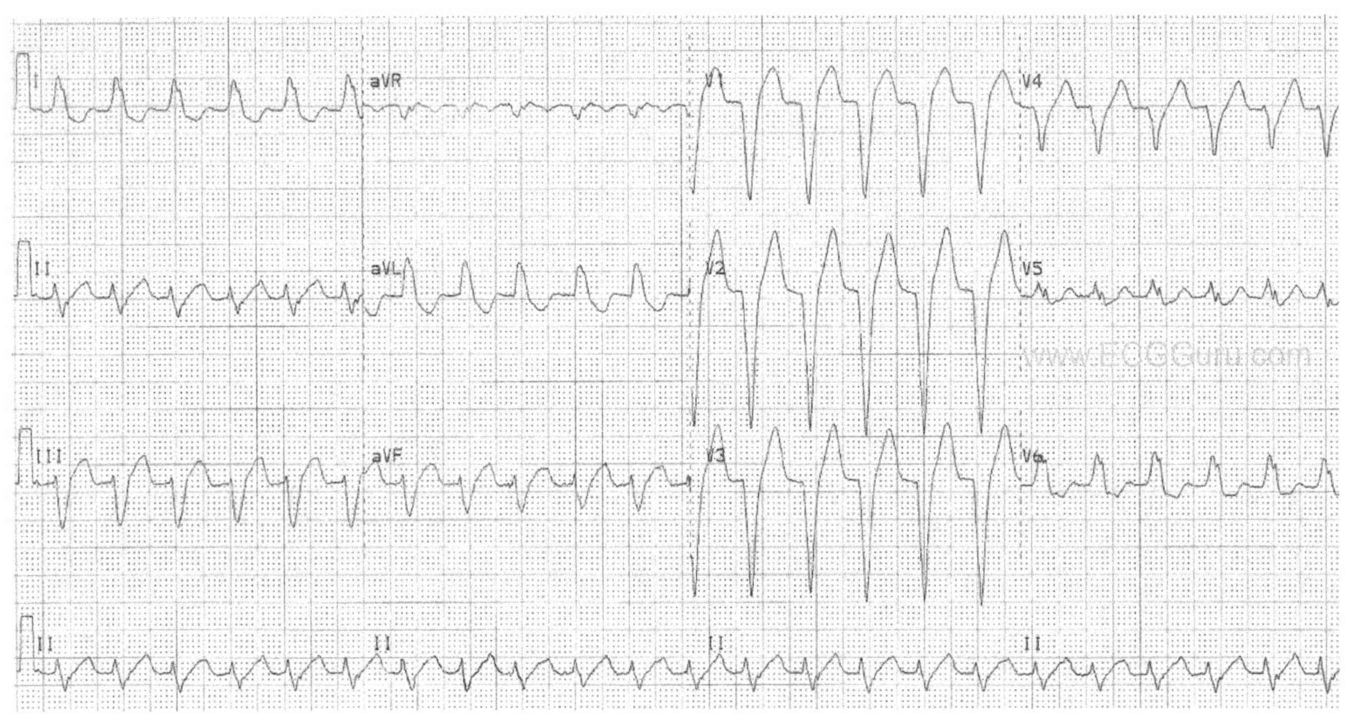

figure 15-13

Chapter 16

The Basel Algorithm

The newest algorithm is the Basel algorithm introduced in 2022. It consists of just three steps. An affirmative answer to *any two* of the three steps diagnoses *ventricular tachycardia*. It is simple and it even has the endorsement and approval of none other than Dr. Pedro Brugada himself. This algorithm is unique because of the first criterion. The first criterion, Step 1, is a *clinical question!* None of the other algorithms or methods ask a clinical question. This step has important implications. Here's why:

Let's say you are presented with a wide complex tachycardia and told nothing about the patient. If you guess ventricular tachycardia knowing *nothing* about the patient – you will be correct 80% of the time! If, however, you are presented with the *same* ECG and told that the patient has *some form of structural heart disease – previous MI, cardiomyopathy with an ejection fraction ≤ 35%, congestive heart failure, or episodes of angina pectoris –* and you then diagnose ventricular tachycardia, you will be correct 95% of the time! **Ninety-five percent!** You will be wrong only five times out of a hundred! So, if the answer to the first question of the Basel Algorithm ("Does the patient have some form of structural heart disease?") is "YES!" then you have already diagnosed ventricular tachycardia with 95% accuracy! What other algorithm or method is that accurate? Let me answer that question for you – "NONE!"

This was a question that was posed as a solution to the problem of distinguishing ventricular tachycardia from supraventricular tachycardia many years ago. To my knowledge, it's never been refuted, but it was never seriously accepted by medical "authorities," either.

> **TIP |** As you quickly learn in medicine, you just can't trust data that isn't complex, confusing, or slightly misleading.

Even Dr. Pedro Brugada was led to wonder how much more accurate the Brugada Algorithm would be if that question were made the first step.

Still, the Basel Algorithm is not 100% accurate, but it is simple, very easy to use while under stress, very quick to arrive at a diagnosis, and about as accurate as the Brugada Algorithm.

Step 1: Presence of *clinical high-risk features* (i.e., evidence of some form of structural heart disease)

Clinical high-risk features mean – specifically - a history of myocardial infarction, a history of congestive heart failure with left ventricular ejection fraction ≤ 35%, or an implanted implantable cardioverter-defibrillator or cardiac resynchronization therapy / defibrillator

Step 2: Lead II time to the first change in polarity > 40 msec

This step may seem like the Lead II R wave Peak Time (Pava) Method – but it isn't. In that method, the cutoff for the "onset to first change in polarity" is ≥ 50 msec. Here, it is > 40 msec (note that the "equal" has disappeared).

> **TIP |** Although the Basel Algorithm uses TWO leads instead of one, *the requirement of a QRS morphology that is amenable to analysis* still holds and, unfortunately, is not always present.

Step 3: Lead aVR time to the first change in polarity > 40 msec

While Step 3 of the Basel Algorithm is said to be similar to Step 2 of the Vereckei Algorithm #1, it is different. In the Vereckei Algorithm #1, there is no mention of the "peak" or "first change in polarity" being more or less than 40 msec. Steps 2 and 3 of the Basel Algorithm mention "time to peak," but later in the original article, the authors specify that "peak" really means "first change in polarity," just as in the Pava method. In the Basel Algorithm, however, "first change in polarity" applies to both Step 2 and Step 3. Here, I have taken the liberty to substitute the words "first change in polarity" for "peak" to avoid confusion.

Will the Basel Algorithm work for you? Try it using the following WCT examples and find out for yourself!

> **REMEMBER! |** You need affirmative answers to at least two of the three steps to diagnose ventricular tachycardia.

Recommended Reading:

Moccetti F, Yadava M, Latifi Y, et al. Simplified integrated clinical and electrocardiographi c algorithm for differentiation of wide QRS-complex tachycardia: the Basel algorithm. *J Am Coll Cardiol EP*. 2022;8(7):831–839.

Let's practice using the Basel Algorithm. With each ECG example, try diagnosing the wide complex tachycardia *with* and *without* the "presence of structural heart disease" in your patient and observe the effect such a clinical question has on the outcome.

Practicing the Basel Algorithm

Basel Algorithm

Step 1: Presence of clinical high risk features (i.e., evidence of some form of structural heart disease)

    a. History of myocardial infarction
    b. History of congestive heart failure with left ventricular ejection fraction ≤ 35%
    c. History of an implanted cardioverter-defibrillator
    d. Cardiac resynchronization therapy-defibrillator

Step 2: QRS in Lead II time from onset to the first change in polarity > 40 msec

Step 3: QRS in Lead aVR time from onset to the first change in polarity > 40 msec

ECG #1

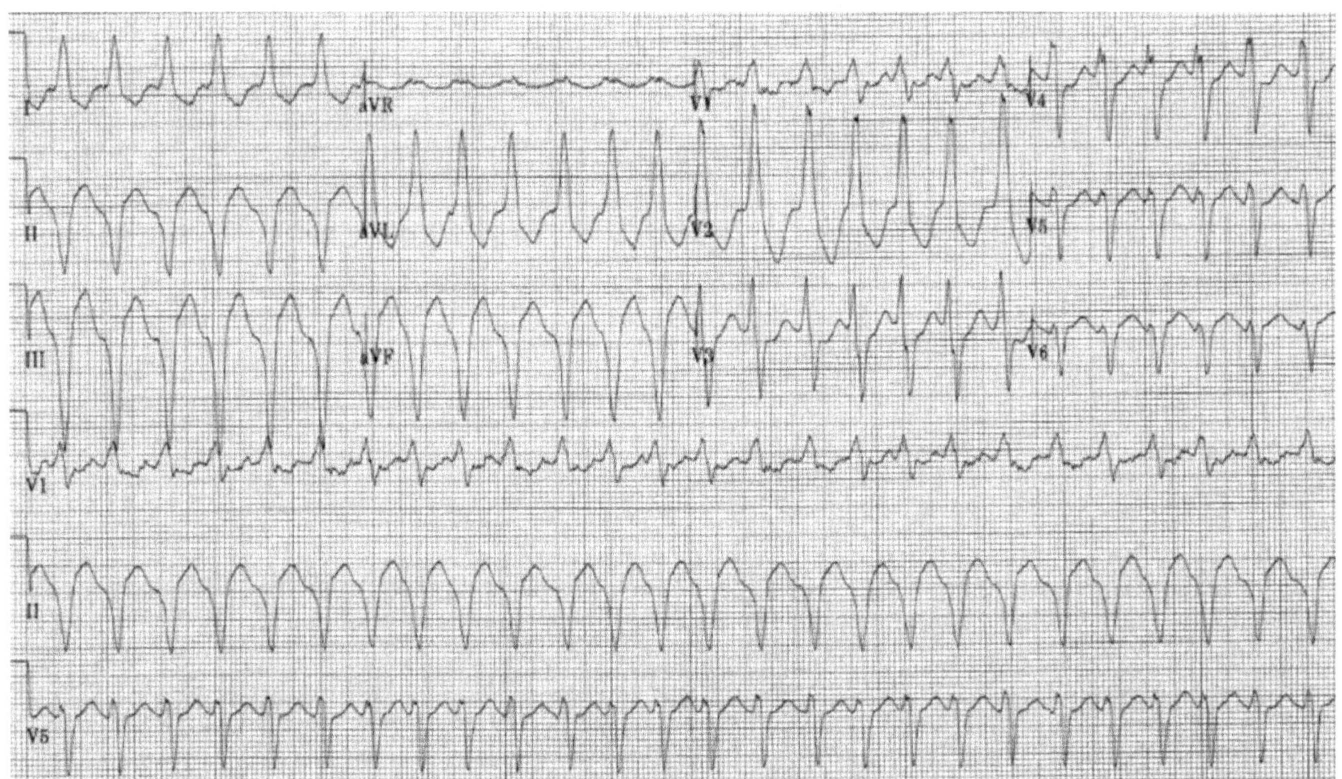

Figure 16–1

Basel Algorithm

Step 1: Presence of clinical high risk features (i.e., evidence of some form of structural heart disease)

   a. History of myocardial infarction
   b. History of congestive heart failure with left ventricular ejection fraction ≤ 35%
   c. History of an implanted cardioverter-defibrillator
   d. Cardiac resynchronization therapy-defibrillator

Step 2: QRS in Lead II time from onset to the first change in polarity > 40 msec

Step 3: QRS in Lead aVR time from onset to the first change in polarity > 40 msec

ECG #2

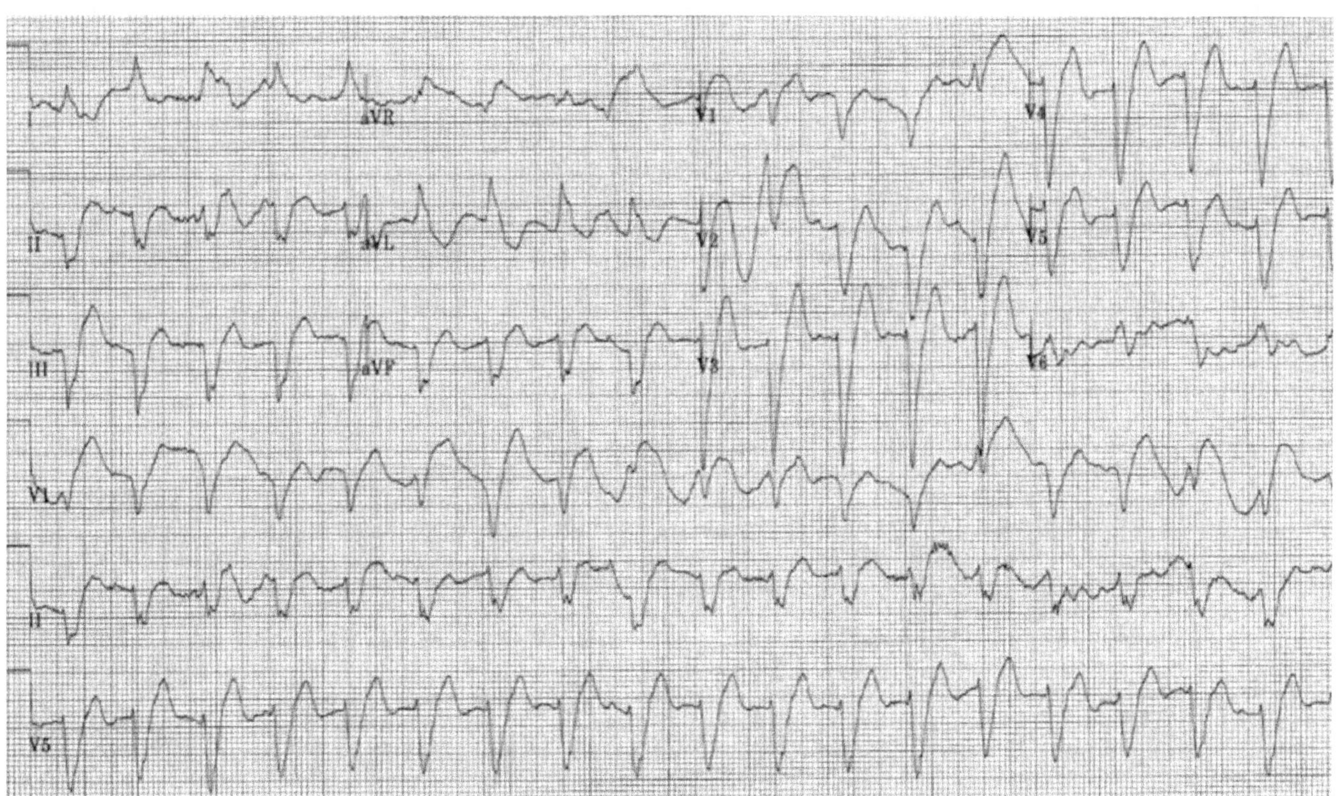

Figure 16-2

Basel Algorithm

Step 1: Presence of clinical high risk features (i.e., evidence of some form of structural heart disease)

    a. History of myocardial infarction
    b. History of congestive heart failure with left ventricular ejection fraction ≤ 35%
    c. History of an implanted cardioverter-defibrillator
    d. Cardiac resynchronization therapy-defibrillator

Step 2: QRS in Lead II time from onset to the first change in polarity > 40 msec

Step 3: QRS in Lead aVR time from onset to the first change in polarity > 40 msec

ECG #3

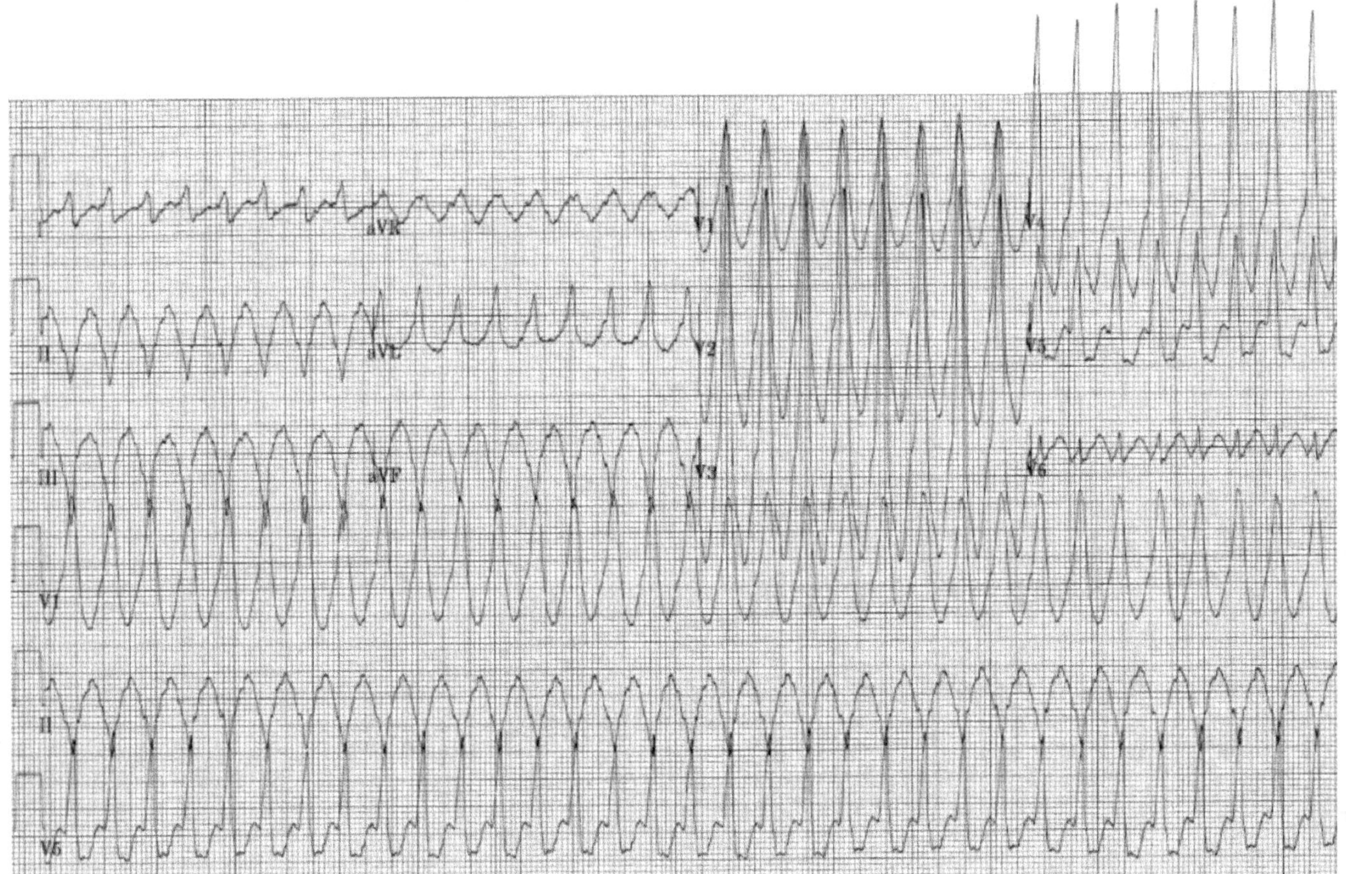

Figure 16-3

Basel Algorithm

Step 1: Presence of clinical high risk features (i.e., evidence of some form of structural heart disease)

    a. History of myocardial infarction
    b. History of congestive heart failure with left ventricular ejection fraction ≤ 35%
    c. History of an implanted cardioverter-defibrillator
    d. Cardiac resynchronization therapy-defibrillator

Step 2: QRS in Lead II time from onset to the first change in polarity > 40 msec

Step 3: QRS in Lead aVR time from onset to the first change in polarity > 40 msec

ECG #4

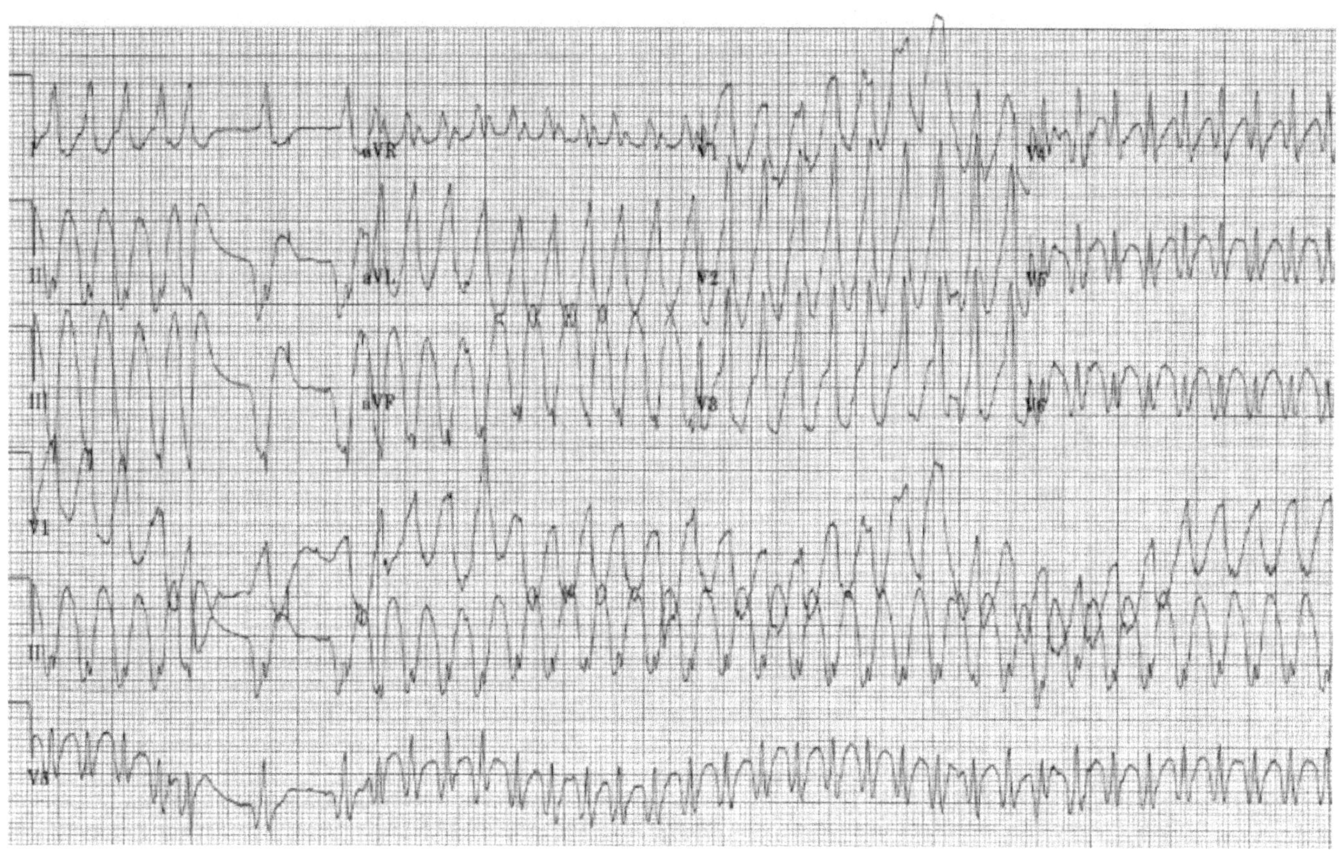

Figure 16-4

Basel Algorithm

Step 1: Presence of clinical high risk features (i.e., evidence of some form of structural heart disease)

    a. History of myocardial infarction
    b. History of congestive heart failure with left ventricular ejection fraction ≤ 35%
    c. History of an implanted cardioverter-defibrillator
    d. Cardiac resynchronization therapy-defibrillator

Step 2: QRS in Lead II time from onset to the first change in polarity > 40 msec

Step 3: QRS in Lead aVR time from onset to the first change in polarity > 40 msec

ECG #5

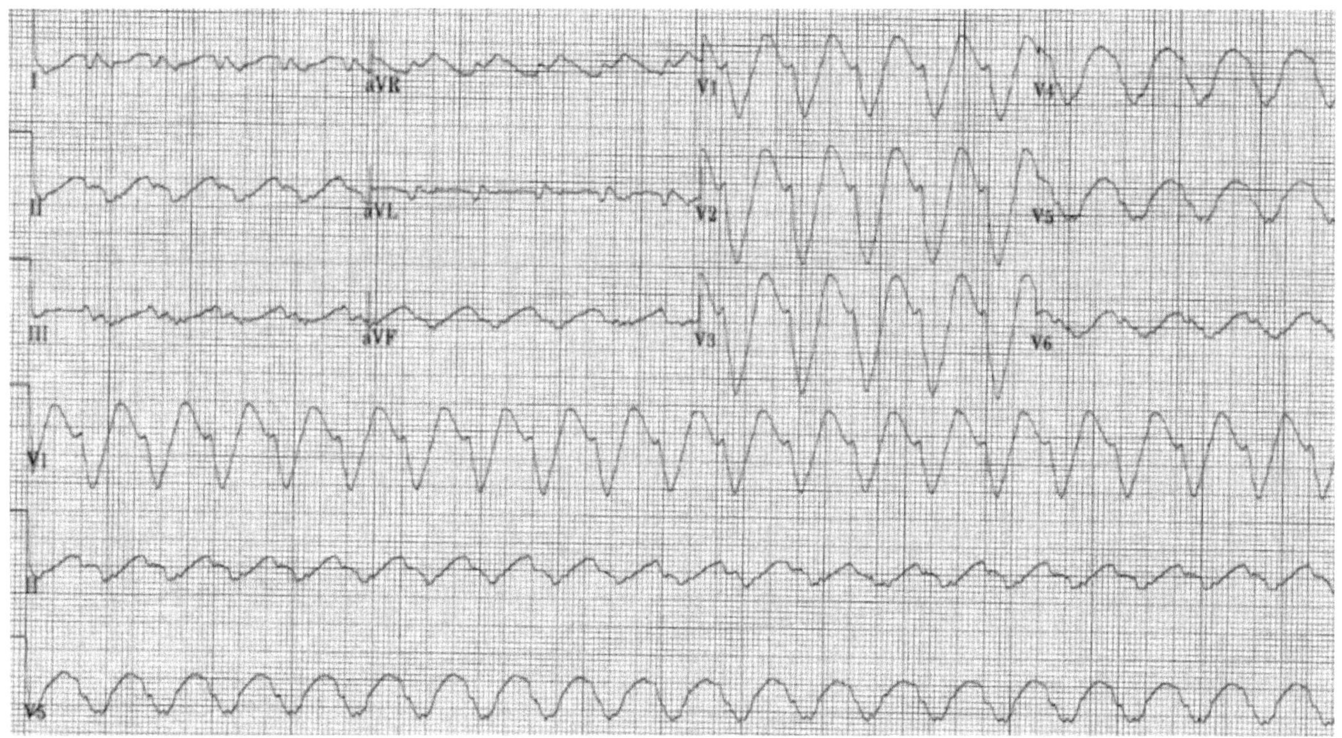

Figure 16-5

Basel Algorithm

Step 1: Presence of clinical high risk features (i.e., evidence of some form of structural heart disease)

    a. History of myocardial infarction
    b. History of congestive heart failure with left ventricular ejection fraction ≤ 35%
    c. History of an implanted cardioverter-defibrillator
    d. Cardiac resynchronization therapy-defibrillator

Step 2: QRS in Lead II time from onset to the first change in polarity > 40 msec

Step 3: QRS in Lead aVR time from onset to the first change in polarity > 40 msec

ECG #6

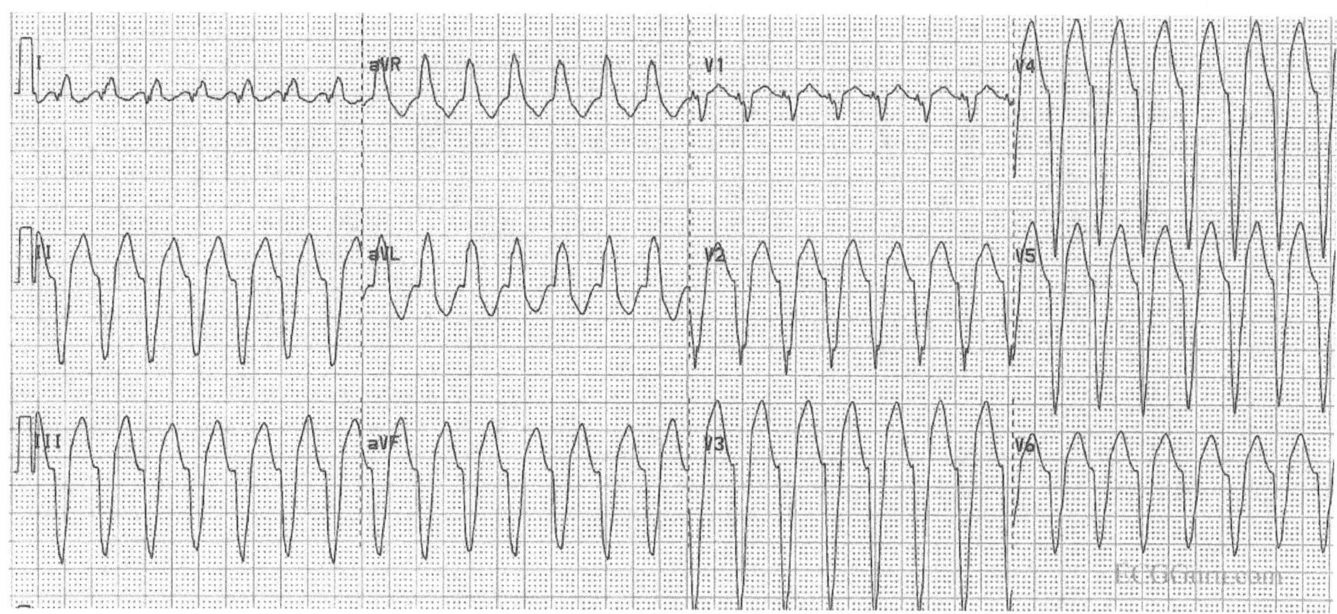

Figure 16-6

Basel Algorithm

Step 1: Presence of clinical high risk features (i.e., evidence of some form of structural heart disease)

    a. History of myocardial infarction
    b. History of congestive heart failure with left ventricular ejection fraction ≤ 35%
    c. History of an implanted cardioverter-defibrillator
    d. Cardiac resynchronization therapy-defibrillator

Step 2: QRS in Lead II time from onset to the first change in polarity > 40 msec

Step 3: QRS in Lead aVR time from onset to the first change in polarity > 40 msec

ECG #7

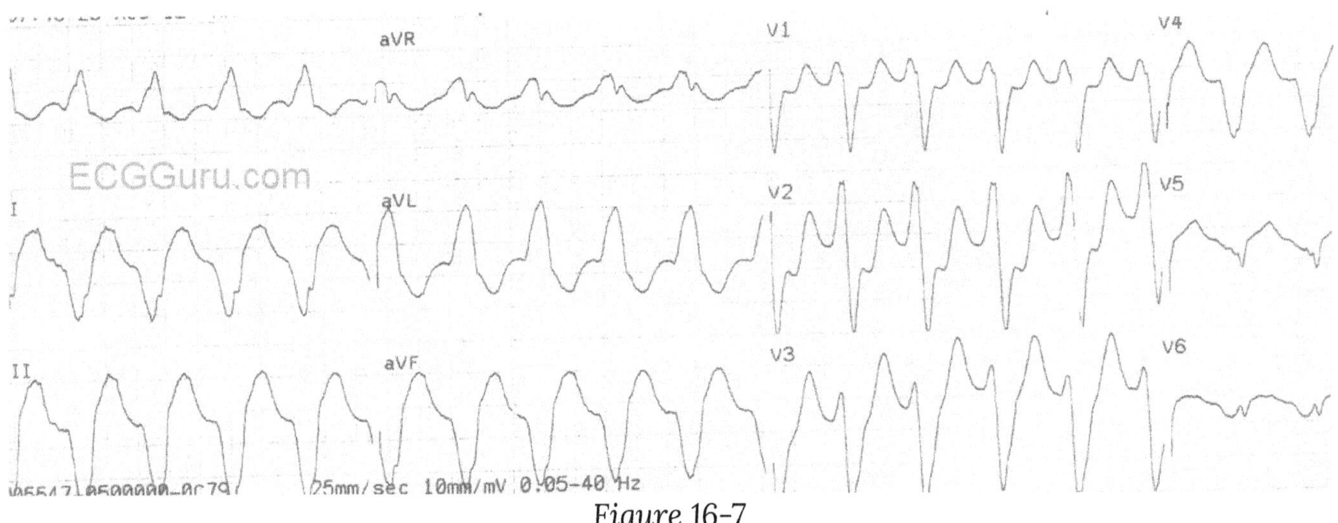

Figure 16-7

Basel Algorithm

Step 1: Presence of clinical high risk features (i.e., evidence of some form of structural heart disease)

    a. History of myocardial infarction
    b. History of congestive heart failure with left ventricular ejection fraction ≤ 35%
    c. History of an implanted cardioverter-defibrillator
    d. Cardiac resynchronization therapy-defibrillator

Step 2: QRS in Lead II time from onset to the first change in polarity > 40 msec

Step 3: QRS in Lead aVR time from onset to the first change in polarity > 40 msec

ECG #8

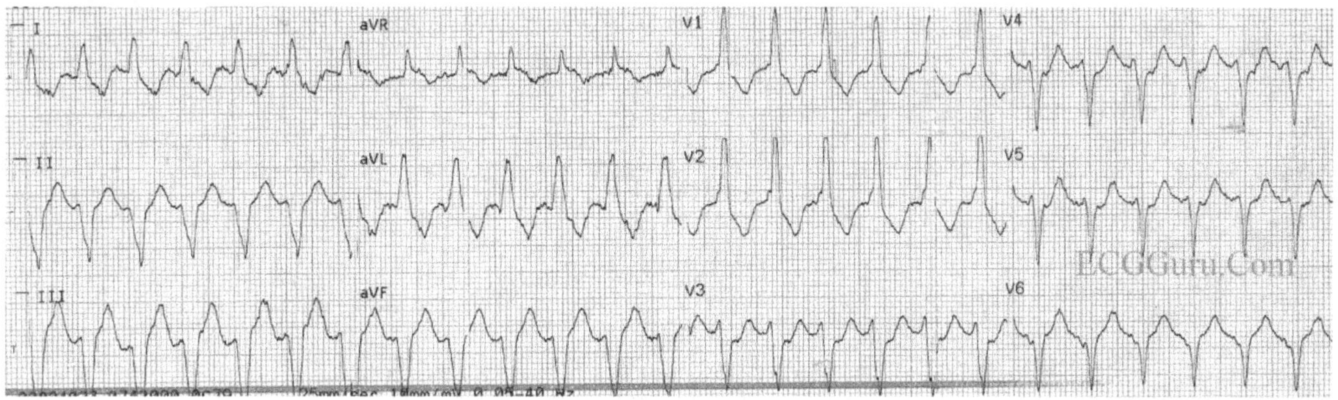

Figure 16-8

Basel Algorithm

Step 1: Presence of clinical high risk features (i.e., evidence of some form of structural heart disease)

a. History of myocardial infarction
b. History of congestive heart failure with left ventricular ejection fraction ≤ 35%
c. History of an implanted cardioverter-defibrillator
d. Cardiac resynchronization therapy-defibrillator

Step 2: QRS in Lead II time from onset to the first change in polarity > 40 msec

Step 3: QRS in Lead aVR time from onset to the first change in polarity > 40 msec

ECG #9

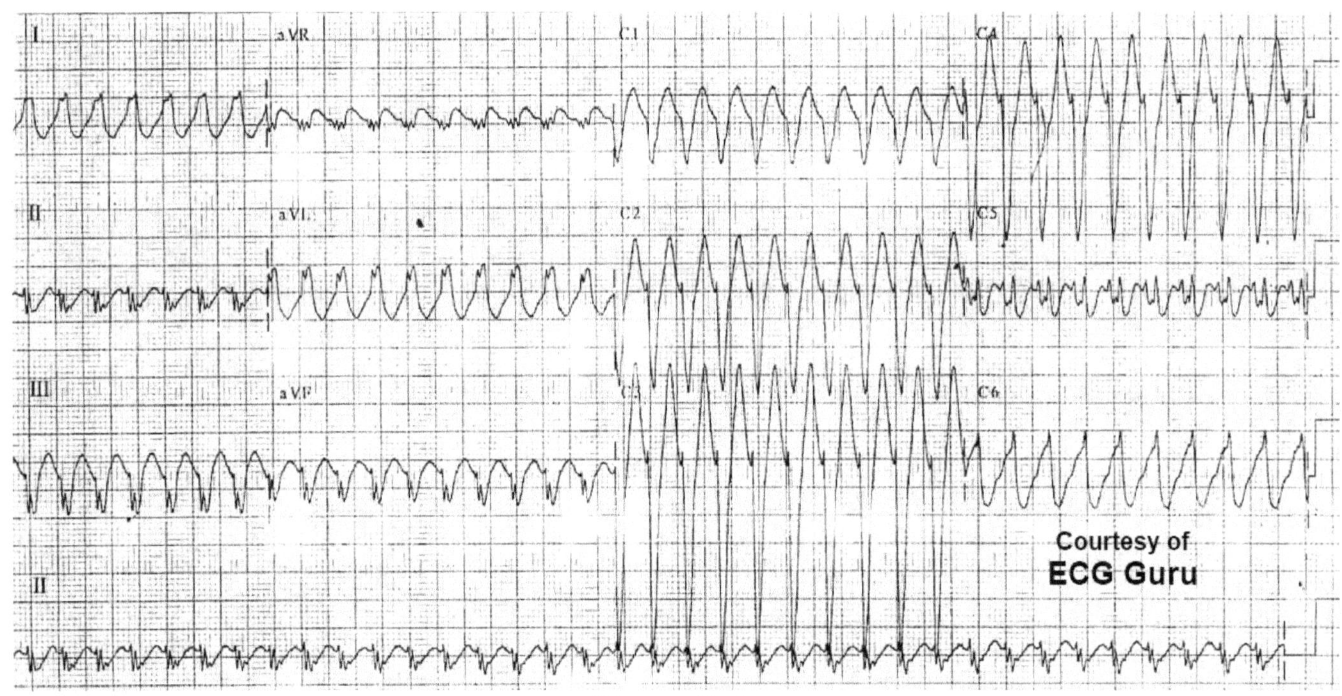

Figure 16-9

Basel Algorithm

Step 1: Presence of clinical high risk features (i.e., evidence of some form of structural heart disease)

    a. History of myocardial infarction
    b. History of congestive heart failure with left ventricular ejection fraction ≤ 35%
    c. History of an implanted cardioverter-defibrillator
    d. Cardiac resynchronization therapy-defibrillator

Step 2: QRS in Lead II time from onset to the first change in polarity > 40 msec

Step 3: QRS in Lead aVR time from onset to the first change in polarity > 40 msec

ECG #10

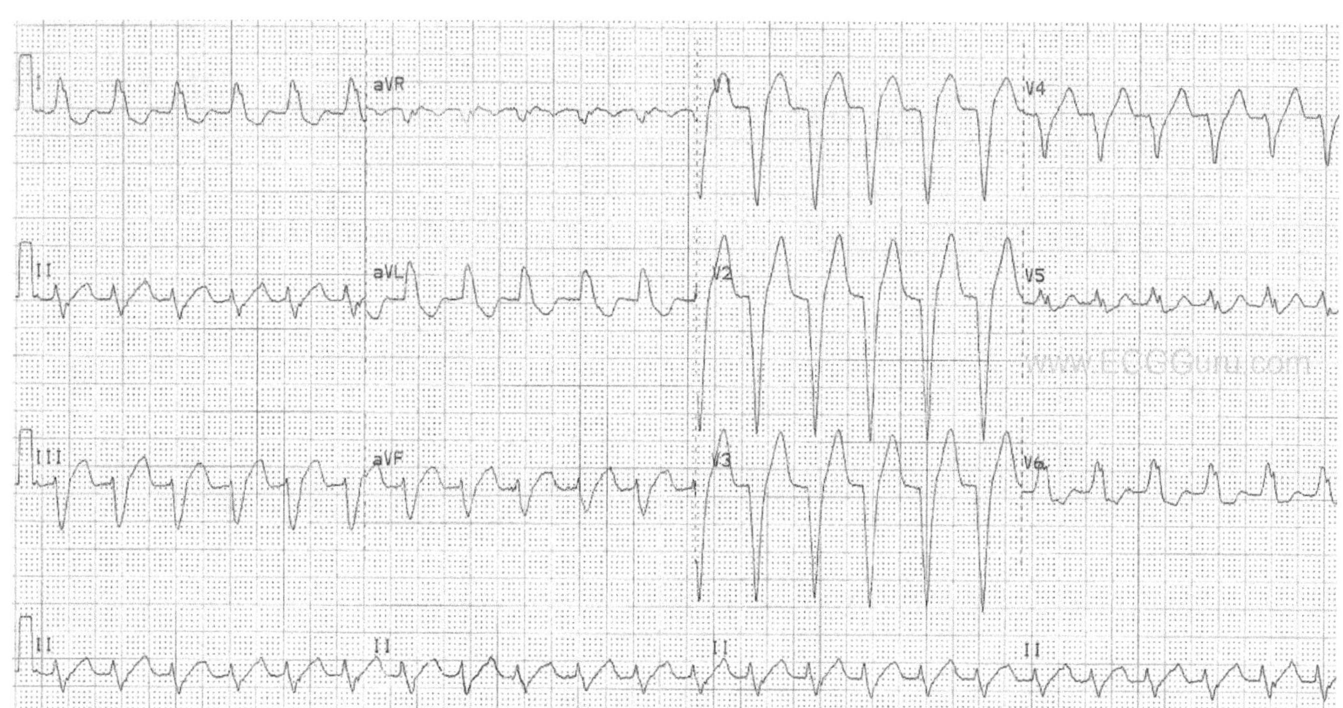

Figure 16-10

Chapter 17

Comparing the Algorithms and Methods

We are going to compare these different algorithms and methods for:

Sensitivity (Sn) / Specificity (Sp)
Accuracy

Method	Sn / Sp	Accuracy
Brugada Algorithm	89.0% / 59.2%[1]	77.5%[1]
Vereckei Algorithm - 1	Note - 1	90.3%[4]
Vereckei Algorithm (aVR) - 2	87.1% / 48.0%[1]	71.9%[1]
Lead II RWPT (Pava)	60.0% / 82.7%[1]	68.8%[1]
Limb Lead Method	66.3% / 59.6[2]	88%[2]
Basel Algorithm	93% / 90%[3]	93%[3]

Table 17-1

1. Jastrzebski M, Kukla P, Czarnecka D, and Kawecka-Jaszcz K. Comparison of five electrocardiographic methods for differentiation of wide QRS-complex tachycardias. Europace. 2012 Aug;14(8):1165-71

2. Chen Q, et al. Simple Electrocardiographic Criteria for Rapid Identification of Wide QRS Complex Tachycardia: The New Limb Lead Algorithm. *Heart Rhythm* (2019)

3. Moccetti F, et al. Simplified integrated clinical and electrocardiographic algorithm for differentiation of wide QRS-complex tachycardia: the Basel algorithm. J Am Coll Cardiol EP. 2022;8(7):831–839

4. Vereckei A. Current algorithms for the diagnosis of wide QRS complex tachycardias. Curr Cardiol Rev. 2014 Aug;10(3):262-76.

Note – 1: No separate validating articles were found for the First Vereckei Algorithm. Validating articles were found for the Second Vereckei (aVR) Algorithm and the results indicated less Sn,

Sp, and accuracy than published in the original article. I have chosen to post no data here since I cannot assume that a validating study would arrive at the same values as the authors.

These are my recommendations:

The Brugada Algorithm

The Brugada Algorithm requires the identification of AV dissociation in Step 3 which is problematic for those with less training and experience in electrocardiography. The original Step 4 has also been difficult for a lot of people regarding memorization. However, the use of the Jones Method of Step 4 makes it easier, faster, and less difficult to remember. The Jones Method for Step 4 of the Brugada algorithm is essentially the same as Step 3 of the First Vereckei Algorithm.

The Vereckei Algorithm #1 (2007)

The first of two Vereckei Algorithms requires the identification of AV dissociation and the calculation of the *ventricular activation velocity ratio*. The ventricular activation velocity ratio is arrived at by dividing the absolute value of the positive or negative voltage achieved during the first 40 msec of depolarization (QRS complex) by the voltage achieved during the last 40 msec of depolarization. Sounds easy enough, but there are a few important caveats:

1. You cannot measure a monophasic R wave or a monophasic QS complex. The measured deflection must be at least biphasic and may have more than just two deflections (Rs or rSR′).

2. There is also the problem of measuring 40 msec. That would be easy enough if the deflection began or ended on one of the vertical grid lines on the ECG paper, but that is often not the case! Magnifying lenses or digital calipers may be required.

The Vereckei Algorithm #2 (2008)

This second iteration of the Vereckei Algorithm is easy for the first three steps. But as mentioned earlier, 50 – 60% of people using this method will eventually find themselves in Step 4.

Lead II R Wave Peak Time (Pava) Method

When you use a method that involves only one lead, you are taking a risk that just one lead will have all the information you need to diagnose or rule out ventricular tachycardia. The lead in question here is Lead II. You have already seen the problems finding a Lead II QRS complex that is amenable to measuring from the onset of the QRS to the first change in polarity.

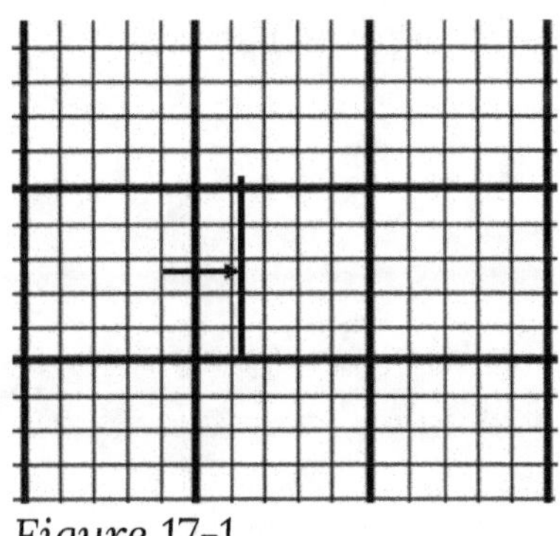

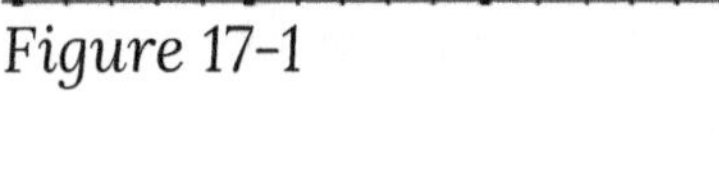

Here is an enlargement of an ECG grid (Figure 17-1). In the middle large square, I have marked off 50 msec from the thick vertical dark line. To measure 50 msec, you must add one small square (40 msec) and 10 msec from the following small square. This diagram is greatly enlarged. How well will you do at normal size (Figure 17-2)...?

Figure 17-1

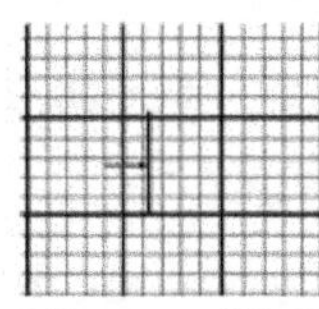

Figure 17-2

What if the first change in polarity is at 52 msec? Will you see it... in the ER... while managing a patient? Before you assume that using just one Lead will be easier, think about whether or not you will be able to make any measurement at all, because if you can't, *you cannot measure in any other lead, either.* And never forget: *you are betting the patient's life on just one lead!*

The Limb Lead (OQL) Method

While the Limb Lead Method may require a bit of familiarity before using it, its main advantages are that 1) you don't have to look for AV dissociation, 2) you don't have to make any measurements or calculations and 3) you aren't going to be affected very much by irregular or unusual QRS morphologies. However, the sensitivity and specificity are somewhat lackluster with an accuracy of about 88% - and this is by their *own* calculations!

The Basel Algorithm

The Basel Algorithm consists of only three steps which are easy to use and easy to remember. PLUS it has the clinical first step which adds sensitivity and specificity – but *only* if the answer is "YES!"

Step 2 is similar to the Lead II R Wave Peak Time (Pava) Method, so it will inherit the problems associated with requiring a QRS that is easily measurable. The same applies to Step 3. Its sensitivity and specificity are very good and it has the endorsement of Dr. Pedro Brugada who participated in the derivation study that produced the famous Brugada Algorithm. However, there are no validation studies as yet.

PEARL | Just because a patient with a wide complex tachycardia is stable at the time of examination doesn't mean they will *remain* stable. Patients with scar-related VT may be stable for a while, but there is a high likelihood that they could crash at any moment.

My Recommendations:

1. The Brugada Algorithm

This algorithm is for *experienced* ECG interpreters. If you are going to be diagnosing wide complex tachycardias, you should be advanced enough to quickly spot AV dissociation when it is present and confident enough to quickly recognize when it is *not* present. Step 4 should be no problem when using the Jones modification (which is essentially the same as Step 3 in the first Vereckei Algorithm). No algorithm or method is more accurate than the Brugada Algorithm by any *independent* validation study.

2. The Basel Algorithm

Although there are no validation studies so far, the Basel Algorithm is easy to use while under stress and comes with an excellent endorsement.

3. The Limb Lead (OQL) Algorithm

Again, there are no independent validating studies. However, it is not a difficult approach to wide complex tachycardias and there are no major caveats other than the usual (see below).

4. Vereckei Algorithm #1 and Vereckei Algorithm (aVR) #2

If you can achieve a diagnosis within the first three steps, then these algorithms are very good and easy to moderate to use – but that's just the first three steps! However, 50 – 60% of the time the diagnosis will depend on the utilization of Step 4 – the *ventricular activation velocity ratio*. This will be too much for the majority of clinicians to handle with the stress and limited time associated with managing a patient with a wide complex tachycardia. With Step 1 of the first Vereckei Algorithm, you will have to search for AV dissociation which will require intermediate to advanced expertise.

5. Lead II R Wave Peak Time (Pava) Criterion

I don't use this criterion as a first-line method for three reasons:

1. I do not feel comfortable making a critical decision based on just one QRS which may be of suboptimal clarity and unreliable if the peak time is anywhere near 50 msec.

2. The required measurement may lead to error.

3. A misdiagnosis is likely to result in diagnosing a ventricular tachycardia as a supraventricular tachycardia which could lead to a very complicated or problematic management.

If the peak time is wide and easily seen as unequivocally greater than 50 msec, then I usually use it to validate the impression that I've already gained by using a different algorithm or method.

Many of these studies will fail when presented with *antidromic AVRT, bundle branch tachycardia, fascicular tachycardia, interfascicular tachycardia*, or some *Mahaim reentrant tachycardias* (*atriofascicular* or *nodofascicular*). The good news is that these tachycardias are either *quite rare* or at least *very, very infrequent*. Regarding antidromic AVRT: WPW syndrome due to an *orthodromic* AVRT, while not very frequent, could hardly be considered rare; WPW due to an *antidromic* AVRT is quite rare. "How rare?" you ask. Many physicians will retire from practice without ever having seen an antidromic AVRT!

Let's Put Things in Perspective...

The majority of supraventricular tachycardias with aberrancy that we are trying to distinguish from ventricular tachycardia will have aberrant conduction primarily due to a *pre-existing, fixed aberrancy* or a *rate-related aberrancy*. Antidromic AVRT will fall way down at the bottom of the list!

Must I use an algorithm or method?

No law says you *must* use one of the algorithms or methods, but if you try managing a patient without doing so and have a bad outcome – you're going to have some very difficult explaining to do. I would recommend that you use one of the algorithms that I discussed – if, for no other reason, than to validate your impression.

A suggestion that I frequently hear is "Why not assume every wide complex tachycardia is ventricular tachycardia and just cardiovert everyone?" I would certainly agree if the patient were unstable – but NOT if the patient is awake, in no acute distress other than complaining of palpitations, and has a tachycardia amenable to medication therapy. Not all ventricular tachycardias are dangerous; some respond quite well to adenosine, amiodarone, sotalol, β-blockers, or verapamil.

Assuming that all WCTs are VT is automatically misdiagnosing and mislabeling up to 20% of your patients. We can do better than that! However, if you are reading ECGs at an introductory level and have little experience interpreting wide complex tachycardias, then I would agree that electrical cardioversion would be the safest form of management *for the patient*. I've always maintained that the greatest danger during a correctly implemented electrical cardioversion will come from a complication of the medication used for sedation and not the 360 J shock.

AN OBSERVATION | During my years as an attending ER physician in various teaching hospitals, I occasionally encountered house staff who felt that just making the patient slightly drowsy was sufficient sedation. It is NOT! I also observed patients being shocked *immediately* after the needle was withdrawn from the IV tubing port and before the medication had taken effect. DON'T DO THAT! As someone who has had the misfortune of receiving a full 360 joules of "Edison medicine" (electricity) *without the benefit of sedation (or warning)*, I can assure you that it is *not* a pleasant experience!

Recommended Reading:

Jastrzebski M, Kukla P, Czarnecka D, and Kawecka-Jaszcz K. Comparison of five electrocardiographic methods for differentiation of wide QRS-complex tachycardias. *Europace.* (2012) 14, 1165–1171 doi:10.1093/europace/eus015.

Vereckei A. Current algorithms for the diagnosis of wide QRS complex tachycardias. *Curr Cardiol Rev.* 2014 Aug;10(3):262-76.

Ventricular Tachycardias Due to Structural Heart Disease

We've studied the major algorithms, methods, and criteria for differentiating supraventricular tachycardias with aberrant conduction from ventricular tachycardia. Now let's discuss ventricular tachycardia specifically.

Ventricular tachycardia is not a *single* dysrhythmia – it's a *collection* of dysrhythmias that have their origin in one ventricle or the other. And they exist along a very wide spectrum of severity: some are rapidly lethal requiring that the patient be cardioverted or defibrillated immediately while some are so benign they require no treatment at all.

There are several different ways to categorize ventricular tachycardias. I am going to begin by dividing them first into two types of tachydysrhythmias:

    1. Ventricular tachycardias due to *structural heart disease*

    2. *Idiopathic* ventricular tachycardias (no structural heart disease)

What is meant by *structural heart disease*? Structural heart disease refers to a *physical alteration of the myocardium* (including the *conduction system*) by a disease process.

    1. Scars due to previous myocardial infarctions, previous surgery, or previous ablations

    2. Fibrosis due to cardiomyopathy or aging

    3. Fibro-fatty deposits in the myocardium due to arrhythmogenic right ventricular cardiomyopathy

    4. Discrete lesions (sarcoid nodules, amyloid deposits, metastases)

The term *idiopathic* in the context of ventricular tachycardia is used a bit differently than its usual context. Normally, idiopathic means *of unknown cause or origin*. That is *not* the case here. In the beginning, physicians began noticing that there were some ventricular tachycardias occurring in people with no prior history of heart disease. The reason for that – *at that time* – was unknown, so those tachycardias were referred to as "idiopathic." Today, we know the origins and causes of these "idiopathic" ventricular tachycardias... but we *still* call them *idiopathic*. It is within this group of ventricular tachycardias that lie some of the most *lethal* and some of the most *benign* tachydysrhythmias.

Let's begin our discussions of ventricular tachycardia with those due to structural heart disease...

1. Ventricular Tachycardia Due to Structural Heart Disease

Ventricular tachycardia in a patient with structural heart disease is almost invariably caused by reentry. What are some of the electrocardiographic characteristics of a reentrant ventricular tachycardia due to structural heart disease, i.e., what is its **Electrocardiographic Signature?**

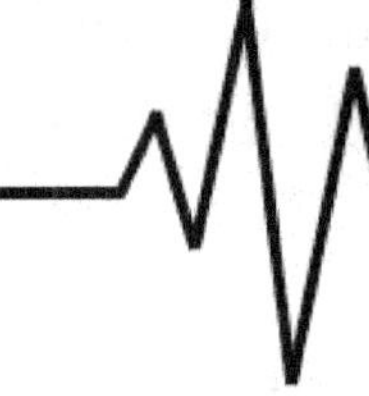

Electrocardiographic Signature

Regularity

Monomorphic QRS Complexes

Wide QRS Complexes (often > 160 msec)

Abnormal Frontal Plane Axis

Regularity

When I was a resident in internal medicine back in the '70s, we were still being taught that ventricular tachycardia was an *irregular* rhythm. That is *partly* true. Several of the idiopathic VTs are indeed characteristically irregular, but extremely few of the reentrant VTs due to structural heart disease are irregular. "If they are reentrant, how can they be irregular?" you ask.

Every reentrant focus has a *reentry circuit* and *entrance and exit pathways* (Figure 18-1). Rarely, a block can develop in the exit pathway – an *exit block*. By block, I am referring to a *Mobitz I* or a *Mobitz II exit block*. Why not a first degree exit block or a third degree exit block? Think about that for a moment. How would you know that one of those were present? You wouldn't!

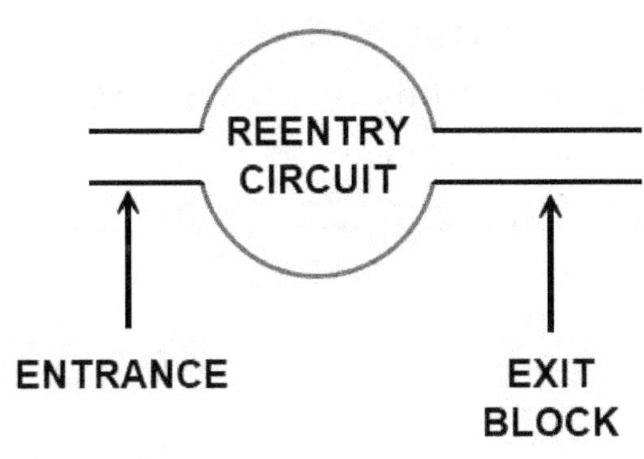

Figure 18-1

The main reason, however, for the idea that ventricular tachycardias were irregular began before there was widespread knowledge of accessory pathways. Many cases of atrial fibrillation using an accessory pathway as a *bystander* pathway (a pathway between atria and ventricles that is not acting as part of a reentry circuit but more like an open door) produced very irregular wide complex tachycardias that were misinterpreted as ventricular tachycardia, like this one (Figure 18-2):

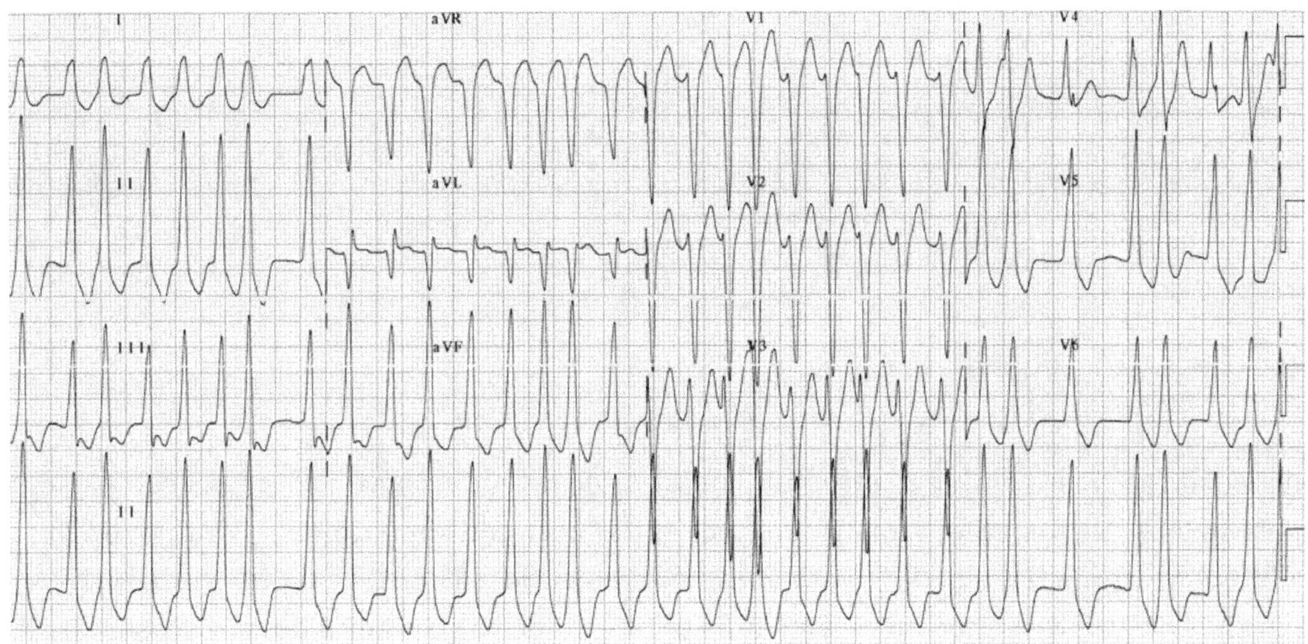

Figure 18-2

Monomorphic QRS Complexes

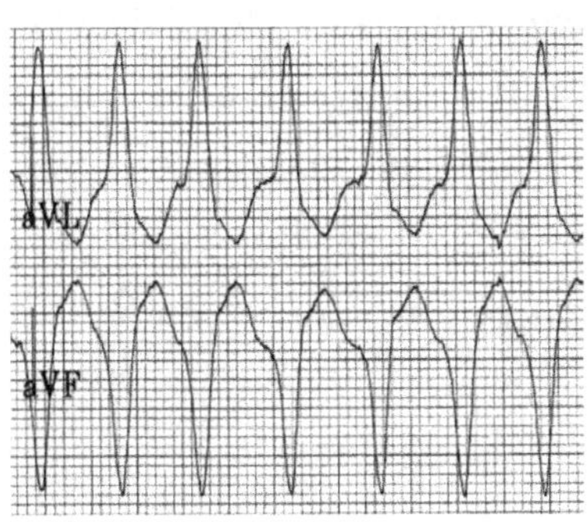

Figure 18-3

Reentrant ventricular tachycardias are almost always *monomorphic*. Now, don't confuse the term *monomorphic* with *monophasic*. *Monomorphic* means that all QRS complexes *within a given lead* will have the same morphology. *Monophasic* means that a QRS complex is either entirely POSITIVE with no q or S wave or entirely NEGATIVE with no R or r′ wave. This is an ABSOLUTE! The two leads (aVL and aVF) (Figure 18-3) on the left BOTH exhibit a *monomorphic* QRS (the QRS is *exactly the same* within each lead – this does *not* include the T wave or baseline!). Also, both leads exhibit *monophasic* QRS complexes – there is one and only one deflection comprising each QRS complex.

I said "almost always" monomorphic. Again, on very rare occasions there may be *more than one exit pathway* which could result in a *different QRS morphology* from the rest of the QRS complexes. But like an irregularity in the rhythm of a reentrant ventricular tachycardia – this will be *very rarely* encountered. Just consider *all reentrant VTs due to structural heart disease to be regular and monomorphic.*

Wide QRS Complexes

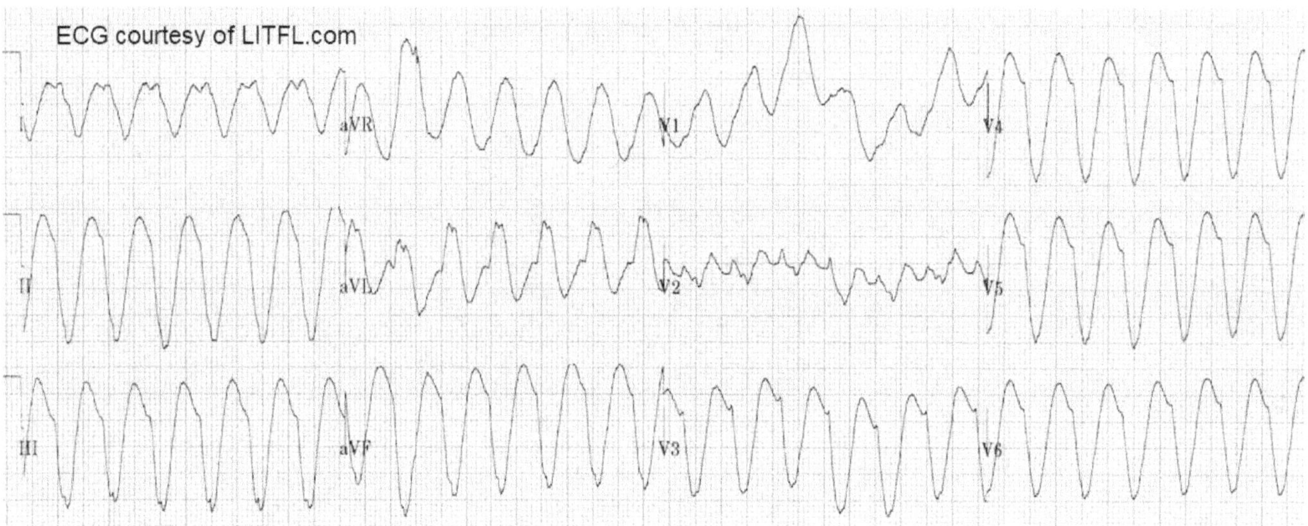

Figure 18-4

Ventricular tachycardias due to structural heart disease tend to have wider QRS complexes (Figure 18-4). Unfortunately, there is no exact cutoff between idiopathic VT, VT due to structural heart disease, and SVT with aberrant conduction. There is a lot of overlap. The wider the QRS, however, the more likely it is to be VT due to structural heart disease. Its main confounder will be an antidromic AVRT which also begins in working ventricular myocardium and can be very wide. Always consider hyperkalemia. One other possibility is sodium channel blocker toxicity. Many non-cardiac drugs have a similar action to the anti-arrhythmic medications: tricyclic antidepressants, some macrolide antibiotics, and even diphenhydramine. Most (though certainly not ALL) idiopathic ventricular tachycardias begin in, or in very close proximity to, the Purkinje system so they will tend to have narrower QRS complexes. I would strongly suggest that if the QRS duration is > 160 msec you narrow your differential diagnosis more urgently to antidromic AVRT, sodium channel blocker toxicity, hyperkalemia, and scar-related ventricular tachycardia.

TIP | To put things in perspective, antidromic AVRTs are rare – not "occasional" or "infrequent," but *rare!* Many physicians will retire from practice without ever having seen one. In my almost 40 years of practicing internal medicine and emergency medicine, I did not personally see one case! So don't be quick to immediately jump to a diagnosis of antidromic AVRT. It will be far down on the list of your differential diagnoses.

A QRS duration > 160 msec may not be diagnostic but it is certainly supportive of ventricular tachycardia. Generally, the more *peripheral* the origin of a ventricular rhythm – the *wider* it will be because it is located remotely from the rapidly conducting His-Purkinje system (HPS). The *closer the origin of a ventricular rhythm is to the septum* – the *narrower* it will be because it is located closer to the rapidly conducting fibers of the HPS. Focal ventricular tachycardias that originate in the epicardium are characteristically wide because it takes time for the impulse traveling cell-to-cell to reach the endocardium and Purkinje fibers. Purkinje fibers are located in the inner one-third of the ventricular wall. In such cases, the initial part of the QRS complex is slurred or widened and may resemble a delta wave.

Frontal Plane Axis

Most SVTs – with or without aberrancy – will have normal axes... *but they don't have to!* Abnormalities within the conduction system can result in right or left axis deviation. For any complex entering the ventricles through the AV node and His-Purkinje system, arriving at an axis in the right upper (northwest) quadrant ("No Man's Land") is essentially impossible without more associated abnormalities of the conduction system or the influence of extracardiac conditions (hyperkalemia, sodium channel blocker toxicity). A focus of reentry in the apex of one of the ventricles, however, can easily result in a mean QRS axis in the right upper quadrant. Such an axis during a wide complex tachycardia is an excellent indicator of ventricular tachycardia, though not without exceptions. Remember: that is the basis for the Second Vereckei (aVR) Algorithm or Step 1 of the Limb Lead Method.

Ventricular tachycardias originating from the superior portion of the ventricle will have an *inferior axis* – that means that the QRS complexes in the inferior leads will consist of tall R waves indicating that the origin of the impulse is located superiorly. Ventricular tachycardias originating in the lower, apical region of the ventricle will have a *superior axis* – which means that the inferior leads will have deep S waves. Tachycardias that originate in the left free wall will manifest dominant S waves in Leads I and aVL because the impulse is traveling *away* from the positive poles of those leads and often a right (or rightward) mean QRS axis because the impulse is traveling *toward* the right. An impulse that originates in the *upper* septal (*basal septum*) will manifest dominant R waves in Leads I and aVL because the impulse is traveling toward those leads. There will be a left (or leftward) mean QRS axis because the impulse is traveling to the left.

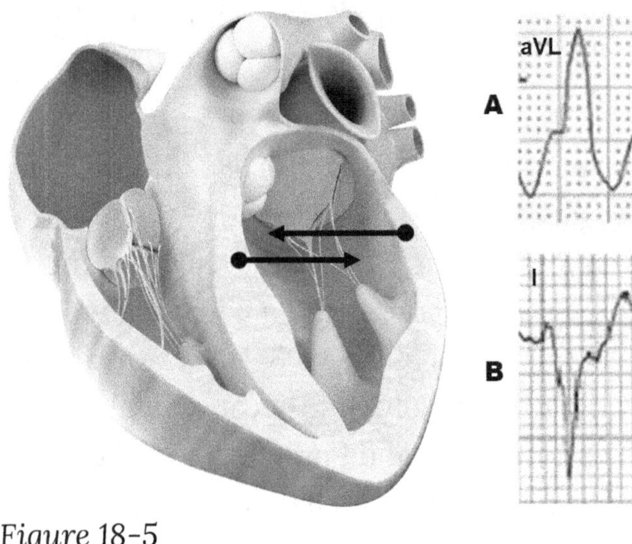

Figure 18-5

As you see in the illustration on the left (Figure 18-5), the impulse that developed in the septum and is traveling towards the electrode for Lead aVL is producing a wide, monophasic R wave (**A**). The impulse that developed in the middle of the left ventricular lateral wall sent a large vector to the right and a smaller vector to the left, which resulted in an rS complex in Lead I (**B**). Had the impulse originated in the epicardium, it could not have sent a vector to the left because there's no myocardium there! It would have traveled exclusively to the right creating a QS complex in Lead I.

TRICK | Here's a trick I learned many years ago. It will help you understand impulses within the ventricles better and make much of what you are learning more intuitive: close your eyes and visualize an impulse moving from the left lateral ventricular wall to the right – with the Hexaxial Reference Grid in the background. If it is moving to the right, it is leaving the area of Leads I and aVL and traveling toward Lead aVR (and possibly Lead III, also). At the same time, imagine a QS complex developing in Leads I and aVL and R waves appearing in Leads aVR and III. You only have to do that a few times before it becomes so intuitive that when you see the QRS in one lead you almost immediately know what other leads should look like.

Reentry: Structural Heart Disease vs. Idiopathic Ventricular Tachycardias

Keep in mind that we are discussing reentrant ventricular tachycardias *caused by structural heart disease*. Sometimes this is referred to as *scar-related* ventricular tachycardia. Reentry, however, can also occur in some of the idiopathic ventricular tachycardias and they, too, will be regular and monomorphic. But here's the difference – almost *all* tachycardias due to structural heart disease are reentrant while that is *not* the case with *most* idiopathic VTs. Most idiopathic VTs are based on triggered activity.

To put things in perspective, if the ECG tracing manifests an RBBB-like pattern, then the ventricular tachycardia originates in the LEFT ventricle. Ninety percent of all ventricular tachycardias are due to structural heart disease and 10% are due to idiopathic ventricular tachycardias. And 90% of all idiopathic ventricular tachycardias originate in the RIGHT ventricle as triggered activity and only 10% originate in the LEFT ventricle. So... of all ventricular tachycardias originating in the left ventricle, less than 1% will *not* be reentrant tachycardias due to structural heart disease.

> **PEARL |** If a ventricular tachycardia has a wide, regular monomorphic pattern with an RBBB-like morphology in Lead V1, think *scar-related* reentrant VT until proven otherwise.

There are fewer reentrant ventricular tachycardias due to structural heart disease originating in the right ventricle. And why is that? It's because there are fewer myocardial infarctions of the right ventricle: the walls are much thinner, they operate against far less pressure and they can augment their blood supply from the intracavitary blood. However, there are foci of fibrosis (same as *scar*), *fat*, and *sarcoid nodules* that can result in the reentrant ventricular tachycardias characteristic of scar-related tachycardias – and which are equally dangerous. Fortunately, these types are very infrequent.

Learning From a Real ECG

Let's take a look at a scar-related ventricular tachycardia and see what we can learn from it (Figure 18-6):

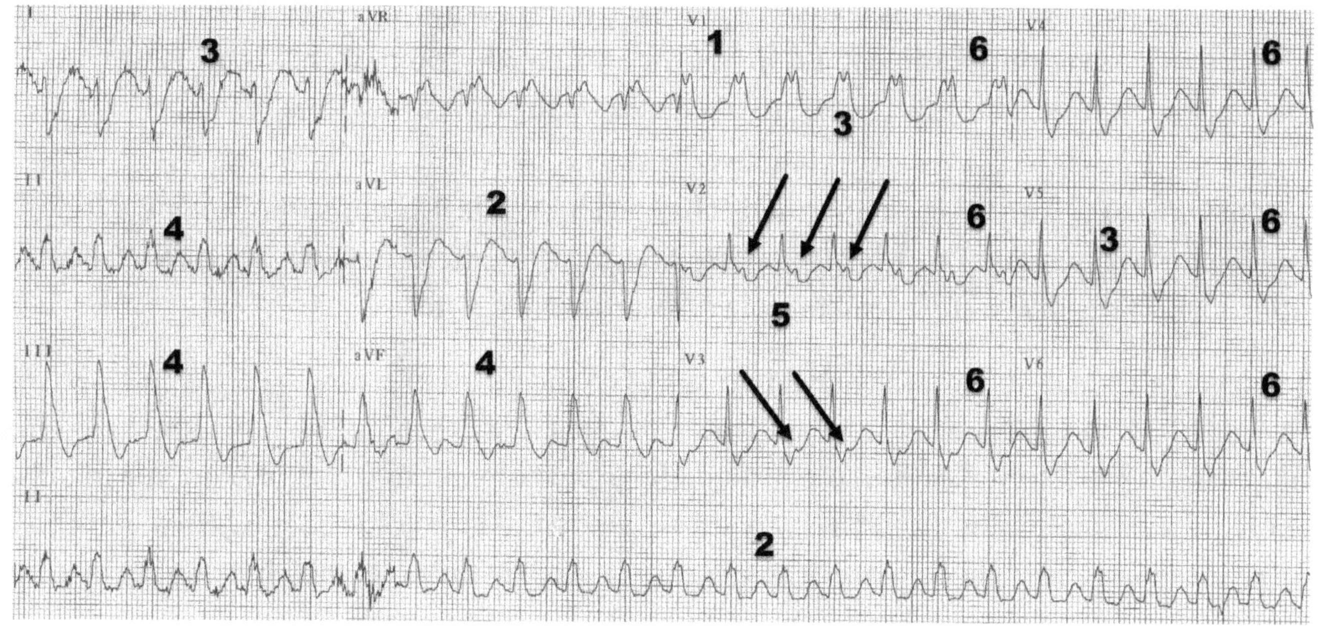

Figure 18-6

What is it about this ECG that would have us favor VT over SVT with aberrancy, even before resorting to one of the algorithms or methods discussed earlier?

This ECG has an RBBB-like morphology in Lead V1 which indicates that the tachycardia is originating in the left ventricle. *Most ventricular tachycardias – and certainly most VTs due to structural heart disease – occur in the left ventricle.* That is because *most myocardial infarctions occur in the left ventricle,* leaving scars that become a substrate for scar-related reentrant VTs.

The tachycardia is *monomorphic* – every QRS *within a lead* is the same as the other QRS complexes *in the same lead* which makes it more likely to be reentrant.

> **PEARL |** Monomorphic ventricular tachycardias are *regular*. Polymorphic ventricular tachycardias are *irregular*. Although this is another "rule of thumb" – there are very few exceptions to this one.

Look at Leads V3 and V4. If you saw only those two leads, would you be impressed that they are part of a wide complex tachycardia? Or would you do as many others do and look only at the narrow R waves and ignore the S waves, which add a lot more width (duration) to the QRS? Lead V1 makes it obvious that this is a wide complex tachycardia.

> **TIP |** It is vitally important that you diagnose a tachycardia – wide or narrow QRS complex – from a 12-lead ECG and *never* from a rhythm strip! Narrow tachycardias may rarely masquerade as wide complex tachycardias (mostly when associated with ST elevation), but it is not difficult for a true wide complex tachycardia to masquerade as a narrow tachycardia – occasionally with disastrous results!

The QRS complex is 170 msec in duration. That's wide! While it is *not pathognomonic for ventricular tachycardia,* it certainly supports limiting our differential diagnosis to VT or antidromic AVRT (and you remember how *rare* antidromic AVRT is).

The inferior leads in the frontal plane on this ECG indicate an inferior axis – the tall R waves in Leads II, III, and aVF are *pointing upward to the origin* of the impulse. Remember: the QRS complexes in the inferior leads in the frontal plane always point to the ORIGIN of the impulse – NOT toward its DESTINATION! They point to where the impulse is coming *from* – not to where it is going! So, if the impulse originates in the upper ventricle, then it must be traveling downward (inferiorly) toward the apex – resulting in an *inferior axis.*

If you look at Leads V2 and V3, you can see small, upright deflections at the *same R-P′ interval* following *every* QRS complex (arrows). This is **ventriculoatrial (VA) association.** An impulse *from the ventricle* enters the atria via the AV node in a retrograde manner. While it seems as though it *should* indicate ventricular tachycardia, believe me – *it does not!* Note that I said an *impulse from the ventricle* and not an impulse *originating* in the ventricle. Certainly, a ventricular tachycardia could produce such VA conduction, *but so could an orthodromic or antidromic AVRT as well as a permanent reciprocating junctional tachycardia (PJRT)!* We know this is not AV dissociation because *there is no dissociation!* Those P′ waves have a *fixed relationship with the previous QRS*. This tells us that the QRS – or *whatever is producing the QRS* – is producing those P′ waves. Could a junctional tachycardia with aberrant conduction produce such a pattern? Yes! But allow me to let you in on a tightly-held secret: most physicians – even those who read a significant number of ECGs every week – will eventually retire from practice without ever having seen a true junctional tachycardia! Granted, they may see a *premature junctional complex* from time to time or a *junctional escape rhythm* – but junctional tachycardias are *very* rare. Who sees them? Cardiologists, pediatric cardiologists especially, and those healthcare providers managing patients who have had *heart surgery for congenital heart disease.* Other than them, very few others. I practiced internal medicine and emergency medicine for almost 40 years – many of those years at the hospital for the Texas Heart Institute – and I *never* encountered one true junctional tachycardia during my years of practice. I saw premature junctional complexes, idiojunctional (idionodal) rhythms, and junctional escape rhythms – *but no junctional tachycardias!* Be aware that many people refer to AVNRT and AVRT as "junctional tachycardias." That is NOT correct!

> **PEARL |** PACs are much more common than PJCs. If you think you are seeing a PJC – and you certainly will, from time to time (they may be infrequent but they aren't *rare*) – be certain that you aren't seeing a PAC with a hidden P′ wave.

The precordial transition appears to occur before Lead V1, so it is definitely a very early transition. The R/S ratio does appear to be decreasing.

> **PEARL |** The *earlier* the transition, the *further to the left* (or posterior) the origin of the rhythm. The *later* the transition (at or after Lead V4), the *further to the right* (or anterior) the origin of the rhythm. If the precordial transition occurs before Lead V1, the origin of the ectopic focus is likely in the free wall of the left ventricle. If the precordial transition is after Lead V6, the ventricular focus is likely in the free wall of the right ventricle.

Since this precordial transition occurred *before* Lead V1, the origin of the rhythm is very leftward (posterior), which concurs with our diagnosis of a tachycardia originating in the left ventricle.

Without looking back at the ECG (Figure 18-6), and – remembering what was just said about the precordial transition suggesting an origin in the free wall of the left ventricle – what should Lead I look like if the ectopic focus were in the endocardium of the free wall? In the epicardium of the free wall? If it is in the endocardial layer, Lead I should manifest an rS complex; if it is in the epicardium, Lead I should manifest a QS complex. *Now* look at the ECG.

PEARL | Under normal conditions, during sinus rhythm, the first ventricular activation occurs on the left side of the interventricular septum. Given that, the normal precordial transition is between Leads V3 and V4, both leads inclusive. So during a WCT, if the precordial transition is on or between those leads, the ectopic focus is going to be on the septum – likely on the left side.

2. Arrhythmogenic Cardiomyopathy (AC, formerly ARVC/D)

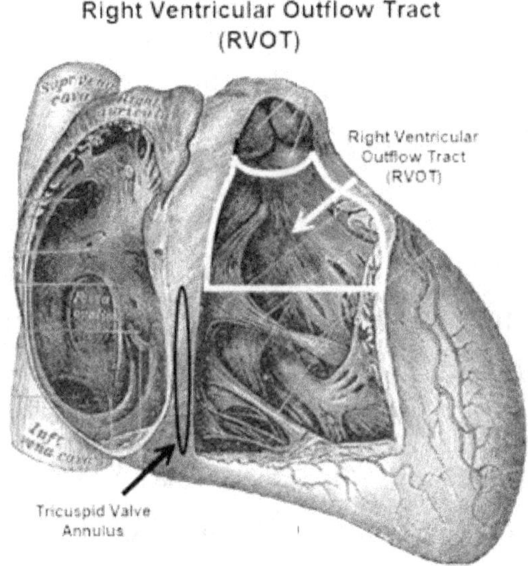

Figure 18-7

Here is a very important PEARL that I want to emphasize at this point:

PEARL | When we compare the magnitude of two QRS complexes, for example, we typically compare the height of the R waves or the depth of the S waves. Please understand that such observations are nothing more than *rough approximations*. What we *should* be comparing is the algebraic summation of all areas within the deflections comprising the QRS – both *positive* and *negative*. Now don't panic and make this more difficult! What you need to be alert to is that when there is a relatively tall but very thin R wave and a shallow but very wide S wave, the QRS is likely a *negative* deflection. It doesn't matter which deflection is taller or deeper – **it's the area within the deflection that matters most!**

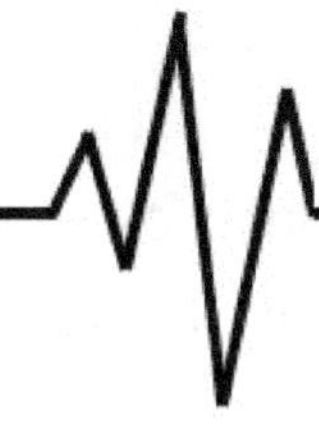

Electrocardiographic Signature

Left bundle branch-like pattern in Lead V1

Usually a superior axis in the frontal plane (but occasionally an inferior axis)

Epsilon waves, seen only in 10% to 37% of cases - but pathognomonic

QRS duration in Lead I > 120 msec

R wave peak time > 80 msec in one or more leads

QRS notching in one or more leads

Precordial transition at Lead V6 or later

Since the term ARVC/D is still in use, I will use both AC and ARVC/D. You may never have heard of this particular cardiomyopathy (formerly known as *arrhythmogenic right ventricular cardiomyopathy/dysplasia*, or ARVC/D) but if you want to know anything about ventricular tachycardias, you must know about THIS one! Here's why: in the next chapter you will learn about *idiopathic ventricular tachycardias* and that some ventricular tachycardias are *benign* (yes, you read that correctly!) and that some don't even require any treatment (yes, you read that correctly, also!). Those benign ventricular tachycardias reside mostly in the *outflow tract of the right ventricle* (Figure 18-7), from the pulmonic valve leaflets to the top of the tricuspid valve annulus, (i.e., the upper part of the right ventricle) *mostly on or immediately adjacent to the upper septum*, even though it includes the full circumference of the upper right ventricle.

Arrhythmogenic cardiomyopathy is a potentially lethal ventricular tachycardia due to structural heart disease that also resides mostly in the right ventricle. But most of the time it originates in the *lower* right ventricle, around the apex, and especially the lateral free wall below the RVOT. So, there are two types of ventricular tachycardias in the right ventricle – a *benign* VT that originates in the *upper* part of the ventricle and a *malignant* VT that develops in the *lower* part of the right ventricle. (Note: there are other types of structural heart disease in the right ventricle other than AC, such as sarcoidosis.)

An impulse originating in the *upper, benign* area will travel *downward* toward the inferior leads (II, III, aVF) which will result in *tall R waves* in those leads, pointing UP toward the origin of the impulse. On the other hand, an impulse originating in the *lower, more lethal apical area* will travel *upward* and away from the inferior leads (II, III aVF) which will result in *deep S waves* in those leads, causing them to point DOWN toward the apex and the origin of the impulse.

So, at this point things appear pretty clear and simple, at least in the presence of ventricular tachycardia with an LBBB-like pattern in Lead V1 (indicating origin in the right ventricle): if the QRS complexes in the inferior leads are tall R waves, then the ventricular tachycardia is benign; but if the QRS complexes in the inferior leads are deep S waves, then the ventricular tachycardia is very dangerous.

I truly wish that were so! I really do!

Unfortunately, rarely, the malignant arrhythmogenic cardiomyopathy can also originate in the upper part of the right ventricle (right ventricular outflow tract, or RVOT) and present with an LBBB-like morphology and an inferior axis (tall R waves) in the inferior leads. It will look very much like the benign type of ventricular tachycardia. But... some differences can help distinguish one from the other when the arrhythmogenic cardiomy-opathy originates from the right ventricular outflow tract. I discuss how to do that in Chapter 23, "Look-Alike WCTs and How to Distinguish Them..."

Arrhythmogenic cardiomyopathy is a genetically inherited disorder. It is present even in the fetus. It specifically affects the gene that produces *desmosomes* – the tiny fibrils that hold myocytes together in groups. If the desmosomes are defective, the individual cells begin to separate and the space that develops between them fills with fibrin and fat. This begins in the right ventricle and the right ventricle is primarily affected. However, the cardiomyopathy can also affect the left ventricle and both ventricles can be involved simultaneously. That's why the words "right ventricular" were taken out of its original name (arrhythmogenic ~~right ventricular~~ cardiomyopathy).

The little foci of fat and fibrin distributed throughout the ventricular walls are non-con-ducting, forming barriers that can slow conduction through the ventricle. This is a great substrate for reentrant ventricular tachycardia *due to structural heart disease!*

There are two characteristic findings for arrhythmogenic cardiomyopathy visible *only* during *sinus rhythm*: post-depolarization deflections called *epsilon* (ε) *waves* and T wave inversions in Leads V1 – V3 (usually accompanied also by T wave inversions in the inferior leads) which may also *occasionally* be seen during the tachycardia. Epsilon waves are *pathognomonic* – specificity is excellent (100%) but sensitivity is poor (between 10 – 37%). The T wave inversions are fairly specific but are also shared with *acute pulmonary emboli* and *juvenile T wave inversions*. Again, these are findings *only during sinus rhythm*.

What does ARVD/C look like *during sinus rhythm*?

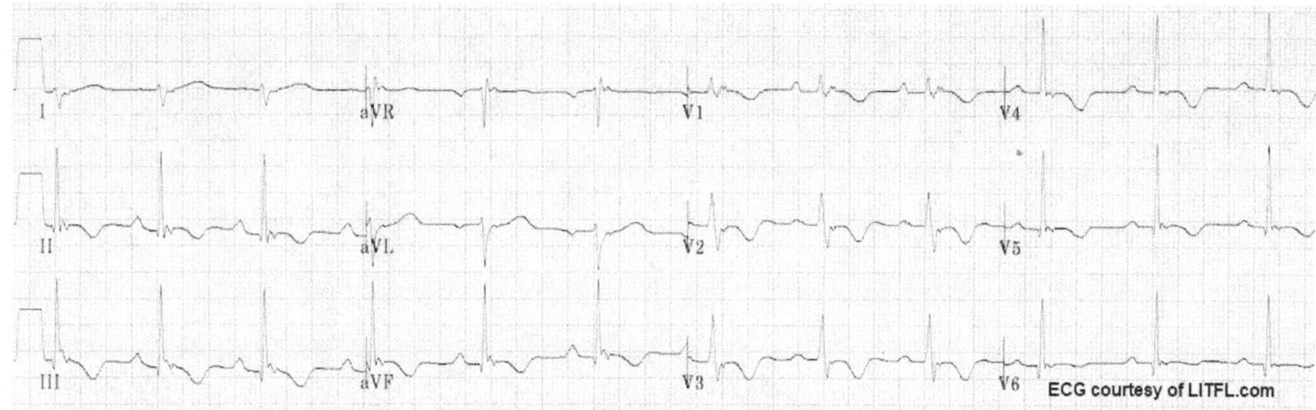

Figure 18-8

As you see in Figure 18-8, there is T wave inversion not only in Leads V1 – V5 (*most notably in V1 – V3*) but also T wave inversion in the inferior leads. There are also epsilon (ε) waves present which are pathognomonic for ARVD/C but not usually present. Some articles state that they are only present in the right precordial leads, but, in my experience, I have seen them in the inferior frontal plane leads as well. Here is an example enlarged from this ECG (Figure 18-9):

The arrows indicate the epsilon waves which are *post-depolarization* deflections – like J waves – and *not part of the QRS complex*. Sometimes the epsilon waves appear at the J point; at other times, the epsilon wave may be slightly separated from the J point. In my classes, I refer to that as a bit of "daylight" between the J point and the epsilon wave.

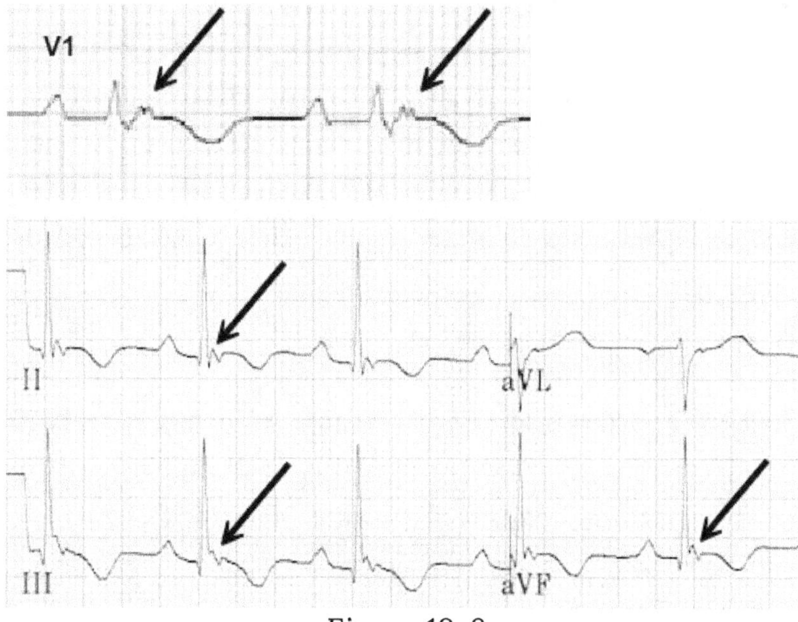

Figure 18-9

Here is what arrhythmogenic cardiomyopathy (AC) looks like during ventricular tachycardia (Figure 18-10):

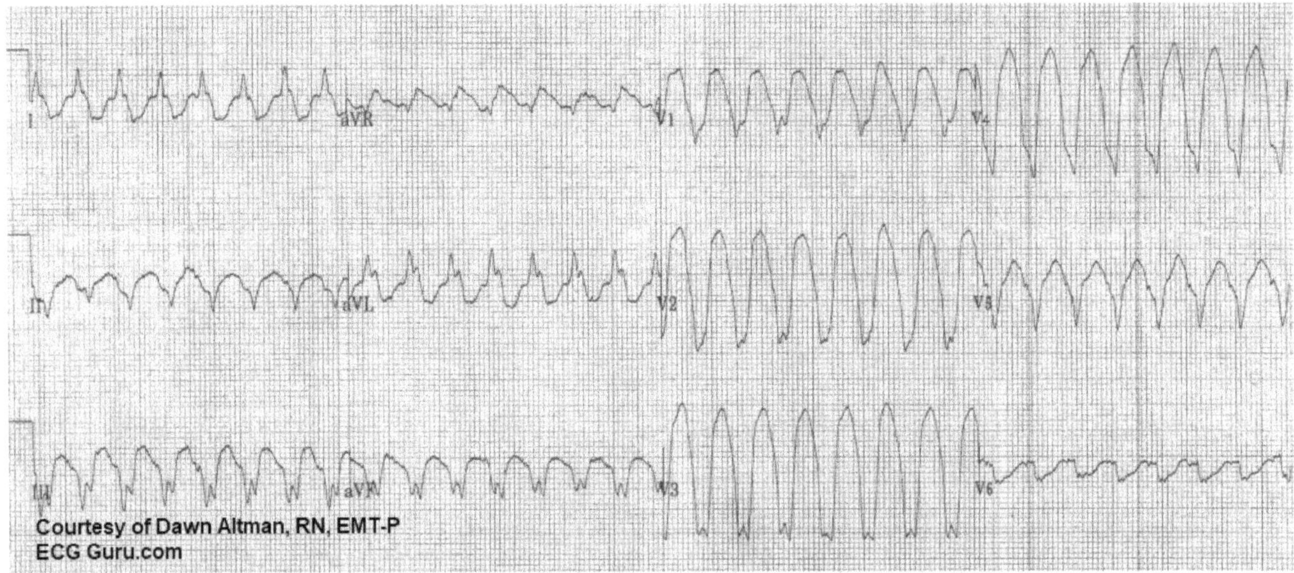

Figure 18-10

This has a typical signature for a tachycardia coming from the right ventricular apex – AC's own neighborhood! There is a **LBBB-like morphology in Lead V1** indicating an origin in the right ventricle. What else indicates a right ventricular origin? **The precordial transition occurs very late** – probably beyond Lead V6! You will likely not see epsilon waves or right precordial T wave inversions *during* ventricular tachycardia. The big hint, however, that this is likely due to arrhythmogenic cardiomyopathy is the **superior axis** manifested by the dominant S waves in all three inferior leads. This is a reentrant tachycardia (How do we know that it's reentrant?) in a patient with structural heart disease (AC is *structural* heart disease!). What is the likelihood that this ECG is from a patient with AC? Very good! Ventricular tachycardias coming from the right ventricle are uncommon in general. You can find a lot of them online because when someone finds one, they immediately post it. This tachycardia is coming from below the right ventricular outflow tract and that points to AC. Could another kind of ventricular tachycardia be occurring here? Possibly, but this is very characteristic of arrhythmogenic cardiomyopathy. It is managed according to ACLS protocols.

The Fontaine Leads

To maximize the effort to record epsilon waves, which are present only 10 – 37% of the time, we can rearrange the electrodes for the frontal plane leads and record three *new* leads: F1, F2, and F3. These are the Fontaine Leads (F=Fontaine) (Figure 18-11):

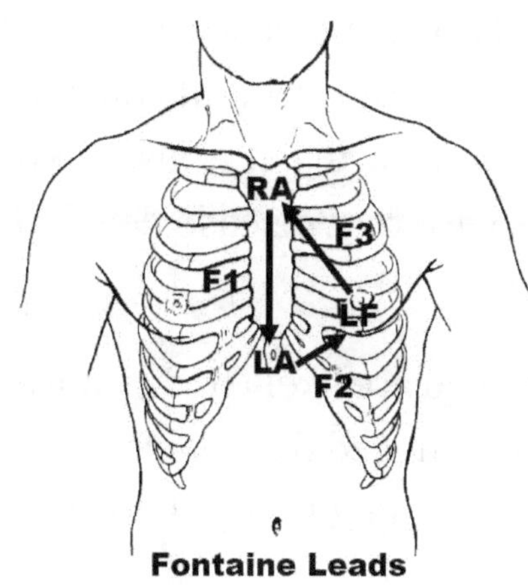

Figure 18-11

The right arm (RA) electrode is placed over the manubrium.

The left arm (LA) electrode is placed over the xiphoid process.

The left foot (LF) electrode is placed in the same position as lead V4. (Note: you cannot use the normal precordial electrode wire for V4; you must attach the left foot electrode wire to the V4 electrode on the chest wall.)

In contrast to the Lewis lead – which is just one lead and is read in Lead I – there are THREE Fontaine leads, so we must name them...

F 1 – Read this in Lead I on the ECG tracing

F 2 – Read this in Lead III on the ECG tracing

F 3 – Read this in Lead II on the ECG tracing

Careful! The number of the Fontaine lead does not necessarily correspond to the number of the limb lead (F2 is Lead III and F3 is Lead II).

When you record the Fontaine leads, the paper speed should be increased to 50 mm/sec and the voltage set at 20 mm/mV. Use a filter setting of 40 Hz.

Epsilon waves are *positive* deflections (never *negative*) appearing at the end of the QRS complex, sometimes slightly separated from the J point – but only by milliseconds. They are very ragged-appearing, so you shouldn't confuse them with retrograde P′ waves. They are considered evidence of the delayed activation of living myocytes scattered among the nodules of fat and fiber located throughout the ventricular walls and are pathognomonic for arrhythmogenic cardiomyopathy.

NOTE | The epsilon wave in Lead V1 of Figure 18-9 may give the impression of greater separation from the QRS – but that's only because the QRS ends with an S wave. The epsilon wave is still located at the J point!

3. Bundle Branch Reentrant Tachycardia (BBRT)

Bundle branch reentrant tachycardia (BBRT) is one of the most lethal of all ventricular tachycardias. While it has been reported in patients without any structural heart disease, which would qualify it as an *idiopathic* ventricular tachycardia, it is almost always associated with dilated cardiomyopathy (ischemic and non-ischemic) or valvular heart disease, which also makes it a ventricular tachycardia due to structural heart disease. Non-ischemic dilated cardiomyopathy is the most common substrate for bundle branch tachycardia. It is also seen in patients with *myotonic dystrophy* in which a minority of patients with that disease develop a progressive degeneration of the ventricular conduction system.

Bundle branch reentrant tachycardia is not a tachydysrhythmia that you are likely to diagnose in the emergency department or critical care unit. Generally, it is diagnosed during electrophysiological testing. However, there are a few hints that you are dealing with this very dangerous dysrhythmia.

PEARL | The impulse traveling down the descending pathway will activate the ventricle on that side first. If the right bundle branch is the descending pathway, then the activation of the right ventricle first will result in a LBBB pattern. So, the type of bundle branch block pattern in Lead V1 will indicate the descending pathway.

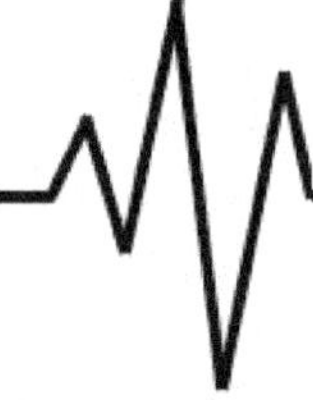

Electrocardiographic Signature

LBBB morphology in Lead V1 (very, very rarely a RBBB morphology)

Monomorphic, usually exhibiting classic LBBB (or rarely, RBBB) morphology

Prolonged PR interval (an ECG while the patient is in sinus rhythm is needed to see this)

Very rapid rates - usually > 200 beats/minute and sometimes approaching 300 beats/minute

There are three types of BBRT (Figure 18-12):

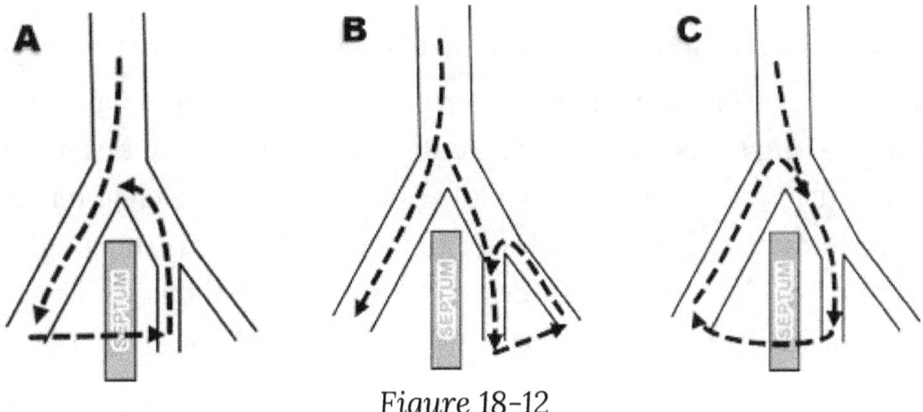

Figure 18-12

The first type, of course, is **Type A** in which the bundle branch tachycardia uses the right bundle branch as the antegrade limb of the tachycardia circuit. Based on Diagram A, it is apparent that the only time the tachycardia impulse is *not* in the rapidly conducting fibers of the His-Purkinje system is at the lower turnaround point where it must cross the working myocardium of the interventricular septum to access the posterior fascicle and ultimately, back up to the common left bundle branch. Thus, it is easy to see why these tachycardias are so rapid. There are no conducting pathways crossing the interventricular septum transversely (from right to left or left to right); all transseptal conduction is cell-to-cell.

What do you think would happen if – hypothetically – instead of the lower turnaround point being slowly-conducting septal myocardium, it was composed of more rapidly-conducting Purkinje fibers? Do you think it could push the heart rate close to 300 beats/minute... or even faster? The bundle branch tachycardia would likely automatically extinguish itself! **The slower-conducting myocardial cells in the septum delay conduction long enough for the rest of the circuit to repolarize and be available to conduct the next impulse.**

> **PEARL |** Every reentry circuit must provide a delay at some point in the circuit – no matter how slight – to allow for repolarization to be completed and refractoriness caused by the previous impulse to end. Otherwise, the impulse would run into the refractoriness of the previous beat and the tachycardia would automatically self-terminate. A dilated cardiomyopathy increases the length of the tachycardia circuit which helps sustain the reentrant mechanism, and disease within the conduction system causing slowing at some points will also provide some delay and help sustain the tachycardia.

The next type of bundle branch tachycardia is **Type C**, in which the antegrade limb is the left common bundle and (usually) the posterior fascicle since it runs along the left side of the septum. It is very similar except that the QRS morphology in Lead V1 exhibits a RBBB morphology. Type C is very rare.

Type B is not based on a circuit involving the major bundle branches, but instead, it utilizes the posterior and anterior fascicles. This is referred to as an *interfascicular* tachycardia. Again, one might think that this tachycardia would be extremely fast, but it, too, is somewhat rate-restricted: it must be slow enough to allow time for both fascicles to repolarize to avoid running into refractory fibers. The lower turnaround point is the length of working myocardium between the bases of the anterior and posterior papillary muscles, which serves to add some delay within the reentry circuit and allow completion of repolarization.

Both **Type A** and **Type C** send retrograde impulses up the His bundle to the atria.

You may have been wondering, "How does a reentrant circuit *that includes a bundle branch that is blocked* support reentry?" The answer lies in the next PEARL:

> **PEARL |** This is a ventricular tachycardia. Bundle branch blocks are "blocks" only when the impulse has conducted down the His bundle and entered the ventricles from a supraventricular origin – either atrial or junctional. When a bundle branch block *pattern* appears during an *ectopic* ventricular tachycardia, it is an indication of the *origin* of the dysrhythmia and *not* a manifestation of a block!

In addition to dilated cardiomyopathy and valvular heart disease, there must be *concurrent disease in the ventricular conducting system.* This may also allow sufficient conduction delay to maintain the reentry circuit.

Bundle branch reentrant tachycardia will respond to D/C cardioversion but you must remember that *the substrate that precipitated and maintained the tachycardia is still present!* Nothing you have done has changed that! Medications neither prevent nor terminate this type of ventricular tachycardia. Ablation is the first line of permanent treatment and is accomplished by ablating the right bundle branch!

> **PEARL |** You may have noticed that the word "ventricular" is not usually included in the name of this tachycardia. And there is a reason for that: *there are no bundle branches in the atria!* The same will apply to another ventricular tachycardia we will discuss later – *fascicular* tachycardia. Again, why must we say "ventricular?" There are no fascicles of the left bundle branch in the atria!

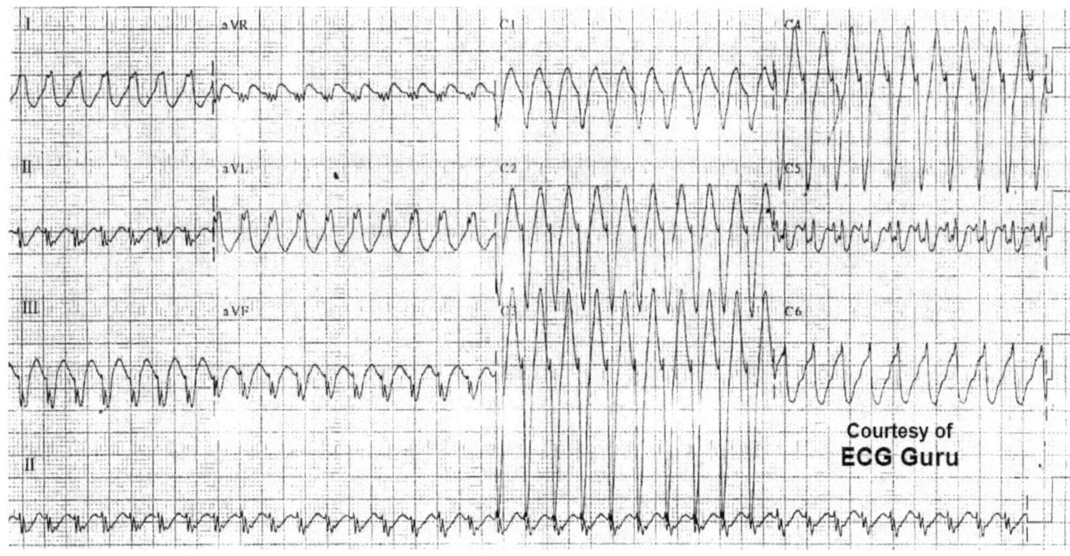

Figure 18-13

Here is a 12-lead ECG (Figure 18-13) that *may* represent a bundle branch reentrant tachycardia. Recall that *the actual diagnosis is made following electrophysiologic testing*, but this is exactly what it looks like on paper.

Again, note that the left bundle branch block pattern in Lead V1 does not suggest that there is any problem with the left bundle branch. It appears because the right bundle branch is activating BEFORE the left bundle branch. On paper or on a monitor, that gives the impression of a bundle branch block when none is present.

How does it do that? There is something that a *left bundle branch block* and an *ectopic beat in the right ventricle* have in common: *they both result in the activation of the right ventricle BEFORE the left ventricle!*

An Exercise to Check Your Understanding

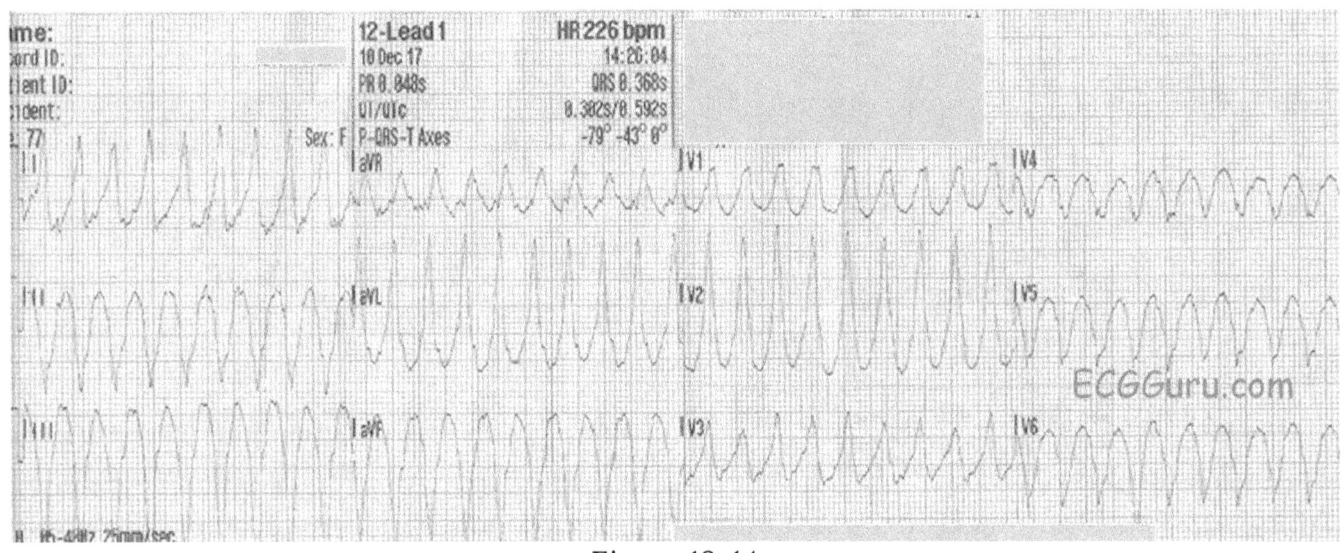

Figure 18-14

How many signs of ventricular tachycardia due to structural heart disease do you see on this ECG? (This isn't a trick! It really is due to structural heart disease.)

(Suggestions following the "Recommended Readings.")

Recommended Reading:

Corrado D, MD, Link MS, MD, Calkins H, MD. Review Article: Arrhythmogenic Right Ventricular Cardiomyopathy. *N Engl J Med.* 2017;376:61-72. DOI: 10.1056/NEJMra1509267

Corrado D, Basso C, Thiene G. Arrhythmogenic right ventricular cardiomyopathy: diagnosis, prognosis, and treatment. *Heart.* 2000;83:588±595.

Jastrzębski M, Moskal P, Kukla P, Fijorek K, Kisiel R, Czarnecka D. Specificity of wide QRS complex tachycardia criteria and algorithms in patients with ventricular preexcitation. *Ann Noninvasive Electrocardiol.* 2018;23:e12493.

Kusa S, MD et al. Bundle Branch Reentrant Ventricular Tachycardia With Wide and Narrow QRS Morphology. *Circ Arrhythm Electrophysiol.* 2013;6:e87-e91.

Wijnmaalen AP. ECG Identification of Scar-Related Ventricular Tachycardia With a Left Bundle-Branch Block Configuration. *Circ Arrhythm Electrophysiol.* 2011;4:486-493.

de Riva M, MD, Watanabe M, MD, Zeppenfeld K, MD. Twelve-Lead ECG of Ventricular Tachycardia in Structural Heart Disease. *Circ Arrhythm Electrophysiol.* 2015;8:951-962.

Roberts JD, MD et al. Bundle Branch Re-Entrant Ventricular Tachycardia – Novel Genetic Mechanisms in a Life-Threatening Arrhythmia. JACC: *Clinical Electrophysiology.* Vol. 3, No. 3, 2017; 276-288.

Suggested Responses to Exercise (Figure 18-14):

1. Origin in left ventricle (more MIs provide more substrate for VT)

2. Wide QRS complexes (suggests slow conduction through working myocardium))

3. Regular rhythm (suggestive of reentry)

4. Monomorphic

Chapter 19

The "Benign" Idiopathic Ventricular Tachycardias

Idiopathic ventricular tachycardias are those ventricular tachycardias that are not due to any structural heart disease. When the first of this type of tachycardia was discovered, researchers and cardiologists were confused regarding the origin. Thus, they called them "idiopathic," meaning "of unknown cause." As more and more of these very heterogeneous tachydysrhythmias were discovered, progress was rapidly being made in the determination of their origins. Today, we know how these dysrhythmias are produced and yet we still call this group "idiopathic."

While ventricular tachycardias are divided into those due to structural heart disease and those without it (idiopathic), the idiopathic category can be divided into *benign* and *potentially lethal*. Some are due to *triggered activity* while others are due to *reentry*. *Triggered* activity produces both *benign* (RVOT, LVOT) and *malignant* (torsade de pointes) tachycardias and *reentry* produces both *benign* (fascicular) and *malignant* (bundle branch) tachycardias.

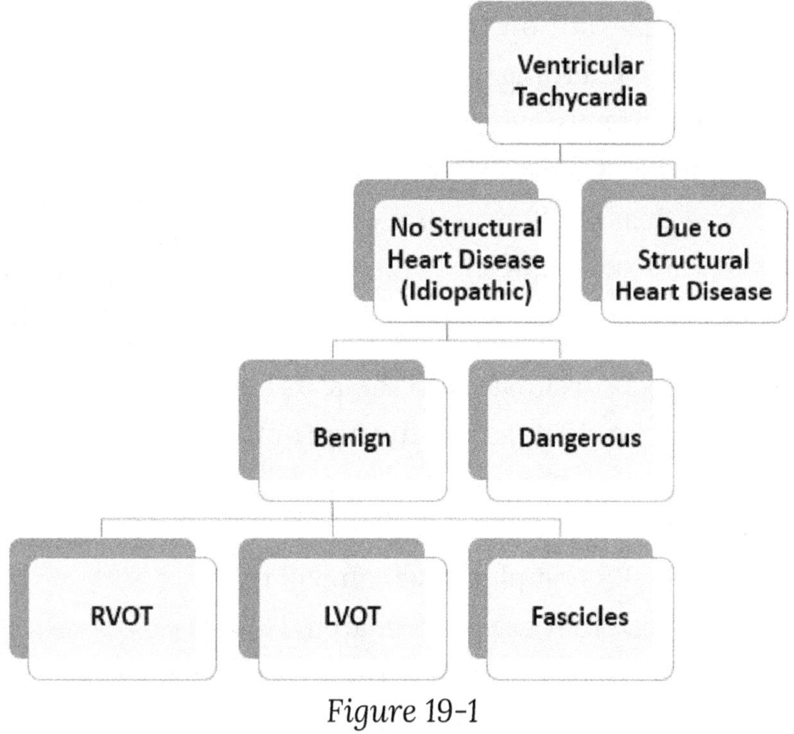

Figure 19-1

The benign idiopathic ventricular tachycardias originate in three places: the right ventricular outflow tract (RVOT), the left ventricular outflow tract (LVOT), and the posterior and anterior fascicles (but mostly the *posterior* fascicle).

Right Ventricular Outflow Tract (RVOT) Tachycardias

Let's begin by demonstrating what the right outflow tract includes (Figure 19-2):

The Right Ventricular Outflow Tract – What Is It and Where Is It?

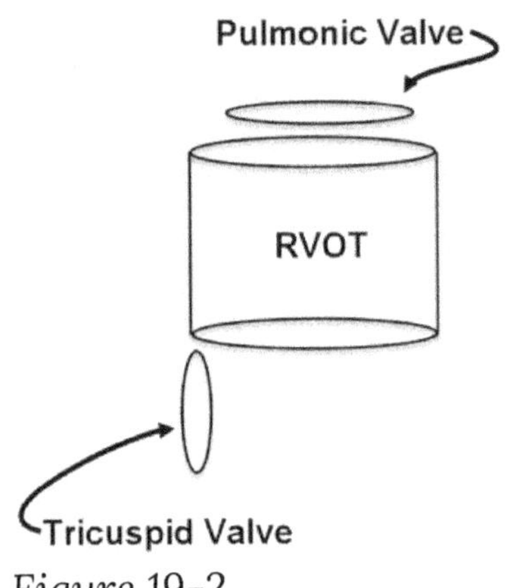

Figure 19-2

The RIGHT Ventricular Outflow Tract (RVOT) is that area bounded superiorly by the pulmonic valve and inferiorly by the top of the tricuspid valve, which itself forms the *inflow tract*. The pulmonic valve and tricuspid valves are oriented at right angles – the pulmonic valve being oriented *horizontally* and the tricuspid valve being *vertically* oriented. The purpose of the schematic diagram on the left (19-2) is to show you that the RVOT extends completely around the right upper ventricle. A more realistic depiction is below (19-3). Although the RVOT is cone-shaped, we think of it as divided into a *right*, anterior, (together, referred to as the *free wall*), *left*, and *posterior* (together, referred to as the *septal*) sides. This can be further simplified to *the posteromedial* ("septal") *area* and the *anterolateral* ("free wall") *area* – a very common designation.

There is also a LEFT ventricular outflow tract which you will learn about later, but here is something you may *not* have anticipated: *part of the RIGHT ventricular outflow tract is located on the LEFT and the LEFT ventricular outflow tract is located on the RIGHT!* (Use this bit of trivia to see if you can win a cup of coffee from your colleagues!)

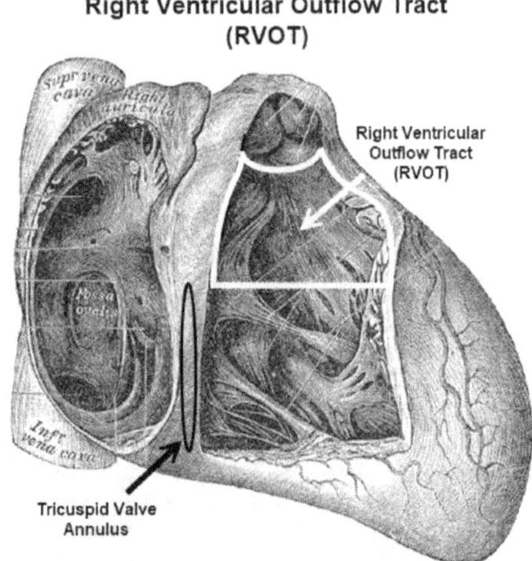

Figure 19-3

TIP | Most of the impulses originating in the RVOT will be on or very near the right side of the septum. They will be closer to rapid-conducting Purkinje fibers (i.e., the bundle branches) and will consequently tend to have better-formed QRS complexes which will tend to be narrower than those that are scar-related. However, they will not be as narrow or well-formed as those QRS complexes of the tachycardias that originate within the Purkinje system!

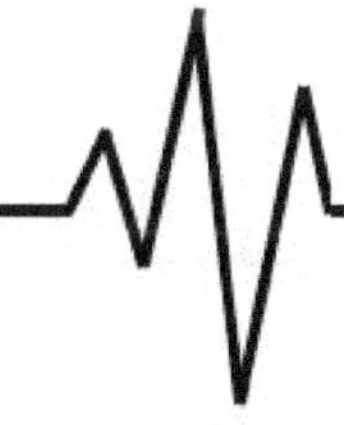

Electrocardiographic Signature

LBBB morphology in Lead V1

Inferior axis (tall R waves in Leads II, III and aVF) in the frontal plane

QRS in Lead I < 120 msec*

Precordial transitions that may be a little earlier (at before Lead V3) than expected for a right ventricular impulse

*The QRS duration in Lead I less than 120 msec is not so much diagnostic of RVOT tachycardia (some can have longer durations), but it serves to differentiate it from its closest "look-alike," the reentrant tachycardia of *arrhythmogenic cardiomyopathy*.

The RVOT has a very unique relationship with the LVOT, which leads to some confusion at times. While the interventricular septum separates the RVOT from the LVOT, we often forget that the septum isn't always a thick, muscular wall like the left ventricular free wall – there is also a thin, membranous section of the first part of the septum at the beginning of the separation into the two ventricles:

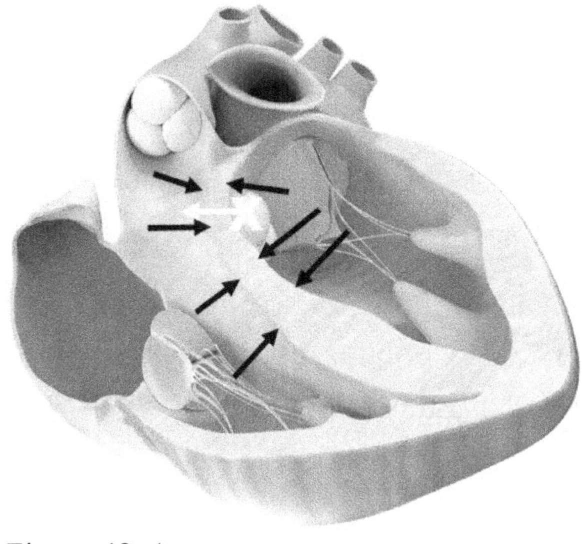

Figure 19-4

This diagram (Figure 19-4) shows the RVOT (R) and LVOT (L) with a gradually thinning septum indicated by the arrows. The interventricular septum is seen dividing the RVOT (R) from the LVOT (L). The *lower part* of the RVOT (which is still in the *upper part* of the right ventricle) is separated from the LVOT by the septum's thick, muscular wall. The *upper part* of the RVOT, however, is separated from the LVOT by a relatively thin membrane. The "X" indicates an ectopic focus in the left ventricular outflow tract (LVOT) that actually exits into the right ventricular outflow tract (RVOT)! This creates the unique paradox in which an ectopic beat originating in the LEFT VENTRICLE presents with an LBBB pattern! So, here's another way to win a cup of coffee from your colleagues: ask them if an impulse originating in the LEFT VENTRICLE can have an LBBB pattern! (Just don't try it on any of your *electrophysiologist* friends – you'll be buying *them* a cup of coffee!)

There are several things to know about RVOT tachydysrhythmias (FYI – the "T" in RVOT refers to "Tract," not "Tachycardia," so it is correct to say "RVOT tachycardia"):

Common Presentation

The patients are typically younger at onset – 20 to 40 years of age – but the tachycardia can continue to recur well into the later years (60's and 70's). The most common complaint is palpitations and occasionally dizziness if the episodes become sustained – rarely syncope. The episodes are usually very short, however – just a few beats and then a spontaneous termination. These can occur many times a day or only occasionally. The greatest danger to the patient is the development of a cardiomyopathy due to persistent episodes called *tachycardia-induced cardiomyopathy*, or TIC (more on that in a moment).

What Causes RVOT Tachycardia?

The tachycardia is caused by *delayed afterdepolarizations* that lead to triggered activity. There is *no prolonged QT interval* and the dysrhythmia is *not related to torsade de pointes*. While these tachycardias are not due to structural heart disease, structural heart disease may be present.

They are considered *benign* (no, that is *not* a typo!). Most treatment is aimed at reducing the annoyance of frequent palpitations. Those patients with a low ectopic burden (infrequent episodes of tachycardia or PVCs) who have no symptoms, or do not consider their symptoms a problem, are sometimes left untreated.

If sustained (a very infrequent occurrence), they will respond quite effectively to *adenosine!* But they also respond to *calcium channel blockers, beta-blockers, amiodarone*, and even (at times) *vagal maneuvers*. Ablation is successful in over 90% of cases and recurrences are few.

While some idiopathic ventricular tachycardias are *benign* (outflow tract tachycardias, fascicular tachycardias) and some are *very dangerous* (torsade de pointes, catecholaminergic polymorphic VTs), **all ventricular tachycardias <u>due to structural heart disease</u> are dangerous and potentially lethal!**

There is a ventricular tachycardia due to structural heart disease that can rarely present in the right ventricular outflow tract and appear very similar to the benign RVOT tachycardias – and that is *arrhythmogenic cardiomyopathy* (see Chapter 18, section on "Arrhythmogenic Cardiomyopathy…). This disease is rare and usually originates in the *apical region* of the right ventricle, but on rare occasions may develop in the RVOT. Distinguishing between these two tachycardias with very different treatments and prognoses is discussed in Chapter 23 ("Look-Alike WCTs and How to Distinguish Them…").

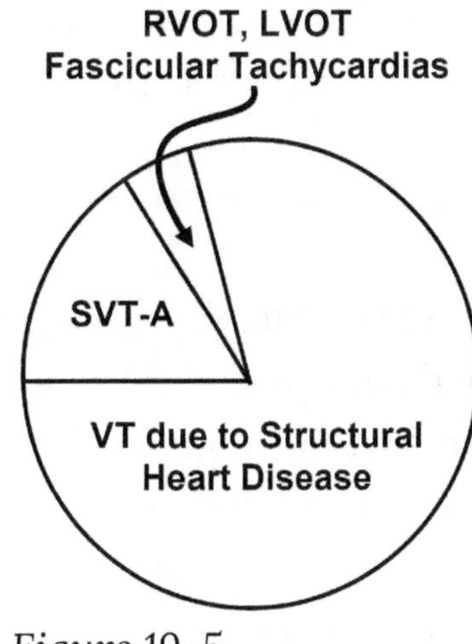

Figure 19-5

Now let's not lose our perspective: idiopathic RVOT tachycardias are *very infrequent*, comprising only 10% of all ventricular tachycardias. RVOTs make up 80 – 90% of all idiopathic VTs (which is 8-9% of all ventricular tachycardias (Figure 19-5). That leaves about 1% for the left-sided ventricular tachycardias. It's easy to find examples of RVOT and posterior fascicular tachycardias on the internet, but that's because when someone encounters one it usually gets posted for all to see. Don't let that distort your concept of the true frequency of these tachydysrhythmias. If you see a lot of heart patients with dysrhythmias you will likely encounter one of them from time to time. The vast majority of ventricular tachycardias that you will manage, however, will be due to *structural heart disease* and they *will* be very dangerous dysrhythmias!

Let's take a look at an RVOT tachycardia ECG...

Right Ventricular Outflow Tract (RVOT) Tachycardia #1

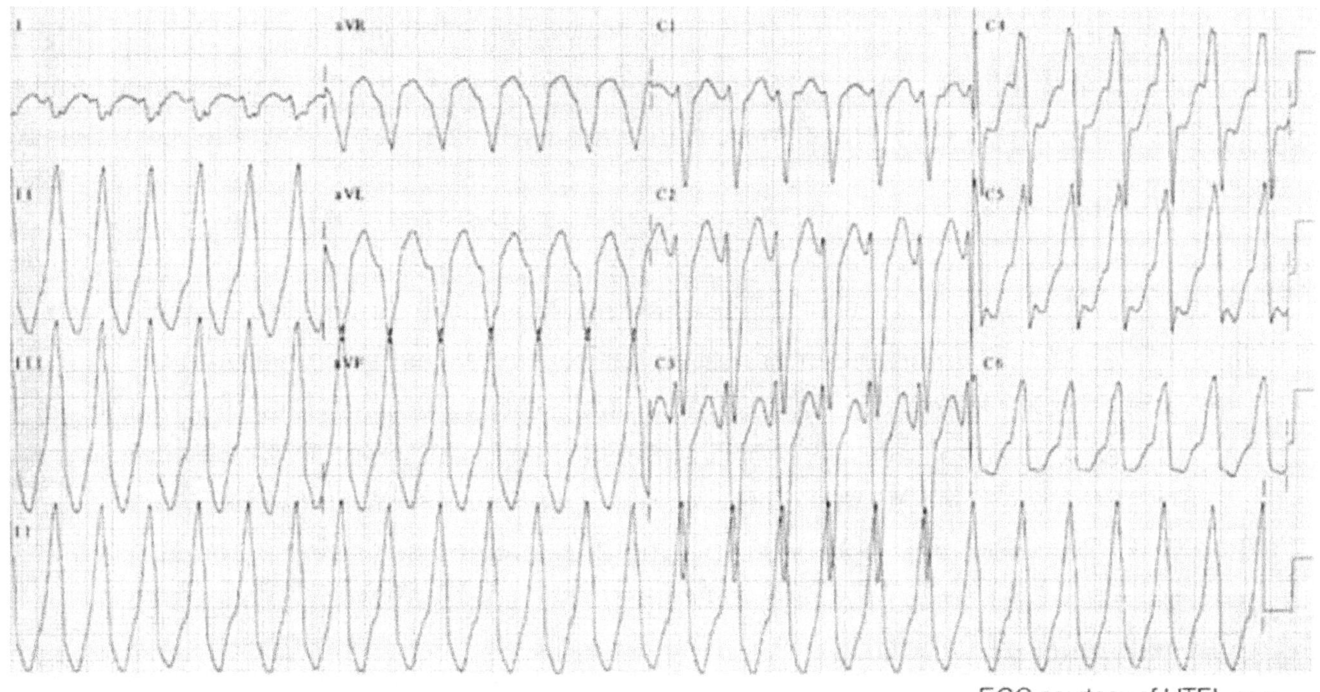

ECG courtesy of LITFL.com

Figure 19-6

There are several things to note about RVOT tachycardias on the ECG tracing (Figure 19-6):

Although they are essentially benign – *they can still look very scary!*

The QRS complexes in the inferior leads (II, III, aVF) consist of tall R waves. This indicates that the origin of the impulse is in the outflow tract. Think of the R waves as *pointing toward the origin of the impulse.*

> **PEARL |** I've never understood why so many authors of textbooks and journal articles insist on listing an "inferior axis" as a requirement for the diagnosis of right ventricular outflow tract tachycardia. The term indicates the *direction* the impulse is traveling. From that, you are supposed to decide where the impulse originated. Why not just look at the QRS complexes in the inferior leads – especially Lead aVF – and say that "the tachycardia originated in the outflow tract"? We need to know the *origin* of the impulse. We don't care *where* the impulse is going – *it's the origin that tells us what we want to know!*

The precordial transition is located at Lead V4 (C4 on this ECG, Figure 19-6). Impulses (vectors) originating in the right ventricle will typically show a precordial transition from Lead V4 onward to Lead V6 and sometimes beyond. Occasionally, in the case of RVOT tachycardias or PVCs, they will transition by Lead V3. A precordial transition at lead V3 or V4 indicates a location on or very near the right side of the upper interventricular septum, a more leftward location but still in the right ventricle. A precordial transition at Lead V6, for instance, could suggest a location of the ectopic focus more rightward within the right ventricle – most likely on the free wall.

> **PEARL |** Do you remember what the RVOT looks like in the *upper* RVOT? (See Figure 17-4) At that point, the interventricular septum is just a thin membrane separating the RVOT from the LVOT. One would expect a focus originating on the LEFT upper septum to have a precordial transition around Lead V3, so why not a focus on the uppermost RVOT in the part that curves around to the LEFT of the LVOT? Therefore, it is not too surprising that an impulse arising in the upper portion of the RVOT may have an earlier precordial transition than expected for a right ventricular structure.

Since RVOT tachycardia is essentially benign, why treat it? The key word here is "essentially." First of all, the palpitations may be very upsetting to the patient. Also, although this rate will be tolerated by someone in good health, imagine if the patient had an aortic stenosis, coronary artery disease, or bad COPD. It won't seem so benign to them! And there is always the threat of **tachycardia-induced cardiomyopathy (TIC)** due to frequent episodes of tachy-cardia. A tachycardia-induced cardiomyopathy can occur in anyone with frequent episodes of tachycardia or even very frequent PVCs (referred to as a *high PVC burden*). If left untreated, the patient's condition will slowly deteriorate, and it will likely eventually prove fatal if untreated. However, there is good news! If the tachycardia or excessive PVCs are treated – generally by *ablation* – the patient can recover their ventricular function *completely* and will return to their pre-cardiomyopathy LV ejection fraction within about 4 – 6 months. TIC can also occur in other tachydysrhythmias – *permanent junctional reciprocating tachycardia (PJRT)* is notorious for causing TIC in children, sometimes fatal.

PEARL | The benign, idiopathic ventricular outflow tract tachycardias are called "benign" because they are extremely unlikely to result in a cardiovascular collapse or sudden cardiac death. There are two issues, however: 1) if the outflow tract VT occurs *too frequently* it could lead to tachycardia-induced cardiomyopathy (TIC), and 2) while the outflow tract VT *itself* is benign, if the impulse finds a scar it can become a *scar-related tachycardia* with all the associated dangers. Don't get confused – the fact that ventricular tachycardia is the benign, idiopathic type due to triggered activity *does not exclude the presence of heart disease.*

Right Ventricular Outflow Tract (RVOT) Tachycardia #2

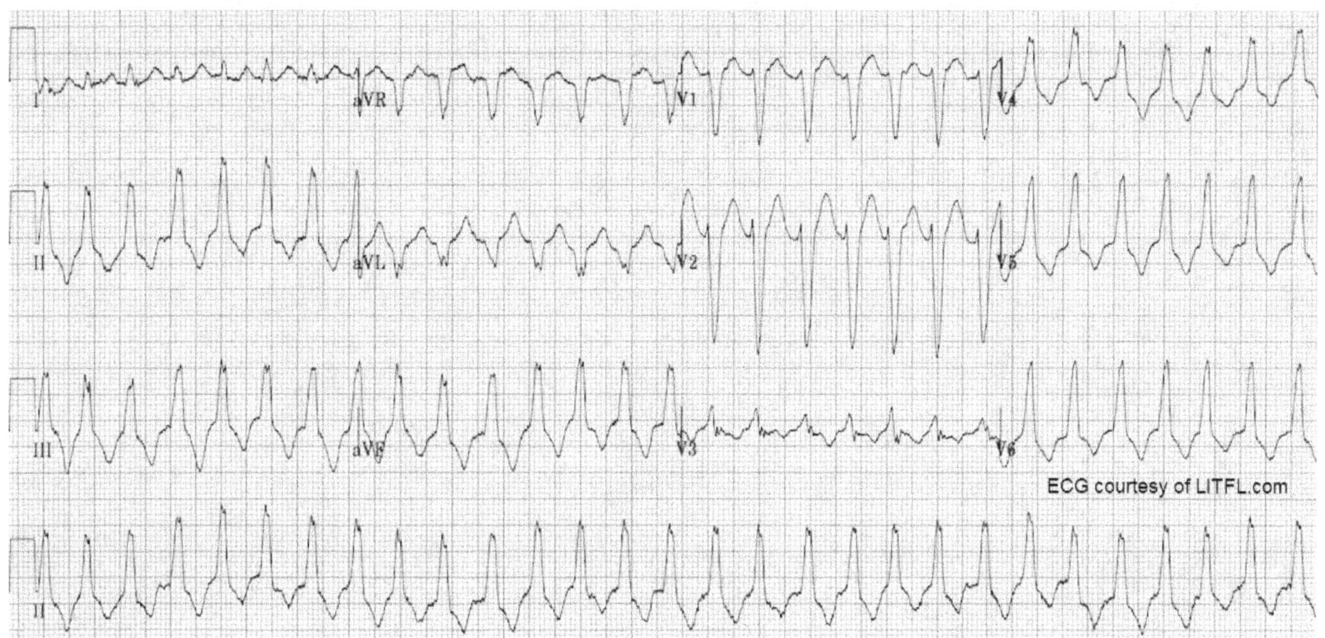

Figure 19-7

Here's a recap of what you learned earlier.

Which leads do you inspect *first* on a wide complex tachycardia 12-lead ECG?

- **Lead V1** – to ascertain in which ventricle the tachydysrhythmia originates

- **Leads II, III, and aVF** – to ascertain the vertical axis of the ectopic impulse (is it coming from the *outflow tract* – usually benign, or the *apex* – never good?)

- **Lead aVR** – to ascertain the presence of an initial R wave and an immediate diagnosis of ventricular tachycardia

In Figures 19-6 and 19-7, the impulse is arising in the RIGHT VENTRICLE because there is a LBBB-like QRS in Lead V1. Turning our attention to Figure 19-7:

There are tall R waves in the inferior leads pointing UP toward the *origin* of the impulse; therefore, the impulse is originating in the outflow tract (upper right ventricle).

There is a *monophasic* QS wave in Lead aVR (the QS complexes themselves are *monomorphic – all exactly the same in Lead aVR*). This unfortunately does not contribute to a diagnosis. A monophasic R wave or a qR in which the q is at least 40 msec in duration would strongly favor ventricular tachycardia – but we don't see that here.

OK… now *where* in the upper part of the right ventricle is the impulse arising? We can see that the precordial transition is between Leads V2 and V3 – *a very early transition for an impulse originating in the right ventricle*. Unless… it is coming from the upper septal area where the septum is more of a thin membrane rather than a thick muscular structure and the RVOT wraps around the aorta to the left. Remember: *the later the precordial transition, the more rightward the impulse origin.* I would suspect this ectopic rhythm is coming from the area of the right *upper* outflow tract.

See how quickly *you* can arrive at a diagnosis of RVOT with this ECG (Figure 19-8). Follow these five steps:

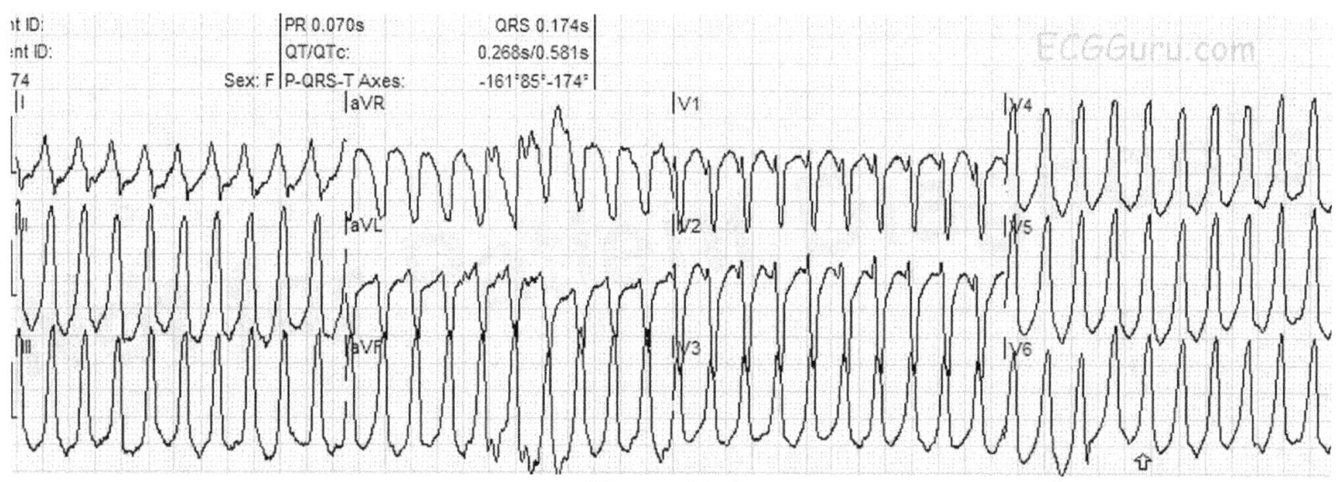

Figure 19-8

1. **Location in the Heart:** Which ventricle?

2. **Location in the Ventricle:** Outflow tract or apex?

3. **Quick Diagnosis:** Is there a monophasic R wave in Lead aVR?

4. **Final Diagnosis:** What is your diagnosis?

5. **Confirmation:** Where is the precordial transition and is it consistent with your diagnosis?

Given the precordial transition, in which part of the RVOT do you suspect the focus is located?

The precordial transition is located between Leads V2 and V3 since Lead V3 is already a monophasic R wave. That is *early* for an impulse originating in the right ventricle. However, it can easily occur if the focus is located *on the upper right interventricular septum* in the upper, leftward portion of the RVOT where the septum is very thin and there is little separation between the RVOT and LVOT.

> **TIP |** If you think the patient has one of the benign idiopathic VTs, be certain that the QRS complexes are 140 msec or less. A wider QRS may be idiopathic, but it should alert you to the likelihood of a scar-related VT and a much more dangerous tachycardia.

Left Ventricular Outflow Tract (LVOT) Tachycardias

This section is short because almost everything said about the RVOT tachycardias applies to LVOT tachycardias. The only copy of a 12-lead ECG of a patient with a documented LVOT tachycardia in my possession is one with an LBBB morphology in Lead V1 – so it looks exactly like an RVOT! Left ventricular outflow tract (LVOT) tachycardias share the same *characteristics*, *treatment*, and *prognosis* as RVOT tachycardias. Their only difference is that the electrocardiographic signature for LVOT tachycardia is usually an RBBB-like morphology in Lead V1. Of course, they both exhibit tall R waves in Leads II, III, and aVF. Whereas idiopathic ventricular tachycardias comprise only about 10% of all ventricular tachycardias, 90% of those occur in the right ventricle and 10% occur in the left ventricle. In the left ventricle, *fascicular tachycardias* (next topic) are by far the most common of the *idiopathic* left ventricular tachycardias, so don't plan on diagnosing an LVOT tachycardia very soon.

> **Interesting Trivia |** Because an ectopic focus high in the left ventricular outflow tract may exit into the right ventricle, an impulse arising in the left ventricle can present with an LBBB morphology in Lead V1. This will never be a concern of yours,

but it is something the electrophysiologist will have to consider prior to an ablation procedure.

TIP | You will sometimes see the term *idiopathic left ventricular tachycardia* (ILVT) as a diagnosis. Although the term includes LVOT tachycardias, it more often refers more specifically to the fascicular tachycardias which are the most common of the idiopathic tachycardias in the left ventricle.

You shouldn't confuse LVOT tachycardias with posterior fascicular tachycardias (by far the most common type of fascicular tachycardia). With the LVOT tachycardias, the QRS complexes in the inferior leads will all be tall R waves; posterior fascicular tachycardias will appear just the opposite: they will have deep S waves in the inferior leads. Also, the fascicular tachycardias will have a sharper, smoother onset of the QRS complexes since they arise in conducting tissue.

Fascicular Tachycardias

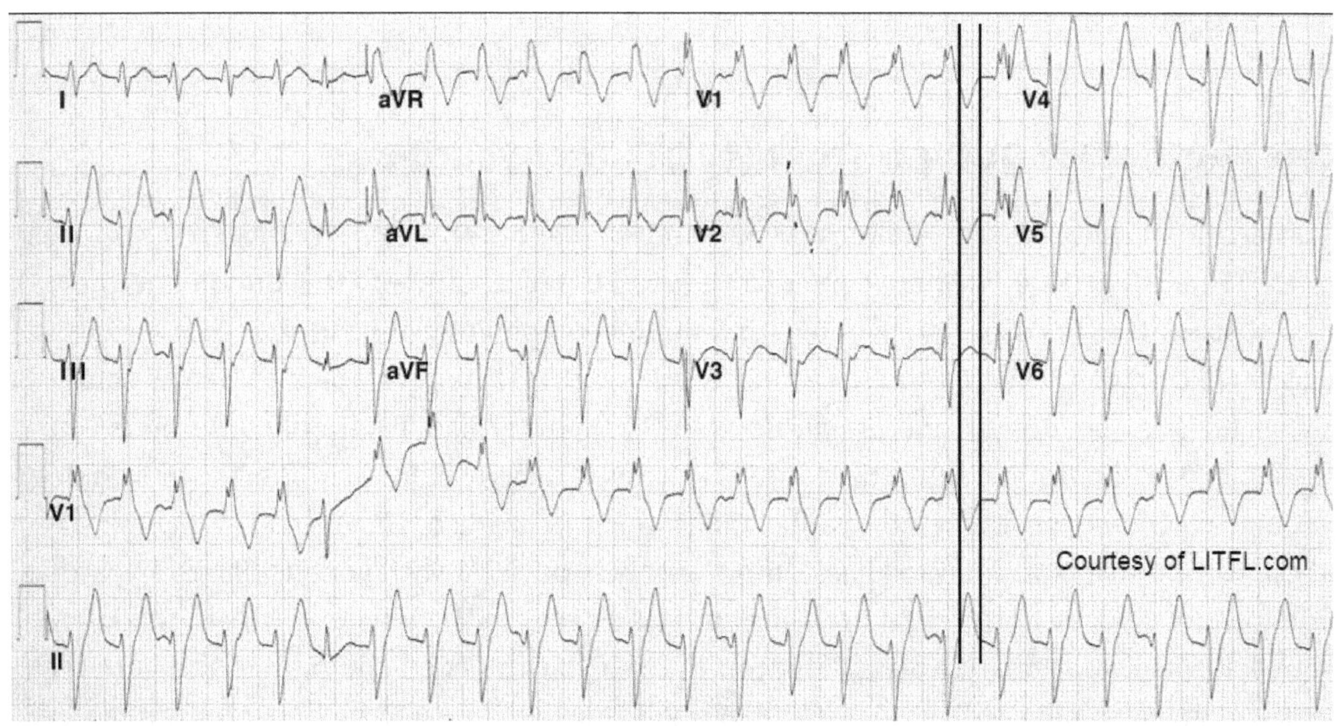

Figure 19-9

Fascicular tachycardias are very interesting because...

1. they are among the "benign" idiopathic tachycardias

2. they are sometimes so narrow they are mistaken for SVTs with aberrancy

3. they respond to verapamil (which adds to mistaking them for SVT-A)

What mechanism drives a fascicular tachycardia? And why does it respond to verapamil when scar-related ventricular tachycardias will develop a profound cardiovascular collapse if given verapamil?

> **PEARL |** Just to keep things in perspective – *posterior* fascicular tachycardias are VERY RARE, but *anterior* fascicular tachycardias are EXTREMELY RARE!

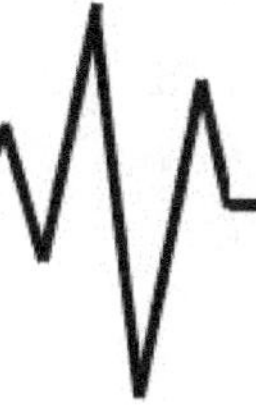

Electrocardiographic Signature

RBBB pattern in Lead V1

Left axis deviation with rS complexes in Leads II, III and aVF, or

Right axis deviation with qR waves in Leads II, III and aVF (Very Rare)

Relatively narrow QRS complexes ($\leq$ 140 msec and usually $\leq$ 130 msec)

R peak time (formerly intrinsicoid deflection) in V1 < 80 msec

Early precordial transition (before Lead V1)

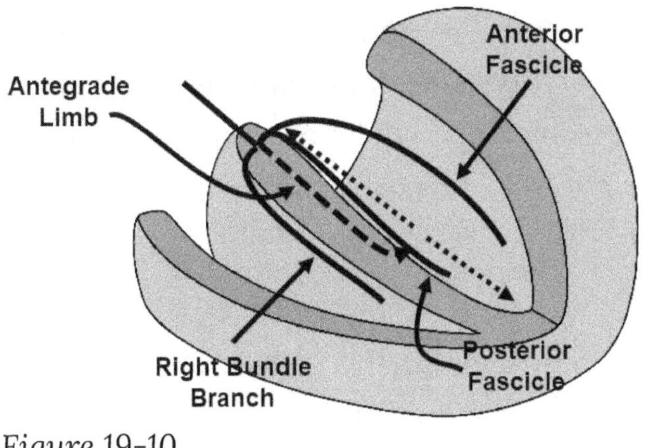

Figure 19-10

Fascicular tachycardias are based either in the *posterior* fascicle (more common) or the *anterior* fascicle (rare). There have been reports of a septal fascicular tachycardia, but that is quite the rarity and you need not concern yourself with it. By far, the most common fascicular tachycardia is the *posterior* fascicular tachycardia. In these tachycardias, the posterior fascicle acts as the *retrograde limb*, and another pathway – still not clearly defined – acts as the *antegrade limb*. The proximal turn-around is the junction of the right and left bundle branches at the end of the His bundle. The distal turn-around is likely somewhere in the septum, between the mid- and apical septum. That is where the antegrade limb joins the posterior fascicle and activates it.

Again, note that the word "ventricular" is not part of the nomenclature here. "Ventricular" is assumed because the posterior and anterior fascicles are not located in the atria.

Look at the diagram of the conducting pathways (Figure 19-10) and locate the *antegrade limb* – it's the arrow with the larger dashes traveling down the middle of the septum. As you can see, it connects with the posterior fascicle *before* its termination at the posterior papillary muscle. At that point, you see two smaller arrows with much smaller dashes. One arrow is pointing proximally and the other, distally. This means that at the point of connection, an impulse travels *proximally* up the posterior fascicle to continue the reentry circuit while, at the same time, another impulse travels *distally* to activate the left ventricle. It should be apparent that the portion of the posterior fascicle conducting *distally* does not participate in the reentry loop – only the portion of the posterior fascicle from the connection with the antegrade limb proximally to the top of the circuit is part of the reentry loop.

> **PEARL |** Because the posterior fascicle is being activated *before* the anterior fascicle, the ECG will have the appearance of an anterior fascicular block (RBBB or RBBB-like morphology in Lead V1 and negative QRS complexes in the inferior leads). But there is no anterior fascicular block present! This is an ectopic tachycardia and QRS morphologies represent either the *origin* of the dysrhythmia or the *order* of activation – not a *block!*

Although there is a reentry circuit, conduction stays mainly within the His-Purkinje system and the QRS complex is often not much wider than if there were an anterior fascicular block. Look closely at the diagram so you can understand the mechanism of the tachycardia.

Now WHY is this ventricular tachycardia responsive to verapamil while verapamil can be so deadly if given to a scar-related ventricular tachycardia? The reason is that the antegrade pathway passes through myocardium that uses the slow L-type calcium channels for initiating the action potential. The functioning of these calcium channels is not based on the activation of the cyclic AMP (cAMP) pathway, so adenosine will have no effect. Of course, verapamil, being a calcium channel blocker, will cause termination of the reentry circuit.

> **PEARL |** The narrowest QRS complexes during ventricular tachycardia are those *very rare* tachycardias that originate in the basal septum and enter both bundle branches immediately and simultaneously. The second most narrow are the *fascicular tachycardias* and in third place are the *outflow tract tachycardias*.

Here is an example (Figure 19-11, next page) of an *anterior* fascicular tachycardia (very rare!)...

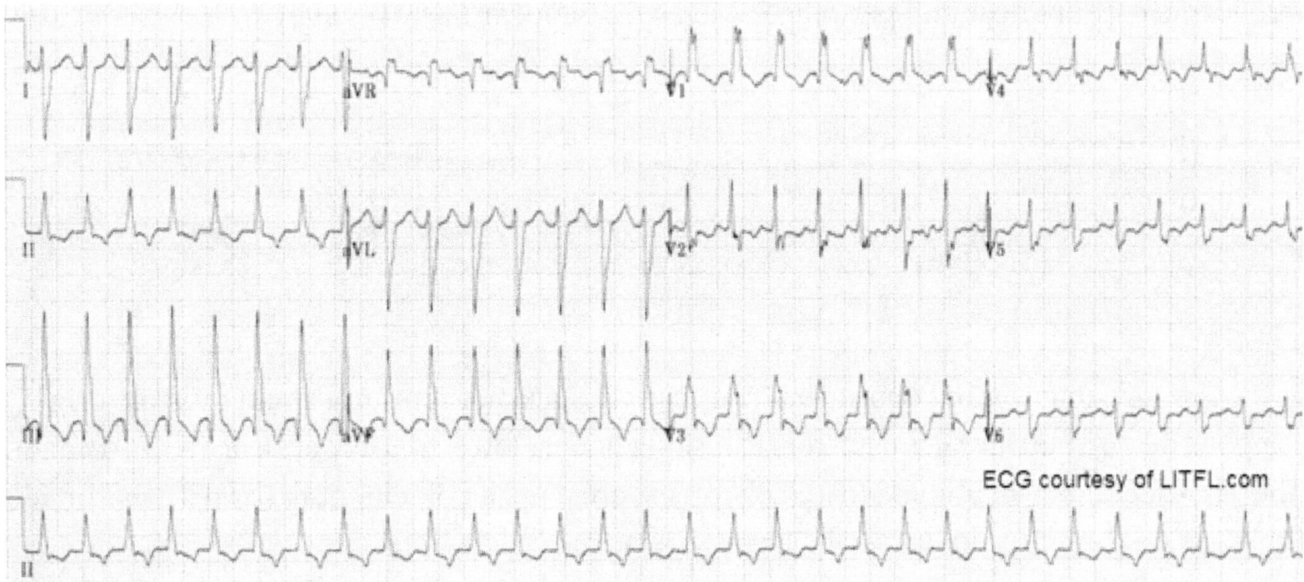

Figure 19-11

Note that there is still an RBBB-like morphology in Lead V1 but now a right axis deviation. The inferior leads manifest an inferior axis with upward-pointing QRS complexes.

"But there's a problem," you exclaim. "That's the same description as an LVOT tachycardia! How can you differentiate an LVOT tachycardia from an anterior fascicular tachycardia?" The answer lies in Chapter 23!

Where is the precordial transition and what does it indicate to you? The precordial transition occurred *before* Lead V1. This indicates that the impulse is originating in the left ventricle, likely more laterally than the area of the interventricular septum. This is in accordance with the distribution of the anterior fascicle (anterolaterally).

> **TIP |** Look for a QRS duration of less than 140 msec and usually less than 130 msec) and an R peak time of less than 80 msec. An RBBB-like morphology and a left axis deviation with a *wide* QRS are very *unlikely* to be a fascicular tachycardia!

> **EXTRA! |** There are signs of AV dissociation in this snippet (Figure 19-12). Can you find them?

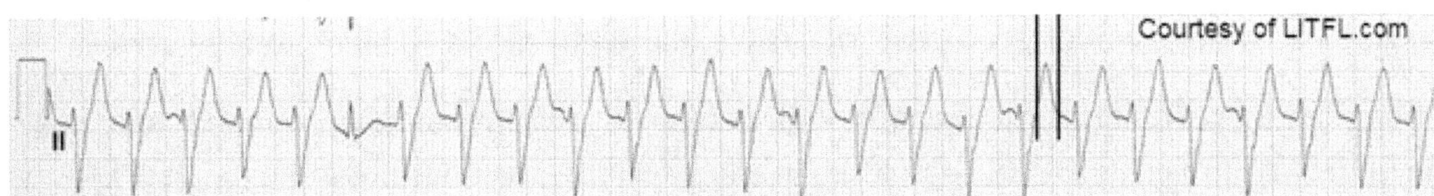

Figure 19-12

There is one capture beat and periodic P waves that appear fairly regularly.

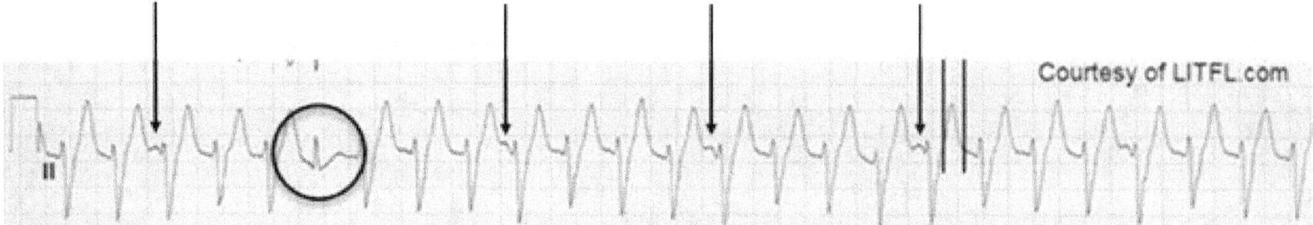

Figure 19-13

The P waves are *upright and appear in Lead II* so they are *not retrograde* and must be orig-inating in the right atrium – most likely the sinus node. However, they appear *regularly* and in the *same location* each time. Most likely this represents a coincidental, fixed isorhythmic ratio between the sinus node and the fascicular tachycardia circuit.

Now please pay attention: here is one of my most *serious* recommendations...

IMPORTANT! | Do NOT give verapamil or any other calcium channel blocker to a patient with a wide complex tachycardia *if you are not absolutely certain of your diagnosis of fascicular tachycardia* nor have any *experience in handling a patient in profound cardiovascular collapse.* While I do NOT feel that ALL patients with a wide complex tachycardia should be *automatically* cardioverted, let me be the first to say that if you aren't confident handling wide complex tachycardias – *but you find yourself in a situation where you MUST!* – a correctly implemented D/C cardioversion is *by far* – BY FAR! – the safest and most efficacious option for terminating the tachydysrhythmia.

One More Thing...

You will often encounter throughout this book my adage "Nothing good comes out of the apex!" And that is true... for *ectopic tachycardias occurring in the presence of structural heart disease.* When the tachycardias begin in the conducting fibers themselves, it's a different matter.

As you may have begun to notice, all negative QRS (rS, QS) complexes in the inferior leads can indicate an origin in the apex of the right or left ventricle, but... all negative complexes in the inferior leads can also indicate a posterior fascicular tachycardia – a *benign* tachycardia.

When the tachycardia fits the description (Electronic Signature) of a fascicular tachycardia, the finding of all negative QRS complexes in the inferior leads does *not* indicate an origin in the apex – it indicates that the posterior fascicle has activated before the anterior fascicle.

So when I say that "Nothing good comes out of the apex," that is in reference to regular, monomorphic ventricular tachycardias due to structural heart disease which are by far the most common tachycardias to originate in the apex.

OK, really... just one last thing to emphasize...

The benign, idiopathic VTs can exist without any evidence of structural heart disease – that's why they are called "idiopathic." On the other hand, *they can also exist in the presence of structural heart disease – although not CAUSED by it*. As explained earlier, what may have begun as a benign tachycardia may "morph" into a very dangerous and lethal tachydysrhythmia if the impulses find an area of scar!

Uhh... did I hear you say you wanted just one more PEARL?

PEARL | A patient with a *wide complex tachycardia* who is stable and in no distress is no proof of an SVT with aberrancy. A patient with a *known ventricular tachycardia* who is stable and in no distress is no proof of a benign, idiopathic tachycardia. A patient with scar-related ventricular tachycardia can appear stable and sometimes in no distress at all. The difference is... the patient with scar-related tachycardia could suffer a cardiovascular collapse at any moment!

Recommended Reading:

Callans DJ, MD, et al. Repetitive Monomorphic Tachycardia From the Left Ventricular Outflow Tract: Electrocardiographic Patterns Consistent With a Left Ventricular Site of Origin. JACC. Vol. 29, No. 5 April 1997:1023±7.

Conti GS, MD et al. Right Ventricular Outflow Tract Arrhythmias: Benign Or Early Stage Arrhythmogenic Right Ventricular Cardiomyopathy/Dysplasia? *Journal of Atrial Fibrillation.* Volume 7: Issue 4; Dec 2014-Jan 2015.

Francis J, MD, Venugopal K, MD, Sudhayakumar N, Khadar SA, MD, Anoop K. Gupta AK MD FACC. Idiopathic Fascicular Ventricular Tachycardia. *Indian Pacing and Electrophysiology Journal.* 4(3): 98-103 (2004).

Kapa S, MD; Gaba P, BS; DeSimone CV, MD PhD, Asirvatham SJ, MD. Fascicular Ventricular Arrhythmias – Pathophysiologic Mechanisms, Anatomical Constructs, and Advances in Approaches to Management. *Circ Arrhythm Electrophysiol.* 2017; 1-14.

Kumagai K, MD. Idiopathic ventricular arrhythmias arising from the left ventricular outflow tract: Tips and tricks. *Journal of Arrhythmia.* 30 (2014) 211–221.

Schiefermueller J. Ventricular Tachycardias in Structurally Normal Hearts - A Case Report and Review of the Literature. *Int J Crit Care Emerg Med.* 4(1); 2018.

Chapter 20

Polymorphic Ventricular Tachycardia I

Torsade de Pointes

Let's begin by seeing how much you may (or may not) already know about **polymorphic ventricular tachycardias** in general...

Are you familiar with this pattern of ventricular tachycardia (Figure 20-1)?

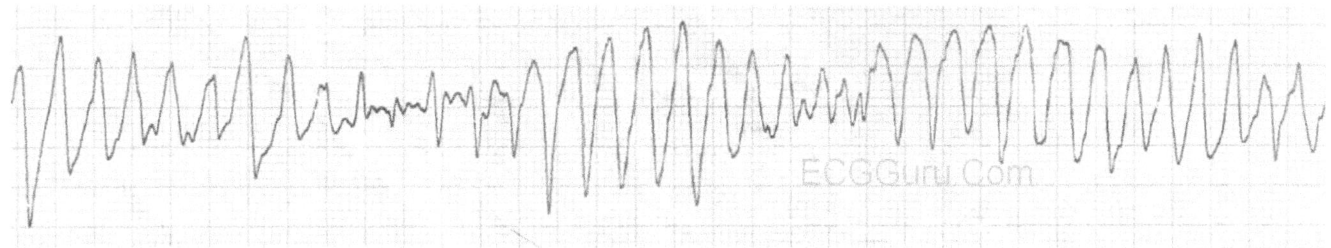

Figure 20-1

Can you identify it?

If you said *torsade de pointes* (TdP) – then you *aren't* familiar with this type of tachydysrhythmia! All that can be said is that it is a *polymorphic ventricular tachycardia* – a much more *general* term. What makes you think this is torsade de pointes? The spindle-shaped episodes in which the polarity changes from negative to positive and appears to "twist" around the baseline? The other polymorphic VTs that have *no connection* to torsade de pointes can look *the same*. Is it because TdP always occurs with a prolonged QT interval? You're *right*, but... can you show me a prolonged QT interval on this rhythm strip? You can't, can you?

The truth is that you don't know WHAT this tachycardia represents for certain *without more information* – and by more information, I mean *significant personal knowledge of this patient and/or a previous ECG recorded during sinus rhythm, preferably at the onset of the polymorphic VT*. In most monomorphic VTs, we study the QRS complexes during the tachycardia to learn more about them. With polymorphic ventricular tachycardias, we need to see the ECG during sinus rhythm to properly diagnose them. There is no need to show you a "documented episode" of torsades de pointes because it would look exactly like what you see in Figure 20-1.

What IS polymorphic ventricular tachycardia?

Ventricular tachycardias can also be divided into *monomorphic* and *polymorphic* based on the morphology of the QRS complexes during the tachycardia. **Monomorphic** ("one shape") means that all the QRS complexes *within a given lead* will look the same, i.e., all the QRS complexes in Lead II will look the same – but they may not look like the QRS complexes in Leads aVR or V1, for instance. Polymorphic ("multiple shapes") means that there are different QRS morphologies within the *same* lead.

Polymorphic VT itself can be expressed in different forms: as...

    1. a simple variations in the QRS complexes:

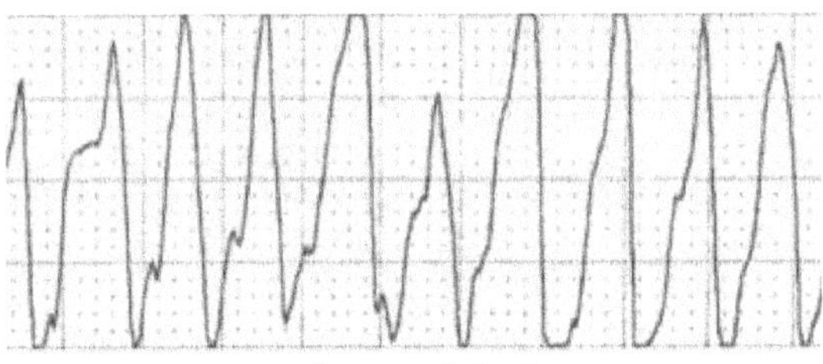

Figure 20-2

2. the iconic spindle-shaped polymorphic VT:

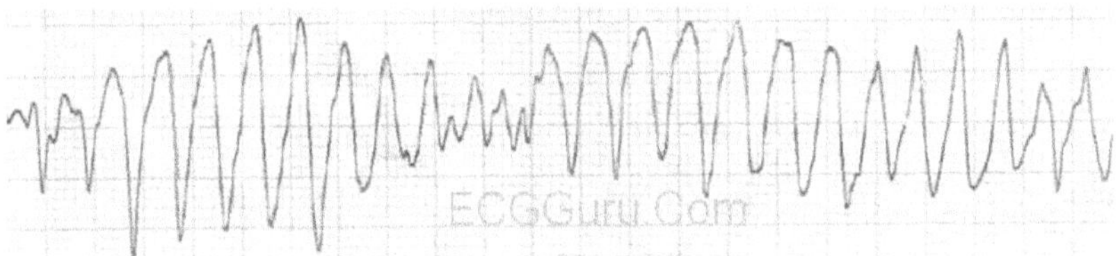

Figure 20-3

3. and bidirectional VT:

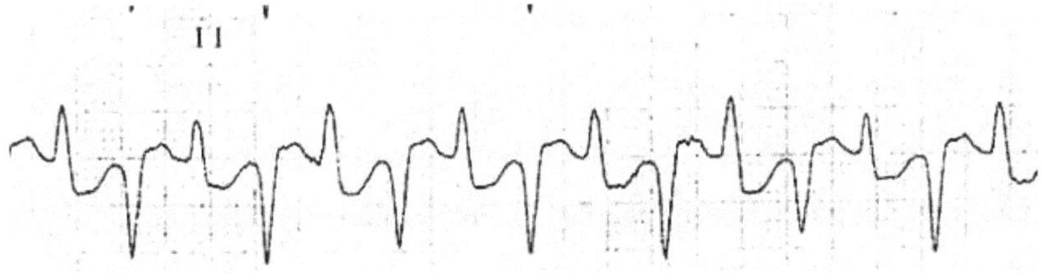

Figure 20-4

Torsade de Pointes

Torsade de pointes is the *only* polymorphic ventricular tachycardia associated with the long QT syndrome. Consequently – as demonstrated in the example that opened this chapter – if you cannot show that the spindle-shaped tachycardia is occurring in the presence of a baseline QTc prolongation, you cannot call it torsade de pointes. It should remain a polymorphic VT until the association with the long QT interval is demonstrated.

What is the **Electronic Signature** for Torsade de Points?

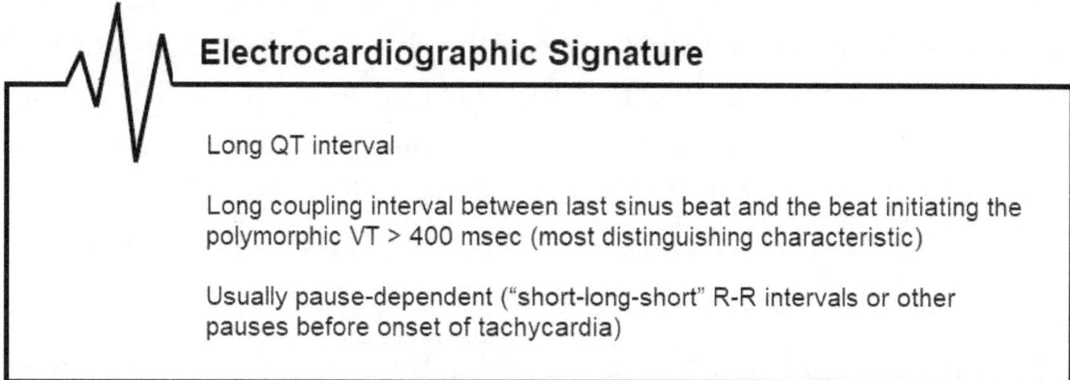

The Origins of Torsade de Pointes

A long QT interval promotes and potentiates torsade de pointes by two methods:

1. prolonged repolarization allows more Ca^{++} to enter the cell during bradycardia and pauses and

2. an increased heart rate that promotes the entry of extra Ca^{++} into the cell.

Let's address each one of these methods...

Prolonging Repolarization

By prolonging repolarization, more Ca^{++} enters the cell during Phase 2 and the myocyte becomes overloaded with Ca^{++}. To remove the extra Ca^{++}, the **sodium–calcium exchanger (NCX)** is activated. This will exchange ONE intracellular Ca^{++} ion for THREE extracellular Na^+ ions. This transport of Ca^{++} out of the cell results in an inward positive Na^+ current. Since *all inward positive currents are depolarizing currents*, this Na^+ current counteracts the outward K^+ currents trying to repolarize the cell. If strong enough, the inward Na^+ current will overwhelm the outward current and an early afterdepolarization occurs. If that early afterdepolarization reaches the threshold potential it will produce a PVC – usually during Phase 3, the T wave. Thus, an "R-on-T" phenomenon occurs. Because the QT prolongation is potentiated by bradycardia and pauses, these LQTS are referred to as *pause-dependent*.

Increased Heart Rate Introducing More Ca^{++} Into the Cell

With some long QT syndromes, a faster heart rate allows for more entry of Ca^{++} into the cell with every heartbeat. These long QT syndromes are potentiated by catecholamines which promote Ca^{++} entry. The extra Ca^{++} entering from the outside may cause a release of even greater Ca^{++} stores within the cell and the resulting Na^{+}/Ca^{++} exchanger goes into action. You know the rest. These LQTS are referred to as *tachycardia-dependent*. Although torsade de pointes is not really considered tachycardia-dependent, it can occur during episodes of acquired LQTS which are tachycardia-dependent due to the "short-long-short" sequence of intervals. The long pause is interjected and the torsade de pointes may then develop.

> **TIP |** Most people think that the Ca^{++} entering the cell is what precipitates excitation-contraction coupling – but it isn't. The Ca^{++} *entering* the cell during Phase 2 is just the "trigger" for the release of truly massive Ca^{++} stores from within the sarcoplasmic reticulum.

Differentiating Torsade de Pointes from Non-torsade Polymorphic VT

It is important to know if you are dealing with a torsade de pointes or a non-torsade polymorphic VT because they have very different causes, very different treatments, and somewhat different prognoses.

To distinguish between torsade de pointes and non-torsade VT we use the fact that there is a QTc prolongation during torsade de pointes but no significant QTc prolongation in non-torsade polymorphic VT.

First – let's understand a very important piece of information:

Both forms of polymorphic ventricular tachycardia can look the same *during* the tachycardia. You may not be able to distinguish one from the other!

Of course, this is regarding types 1 and 2 as shown at the beginning of the chapter. Torsade de pointes *never* presents with bidirectional VT.

To properly distinguish torsade de pointes from non-torsade polymorphic VT, **you will need to see some of the sinus rhythm and the point at which the polymorphic VT was initiated.**

Why sinus rhythm? Is that to see if a prolonged QTc is present?

If the prolonged QTc were significant – over 500 msec, then "Yes!" – that would be enough to make a distinction. However, non-torsade polymorphic VT patients can occasionally have slightly prolonged QT intervals, also. This can lead to an overlap of QT intervals between the two forms of polymorphic VTs. There is a better way to distinguish them...

We use the *coupling interval* of the last sinus-conducted beat and the beat that initiates the polymorphic VT – whether it's torsade or non-torsade.

Important Definition! | A *coupling interval* is the distance from the *onset* of a sinus-conducted QRS to the *onset* of an ectopic QRS that immediately follows it. It *suggests* – but *does not necessarily establish* – a relationship between the two beats.

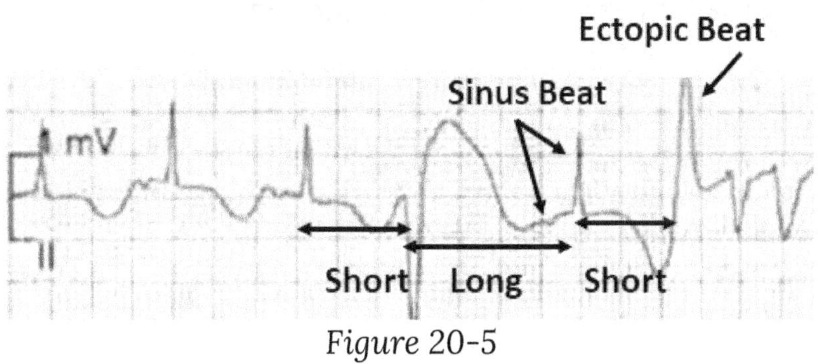

Figure 20-5

The coupling interval that we are interested in is the one that begins with the P-QRS labeled "Sinus Beat" (Figure 20-5). The sinus beat is followed by an ectopic beat at – or near – the end of the inverted T wave, which initiates the tachycardia. Note that the coupling interval is greater than two large squares (400 msec). Note the abnormally enlarged T waves indicated by the dotted arrows. This is typical of the onset of torsade de pointes.

Because of the prolonged QT interval, the coupling intervals for torsade de pointes will be long – at least 400 msec and often a lot longer.

Non-torsade polymorphic VT is not associated with a prolonged QT interval, so a coupling interval at the onset of the tachycardia will be shorter – 400 msec or less.

PEARL | Torsade de pointes will have a longer coupling interval because of the prolongation of the QTc. Since non-torsade polymorphic VT is not associated with a significantly prolonged QTc, its coupling interval will be shorter.

So, in a "nutshell"...

Coupling Interval > 400 msec: **Torsade de Pointes**

Coupling Interval ≤ 400 msec: **Non-torsade polymorphic VT**

There is a phenomenon called the "short-long-short" R-R interval sequence that is frequently used to differentiate torsade de pointes from non-torsade polymorphic VT. If you refer back to Figure 20-5. you will see the words "Short – Long – Short." There is a first short interval caused by the early appearance of a PVC; then a long interval caused by the post-extrasystolic compensatory pause of the PVC which is followed by a sinus-conducted beat; then a second short interval that occurs when a second ectopic beat appears early, ending the second short interval and precipitating the polymorphic VT.

The "short-long-short" sequence is just a setup for the last coupling interval to occur following a pause. Because it is greater than 400 msec, the tachycardia it initiates is a true torsade de pointes. If you want to do more reading about torsade de pointes, you will hear a lot more about the "short-long-short" sequence.

> **TIP |** The coupling interval is used to distinguish *torsade de pointes* from *non-torsade polymorphic* **VT**. It does NOT differentiate between *congenital* and *acquired* LQTS.

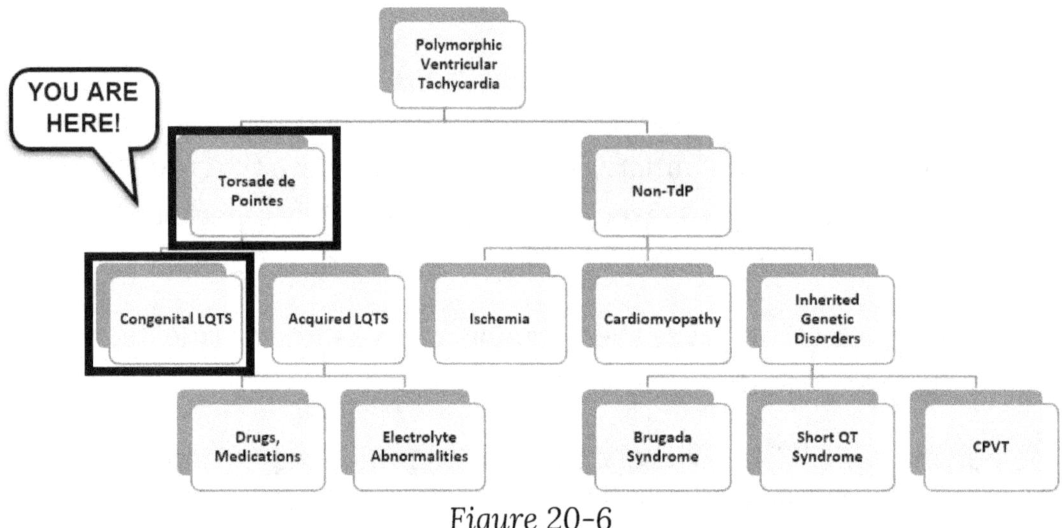

Figure 20-6

Congenital and Acquired LQTS

Because torsade de pointes only appears in patients with some form of the LQTS, let's learn a little more about the congenital and acquired forms.

There are many forms of LQTS – 16, to be precise – and that's just at the time of this writing. Don't worry. Unless you want to be an expert in the field, you don't have to learn any of them.

Congenital LQTS is rare. It is very unlikely that you will have to deal with it – but if you must, it is treated with magnesium sulfate intravenously along with cardioversion/defibrillation if sustained. Just do not give or do *anything* to accelerate the sinus heart rate. Many of the congenital LQTS are potentiated by catecholamines (exercise, emotional stress) which can lead to torsade de pointes.

> **CAUTION! |** The lack of a prolonged QTc on a previous ECG does <u>NOT</u> rule out torsade de pointes – it only rules out *torsade de pointes due to <u>congenital</u> LQTS!* And even then, there are rare exceptions.

A patient may have been on a medication for a long time that is known to prolong the QT interval with no problems; but a case of gastroenteritis, with fever, vomiting, and diarrhea may lower the serum K^+ level to the point that torsade de pointes develops. Thus, **QT-prolonging medication PLUS fever PLUS hypokalemia** (and possibly **hypomagnesemia**) EQUALS **torsade de pointes**.

> **PEARL |** With an acquired LQTS, it may take more than just the QT prolongation to initiate a torsade de pointes.

Acquired long QT syndromes are *pause-dependent*. Exceptions are quite rare, so don't concern yourself with them. Therefore, in addition to defibrillation (when necessary) and intravenous magnesium sulfate, increasing the heart rate will usually get the paroxysms of torsade de pointes under control. Administering intravenous isoproterenol is a good way to increase the heart rate to around 90 – 110 beats/minute until a temporary pacemaker can be placed. Do not, however, give isoproterenol to a patient with a *congenital* LQTS. LQTS 2 and LQTS 3 are pause-dependent, but LQTS 1 is tachycardia-dependent and it is felt to be more common than the other two together.

> **CAUTION! |** Do NOT give or do anything to a patient to accelerate their heart rate if there is any possibility of a congenital form of LQTS.

> **PEARL |** *Magnesium sulfate will not terminate an episode of torsade de pointes*; its efficacy is in **preventing the onset** of another paroxysmal episode once it does stop.

More on Distinguishing Torsade de Pointes from Non-Torsade Polymorphic VT

It is important to distinguish torsade de pointes from non-torsade polymorphic VT. The causes, treatments, and prognoses differ. You cannot treat ALL polymorphic VTs the same way!

I introduced you to the concept of the coupling interval as a distinguishing factor between *torsade de pointes* and *non-torsade polymorphic* VT earlier in this chapter. Now, let's learn a bit more and put that knowledge to practical use!

> **TIP |** I do not want to give you the impression that *torsade de pointes* is dangerous while *non-torsade polymorphic* VT is not. They are *equally* dangerous and potentially lethal. There is *nothing* benign about *any* polymorphic ventricular tachycardia! **They are ALL extremely dangerous due to their tendency to rapidly degenerate into ventricular fibrillation!**

Here is a rhythm strip demonstrating polymorphic ventricular tachycardia. Decide if it represents a torsade de pointes or a non-torsade polymorphic VT. The coupling interval is designated by the line with an asterisk below it.

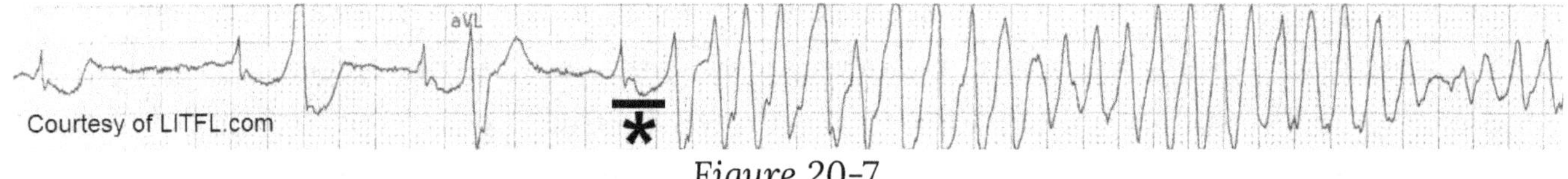

Figure 20-7

Let's take a closer look at that coupling interval. (See how a magnifying lens can help?)

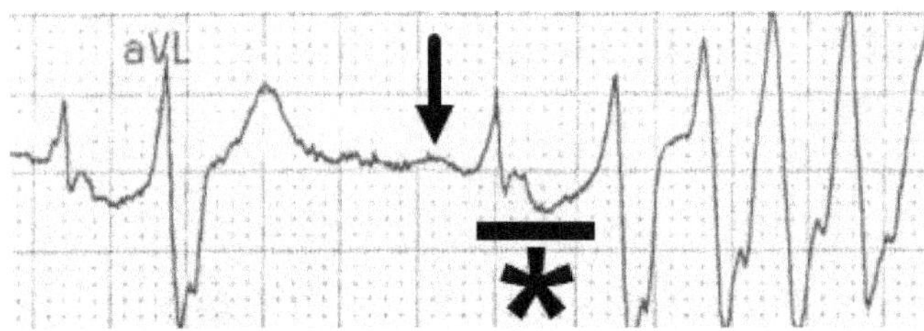

Figure 20-8 Snippet courtesy of LITFL.com

The arrow indicates the P wave of the sinus conducted complex (Figure 20-8). The coupling interval is approximately 280 msec. That's *very short!* Again, please note that the coupling interval is measured from *onset* of QRS to *onset* of QRS – it is *not* measured from R-wave-peak to R-wave-peak! By simply looking at the full rhythm strip (Figure 20-7) you can see that there is no significant QT prolongation (if any at all).

PEARL | You have already heard of the infamous "R-on-T" phenomenon. You may have thought that it was caused by a "random" PVC that just happened to appear on the downslope of the T wave. No, it wasn't "random." That would be an *early afterdepolarization*. Also, the vulnerable period can exist on the upslope of an inverted T wave.

TIP | While torsade de pointes can occur in LQTS 1 due to strenuous exercise, non-torsade VT can also occur due to strenuous activity: catecholaminergic polymorphic VT. Tachycardia-dependent polymorphic VT is not limited to LQTS and torsade de pointes.

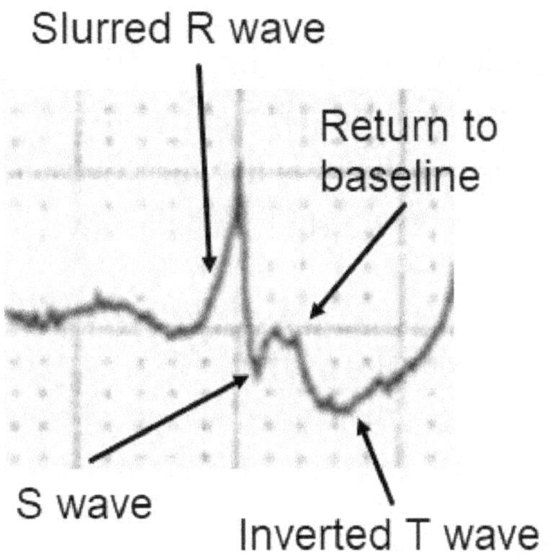

Figure 20-9

Does that sinus-conducted QRS look a little confusing to you? Here is an explanation (Figure 20-9)...

This is a **non-TdP polymorphic ventricular tachycardia**. While the second PVC has provided a pause, it wasn't necessary for the tachycardia to occur. Non-torsade polymorphic VT does not depend on pauses – it is usually caused by acute myocardial ischemia, or occasionally by cardiomyopathy or one of the genetically-transmitted channelopathies (Brugada syndrome, short QT syndrome, or catecholaminergic polymorphic VT). More on this in the next chapter...

The *coupling interval* is an *excellent discriminating factor* between torsade de pointes and non-torsade polymorphic VT. The coupling interval for non-torsade polymorphic VT is shorter because there is no QT prolongation (or just minimal QT prolongation).

PEARL | To put things in perspective: although the coupling interval only needs to be greater than 400 msec for a diagnosis of torsade de pointes, it is *rarely* below 500 msec, and durations in the 600s and 700s are quite common.

Coupling interval ≤ 400 msec: non-TdP polymorphic ventricular tachycardia

Coupling interval > 400 msec: torsade de pointes

Practical Exercises

Here are some examples of coupling intervals leading into polymorphic ventricular tachycardia to help you improve your diagnostic skills. Your ability to...

    1. *locate the correct coupling interval* and

    2. *determine whether it is long or short* (greater than or less than 400 msec, respectively)

...are *essential skills!* Again – we are differentiating torsade de pointes from non-torsade polymorphic VT.

    PEARL | Electrical storms are not unusual with these tachydysrhythmias!

If you can determine whether the polymorphic VT is torsade de pointes or non-torsade polymorphic VT, then you can manage the patient more *effectively,* more *efficiently,* and more *specifically.* Now, try to determine whether the rhythm is *true torsade de pointes* or *non-torsade polymorphic VT.* I have added black marks at the top of the rhythm strips every 200 msec (one large square).

I'll help you with the first one (Figure 20-10). The first R-R interval is representative of the base rate and rhythm.

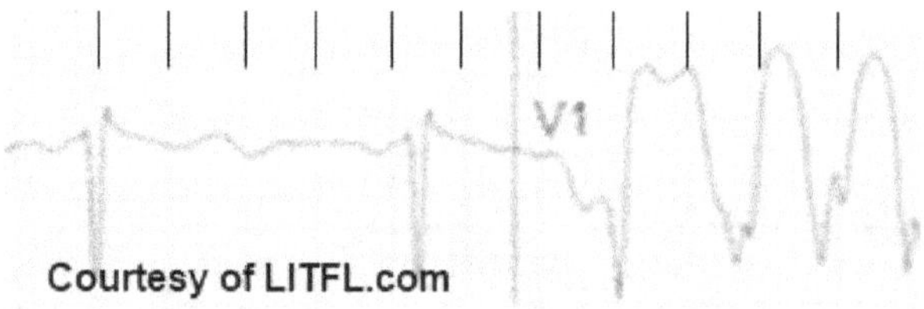

Courtesy of LITFL.com

Figure 20-10

    TIP | The *R-R interval* is measured from the *beginning* of a **QRS complex** to the *beginning* of the next **QRS complex**. The *actual morphology* of the QRS is irrelevant. There does *not* have to be an R wave present.

The third QRS complex (inverted) is *early,* so no matter how "normal" it appears, *it cannot be a sinus beat.* It must be due to an ectopic focus! Remember: the coupling interval is from the *onset* of the last sinus-conducted QRS to the *onset* of the QRS of the *ectopic beat that initiates the tachycardia.* That ectopic beat may or may not be separated slightly from the first beat of the polymorphic VT; regardless, *there will not be another sinus beat between it and the tachycardia.*

Did you note the length of the coupling interval of Figure 20-10? Is it greater than or less than 400 msec? What is your diagnosis? The coupling interval was greater than 400 msec, so you should have diagnosed *torsade de pointes.*

PEARL | Measurement of the coupling interval need not be *exact*. Just remember that two large squares equals 400 msec. Two and one-half large squares equals 500 msec.

TIP | Five hundred is a significant number for torsade de pointes: it rarely appears until the QTc is greater than 500 msec and its coupling intervals are usually more than 500 msec.

Now I want you to assess some more coupling intervals on your own! You will probably need your ECG calipers (you DO have some good calipers, don't you?).

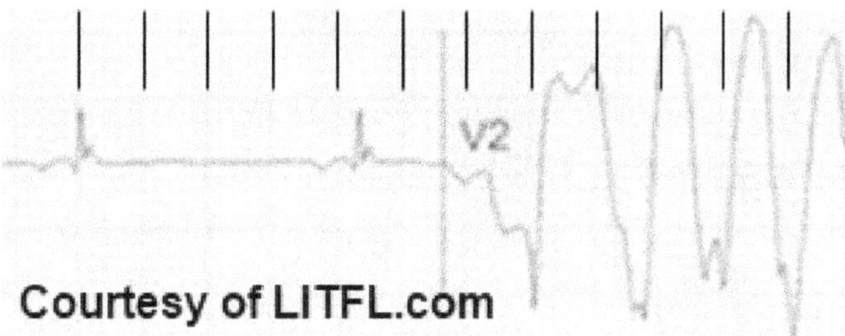

Figure 20-11

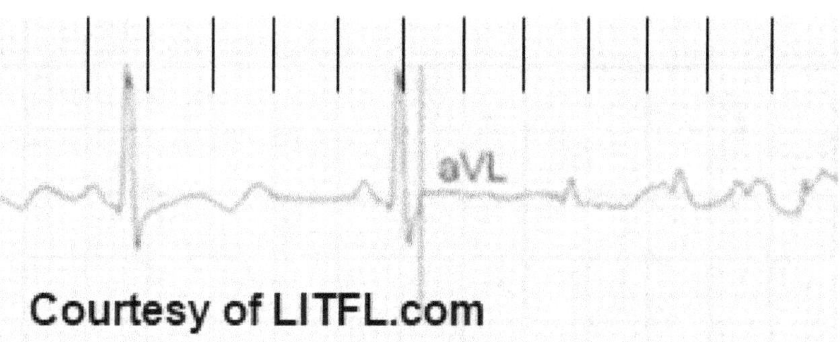

Figure 20-12

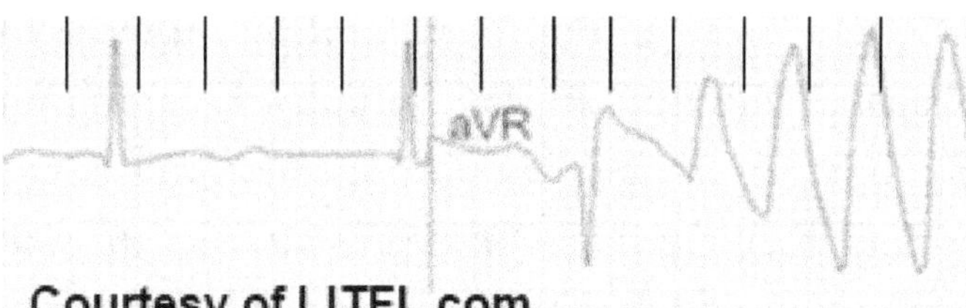

Figure 20-13

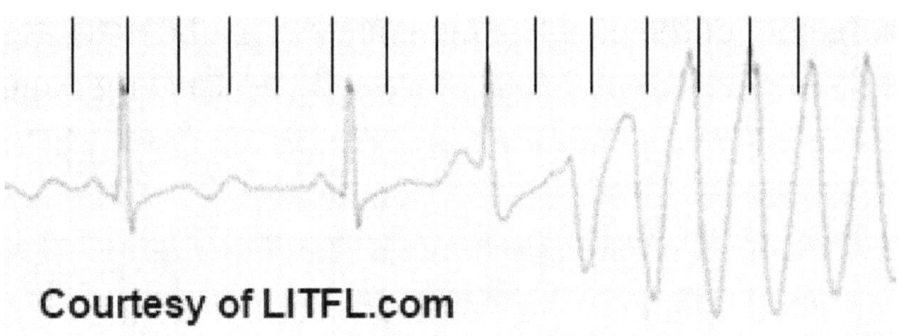

Figure 20-14

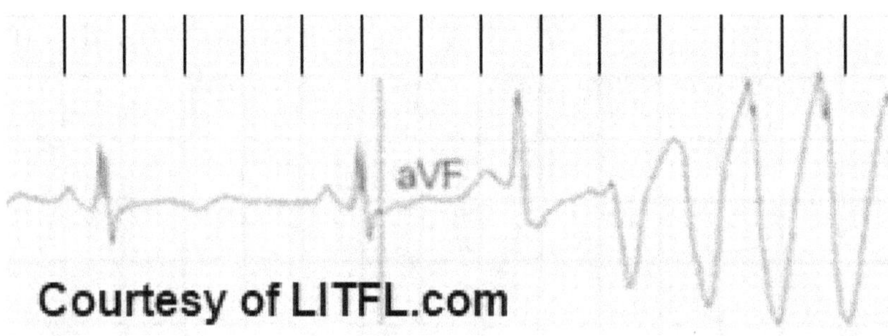

Figure 20-15

Let's take a closer look at Figure 20-15. I've added some notations, so it is now Figure 20-16.

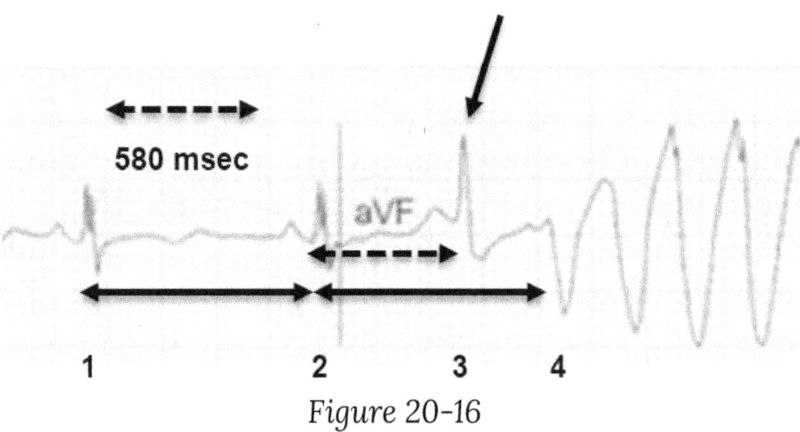

Figure 20-16

Read carefully! I want to make sure you understand this...

The third QRS (Figure 20-16) is an *ectopic* beat because it is *early*. The second QRS is the *last* sinus conducted beat *before* the tachycardia. The **coupling interval** you should measure will be from the **onset of the second QRS (last sinus conducted beat) to the onset of the third QRS (premature ectopic beat)** indicated by the dashed double-headed arrow. **The coupling interval is from the last sinus-conducted QRS to the QRS that initiates the polymorphic tachycardia.** That fourth wide rS complex is not *initiating* the polymorphic VT – it IS the polymorphic VT! **It would not be there were it not for that third (ectopic) beat!**

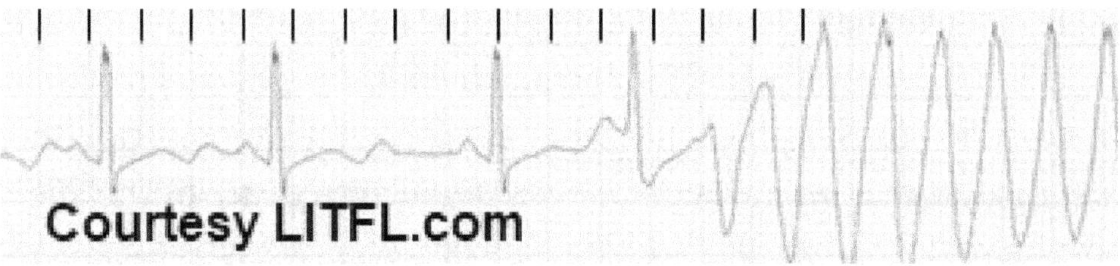

Figure 20-17 (Figure 20-14 repeated)

Figure 20-17 is an example of a true **torsade de pointes**. Again, we have the benefit of seeing some sinus rhythm along with the onset of the tachycardia. The long coupling interval is highly characteristic of true torsade de pointes and based on that, we can make a diagnosis.

Did you happen to notice where the early beat appeared? On the *downslope of the T wave* of the previous beat – the vulnerable period! This is an *early afterdepolarization (occurring during Phase 3 of the action potential)* that reached the threshold potential and resulted in *triggered activity!*

> **PEARL |** Did you also notice that none of the torsade de pointes began as a "spindle-shaped" tachycardia?

Remember: if you have a strip of only the tachycardia, you cannot distinguish between the two tachydysrhythmias (torsade de pointes and non-torsade polymorphic VT). Fortunately, both forms of polymorphic VT tend to be short and paroxysmal, so the chances of catching some sinus rhythm on a rhythm strip as the tachycardia starts and stops are actually pretty good.

> **PEARL | ALL *forms of polymorphic ventricular tachycardia are dangerous and potentially lethal!*** That's because they can degenerate into ventricular fibrillation at any moment!

> **Answers Regarding Figures 20-11 to 20-16 |** They are ALL true torsade de pointes!

Some Advice About Managing Polymorphic Ventricular Tachycardia

Advice #1 | If the patient is experiencing a sustained polymorphic ventricular tachycardia, they will not be stable. Defibrillate immediately and initiate magnesium sulfate 2 gm intravenously! Polymorphic VTs are similar to ventricular fibrillation in that you can't trust the defibrillator to lock onto any R waves to synchronize. If the polymorphic VT is torsade de pointes, the magnesium will help; if it is non-torsade polymorphic VT, it won't help – but it won't hurt, either. So it is always best to start magnesium sulfate even if you aren't sure of the specific type of polymorphic VT!

Advice #2 | *Sustained* episodes of torsade de pointes are infrequent. These tachy-dysrhythmias tend to be very paroxysmal, often not lasting long enough to prepare for defibrillation.

Advice #3 | I often read journal articles in which a physician has a patient with a *sustained* polymorphic ventricular tachycardia, and they terminate it with one shock. I've never been that lucky. My point here is that terminating a *sustained* polymorphic VT may not be as simple as some journal articles and reports may lead you to believe. *Just be prepared for that!* If the patient doesn't cardiovert immediately, don't think you have done something wrong!

Advice #4 | Because of its paroxysmal nature, you will discover very quickly that your goal is not only to *terminate* an ongoing tachydysrhythmia but mostly to *prevent* it from recurring once it has stopped.

Advice #5 | All long QT syndrome patients should be on beta blockers! The *tachycardia-dependent* LQT syndromes are driven by adrenergic input causing the rate to increase, so you want to cool that down as much as possible. The *pause-de-pendent* LQT syndromes depend on the pauses to allow more calcium ions to enter the cell. Since beta-<u>agonists</u> promote calcium entry leading to afterdepolarizations and triggered activity, beta-<u>blockers</u> can help prevent that from happening.

Advice #6 | Shock *if you must* – but do your best to keep DC shocks to an absolute minimum! Cardioversion/Defibrillation greatly increases circulating cat-echolamines (even in the *unconscious* patient) which can, in turn, potentiate the development of torsade de pointes. Giving epinephrine intravenously will do the same thing. Catecholamines increase the heart rate, potentiating tachycardia-dependent torsade. Catecholamines also facilitate the entry of Ca^{++} into the cells thus potentiating pause-dependent tachycardia.

Advice #7 | Giving magnesium IV also helps prevent the entry of both Ca^{++} and Na^+ into the cell. Until a more specific diagnosis is entertained, ALL polymorphic VTs should receive IV magnesium. It will not help the non-torsade polymorphic VTs – but at least it won't hurt, either!

Advice #8 | Do not give magnesium sulfate intravenously and then stand back – waiting for something to happen. **<u>Nothing</u> *is going to happen!*** $MgSO_4$ helps *prevent the onset* of torsade de pointes – but it does not affect a sustained tachycardia in progress. You must stop the tachycardia before magnesium can manifest an effect.

Advice #9 | You must either see the onset of the polymorphic ventricular tachycardia or a previous 12-lead ECG in sinus rhythm to diagnose the type of polymorphic ventricular tachycardia (torsade or non-torsade).

Advice #10 | The coupling interval that occurs at the onset of a polymorphic ventricular tachycardia is the best determinant of *torsade de pointes* or *non-torsade polymorphic* VT. The QT intervals can overlap, but there is much less overlap with the coupling intervals. The coupling intervals are visible *only* during the onset of intermittent episodes of polymorphic VT.

Chapter 21

Polymorphic Ventricular Tachycardia II

Non-Torsade Tachycardias

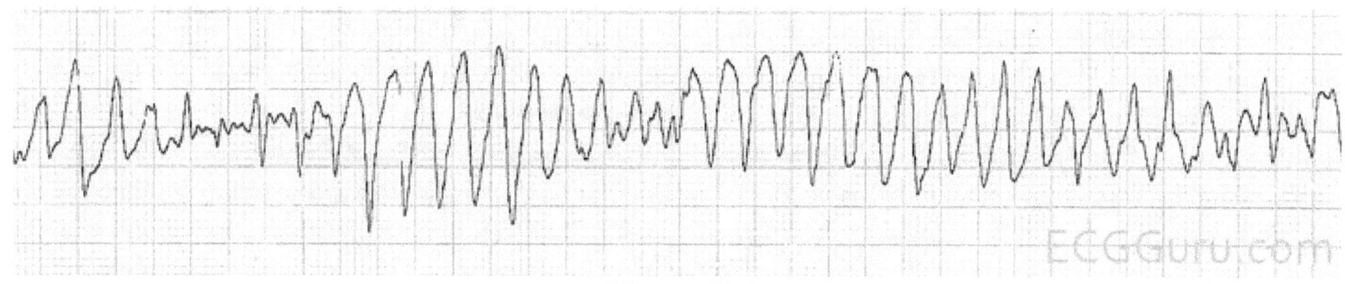

Figure 21-1

Polymorphic means "multiple shapes" and all of these ventricular tachycardias certainly exhibit that. The torsade de pointes and the non-torsade form of polymorphic ventricular tachycardias both exhibit iconic spindle-shaped episodes (Figure 21-1) and catecholaminergic polymorphic ventricular tachycardia occasionally exhibits spindle-shaped episodes in addition to a couple of other forms we will discuss later.

> **PEARL |** As a general rule of thumb, *monomorphic* ventricular tachycardias are *regular*, and *polymorphic* ventricular tachycardias are *irregular*. Most monomorphic ventricular tachycardias are very dangerous rhythms... but a few are benign. ALL polymorphic ventricular tachycardias are very dangerous and potentially lethal!

Non-torsade polymorphic ventricular tachycardia is sometimes called "pseudo-torsade de pointes." However, I prefer **non-torsade polymorphic VT**, and that's the term I will use in this workbook.

It's easy to get lost when you are learning about several new dysrhythmias – they can seem very much alike... a least, superficially. Here are three things to remember:

- All polymorphic VTs are DANGEROUS and potentially LETHAL! ALL of them!

- Patients will not be able to tolerate them for more than a few seconds if sustained before losing consciousness. You will have to be prepared to act quickly.

- Although all can look the same *at times*, they are *very different*.

Again: the only thing they have in common is that all are *extremely dangerous* and *lethal!*

Non-Torsade Polymorphic Ventricular Tachycardia

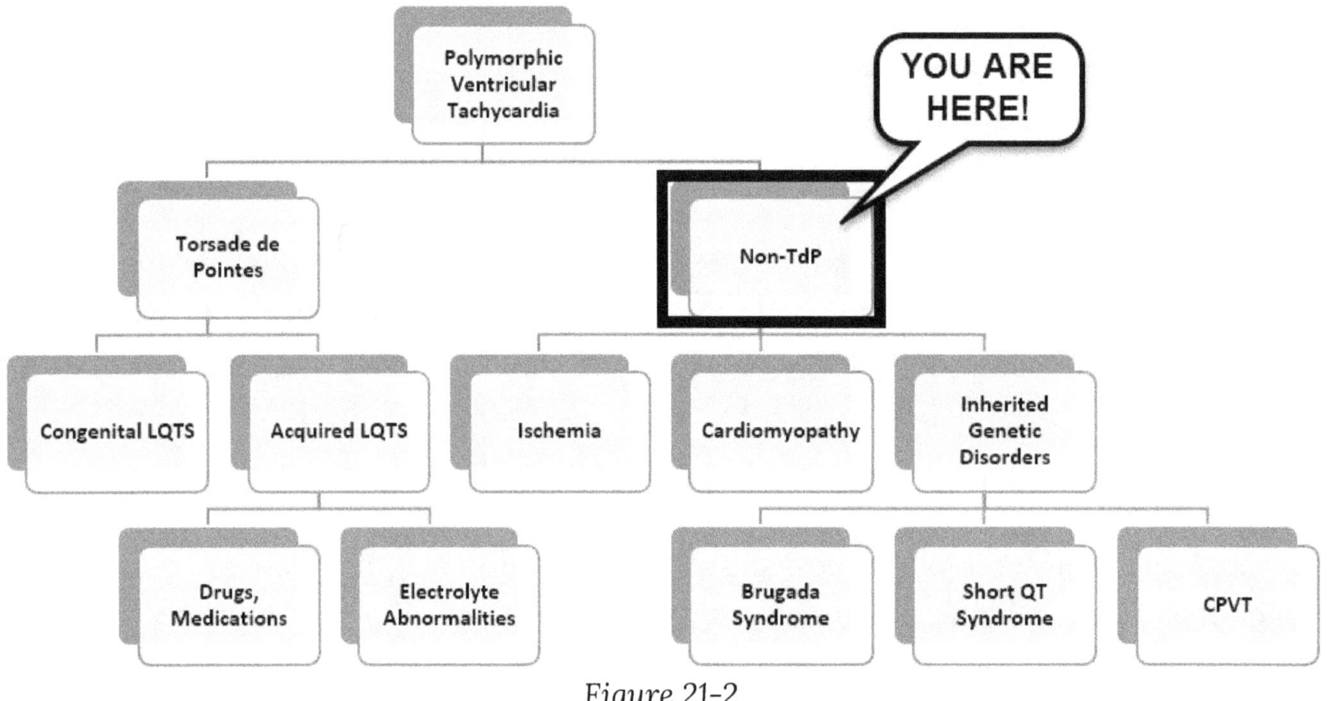

Figure 21-2

There are three basic groups of *non-torsade polymorphic* VTs:

1. **Ischemic**

2. **Cardiomyopathic**

3. **Those due to Inherited Genetic Disorders**

Myocardial ischemia – typically acute, but also chronic – is the *most common cause* of non-TdP polymorphic ventricular tachycardia.

Cardiomyopathies may also produce non-torsade polymorphic VT and include *hypertrophic cardiomyopathy* and *Takotsubo cardiomyopathy*. Hypertrophic cardiomyopathy is the most common source.

Inherited genetic disorders are also a cause of polymorphic ventricular tachycardia. These include the *Brugada syndrome*, the *short QT syndrome*, and *catecholaminergic polymorphic ventricular tachycardia* (CPVT). CPVT may present not only as a non-torsade polymorphic VT – even manifesting "spindle-shaped" episodes, but you will more likely see increased multiform ventricular ectopy (i.e., not spindle-shaped) and/or bidirectional ventricular tachycardia. I will be discussing CPVT at length later in this chapter.

PEARL | ALL *polymorphic VTs are extremely dangerous and potentially lethal, whether torsade de pointes or non-torsade!*

First, the **Electrocardiographic Signature** for *non-torsade polymorphic VT:*

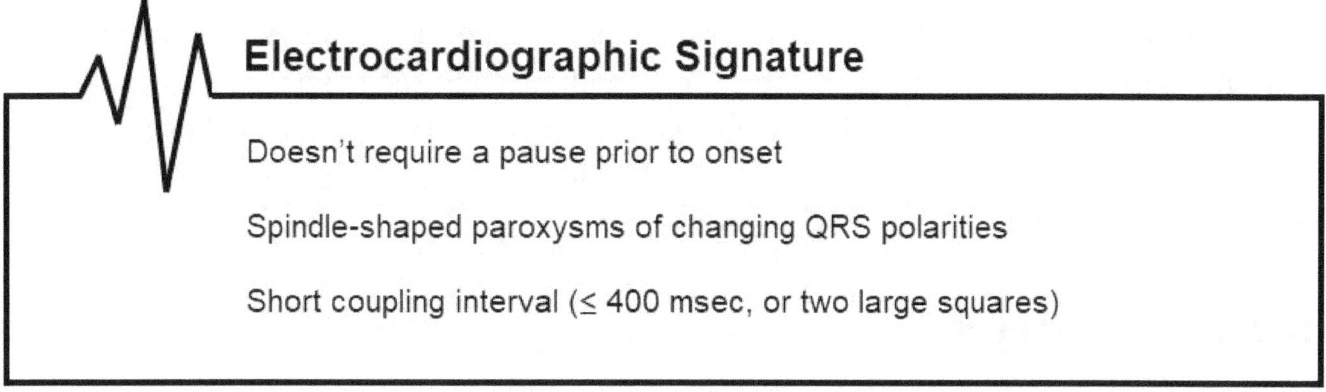

Patients with polymorphic VTs are not going to remain conscious for more than a few seconds after the onset of the dysrhythmia. *Polymorphic VTs are never well-tolerated by the patient* as opposed to idiopathic VTs and even a few monomorphic scar-related VTs.

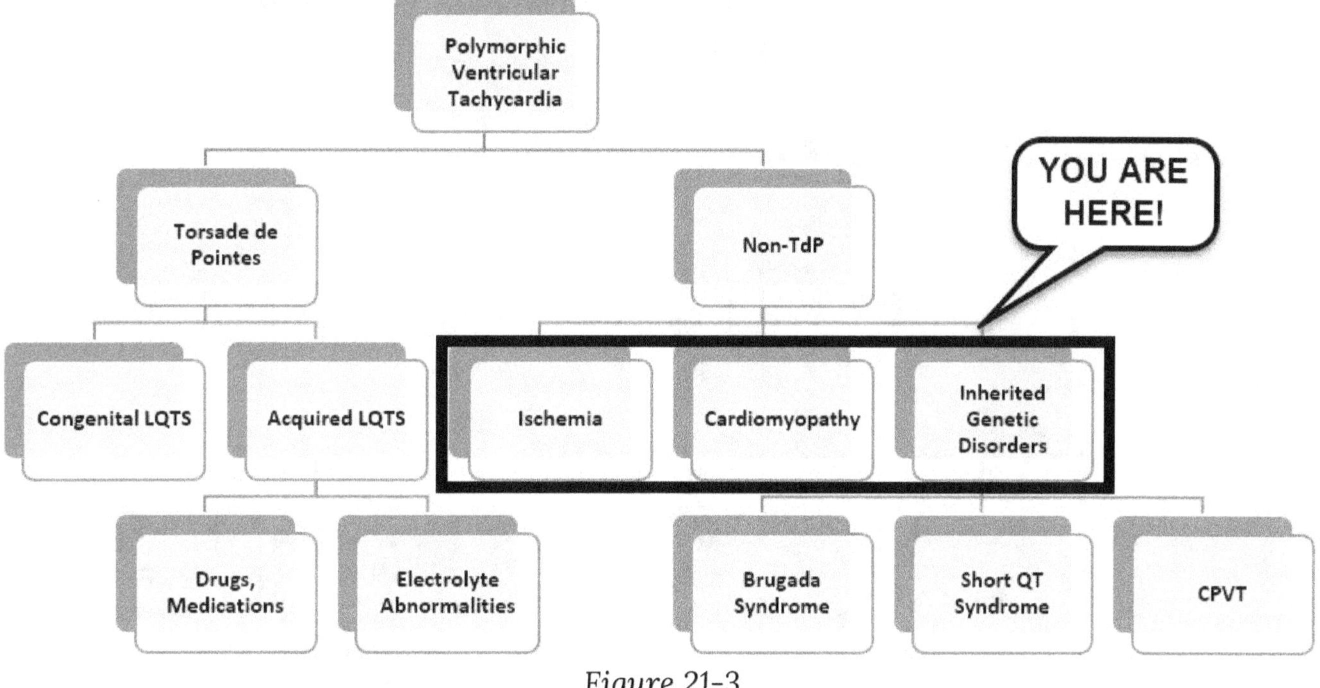

Figure 21-3

ISCHEMIA

The important thing to remember about non-TdP polymorphic ventricular tachycardias is that **the number one cause is ischemia** – usually *acute* ischemia but *chronic* ischemia can do this, also.

While polymorphic VTs, in general, portend a poor extended prognosis, polymorphic VT due to acute ischemia that occurs during the first 12-24 hours of ST elevation surprisingly does not (but only in the long-term – *30-day mortality is still increased*). This is the ventricular tachycardia that strikes *shortly after* the patient is admitted to the hospital for an acute MI (or – too frequently – *before* they have a chance to seek help). The *scar-related monomorphic ventricular tachycardias* that result in increased long-term mortality occur later (weeks to years) – another benefit of early revascularization.

CARDIOMYOPATHIES

While non-torsade polymorphic ventricular tachycardia can complicate several different types of cardiomyopathy – hypertrophic cardiomyopathy, Takotsubo cardiomyopathy, and dilated cardiomyopathy – it appears most frequently in *hypertrophic cardiomyopathy* and is often the cause of sudden cardiac death for these patients. A ventricular tachycardia occurring in the presence of a dilated cardiomyopathy is more likely to be a bundle branch tachycardia – monomorphic but equally lethal!

INHERITED GENETIC DISORDERS

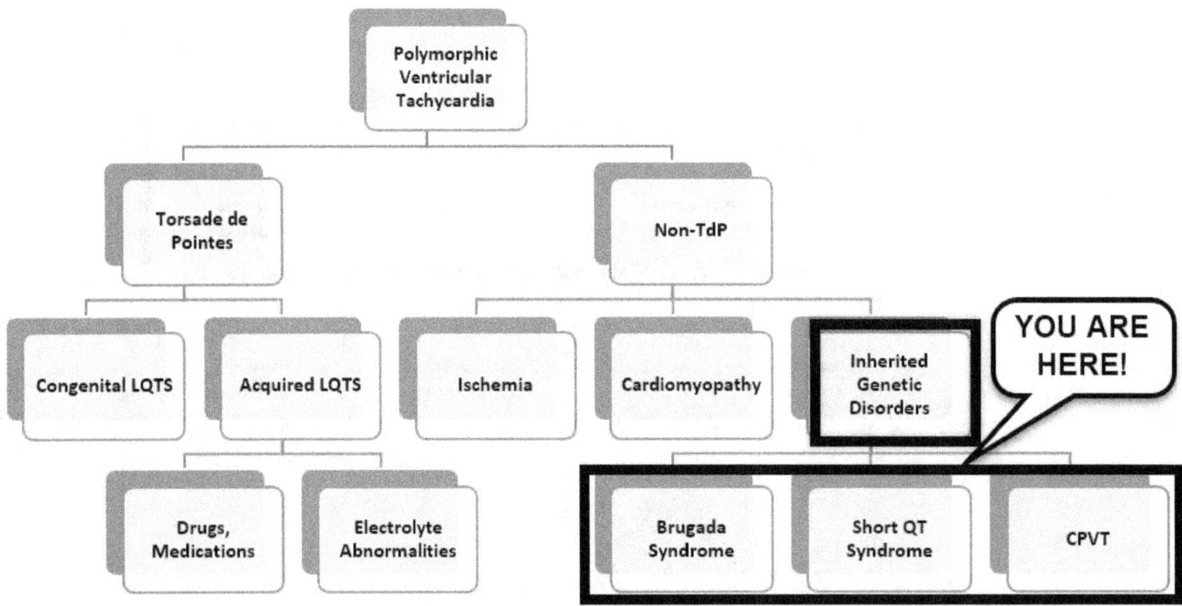

Figure 21-4

There are three inherited disorders – all of which involve the management of calcium within the myocyte:

1. the Brugada syndrome,

2. the short QT syndrome and

3. catecholaminergic polymorphic ventricular tachycardia.

Brugada Syndrome

Brugada syndrome has a predilection for young males, often appearing in their early twenties. It typically occurs at night while at rest. Although most presenting symptoms are episodes of dizziness or syncope, sudden cardiac death may also be the first manifestation of the disorder. Non-torsade polymorphic ventricular tachycardia (Figure 21-5) is the primary tachydysrhythmia; monomorphic VT occurs very rarely.

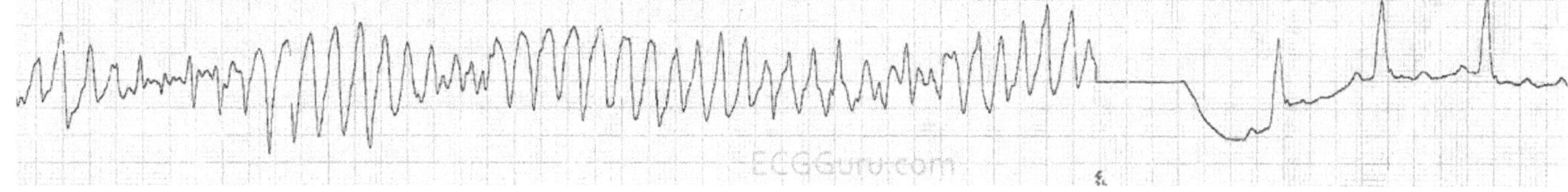

Figure 21-5

Figure 21-5 is an example of what a polymorphic VT associated with the Brugada syndrome looks like. The baseline ECG of the Brugada syndrome has a characteristic appearance in Leads V1 and V2 (Figure 21-6). It was initially thought that the QRS morphology was an RBBB, but we now know that it is actually a J wave.

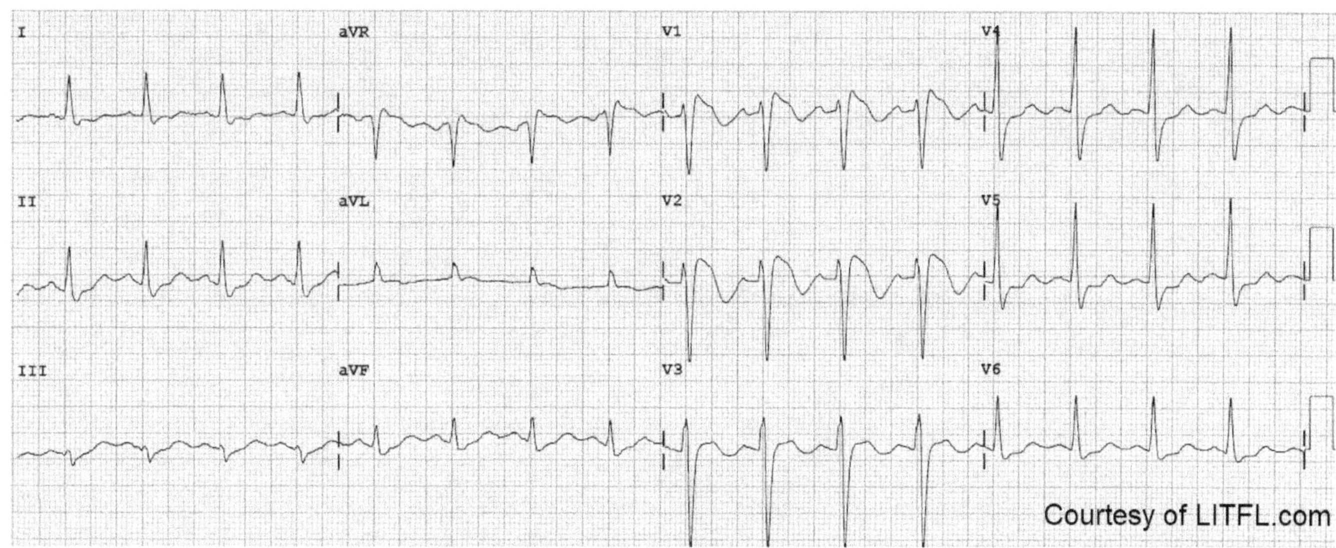

Figure 21-6

For more information regarding the Brugada syndrome and other inherited genetic disorders, check the references at the end of this chapter and in the bibliography at the end of the workbook.

Short QT Syndrome (SQTS)

Short QT syndrome is exactly what it sounds like – a condition resulting in a short QT interval that predisposes to a non-torsade polymorphic ventricular tachycardia. It is due to gain-of-function mutations in the K^+ channels and loss-of-function mutations in the Ca^{++} channels.

It is defined – in *absolute* terms – as a QTc < 330 msec… OR as a QTc < 360 msec AND a history of cardiac arrest, syncope, family history of sudden cardiac death (age 40 or younger), or a family history of SQTS.

> **PEARL |** K^+ channels are responsible for *shortening* the duration of repolarization (Phases 2 and 3 of the action potential) and the Ca^{++} channels are responsible for *prolonging* Phase 2 of the action potential (the ST segment).

Like the Brugada syndrome, the short QT syndrome has a very characteristic ECG appearance (Figure 21-7):

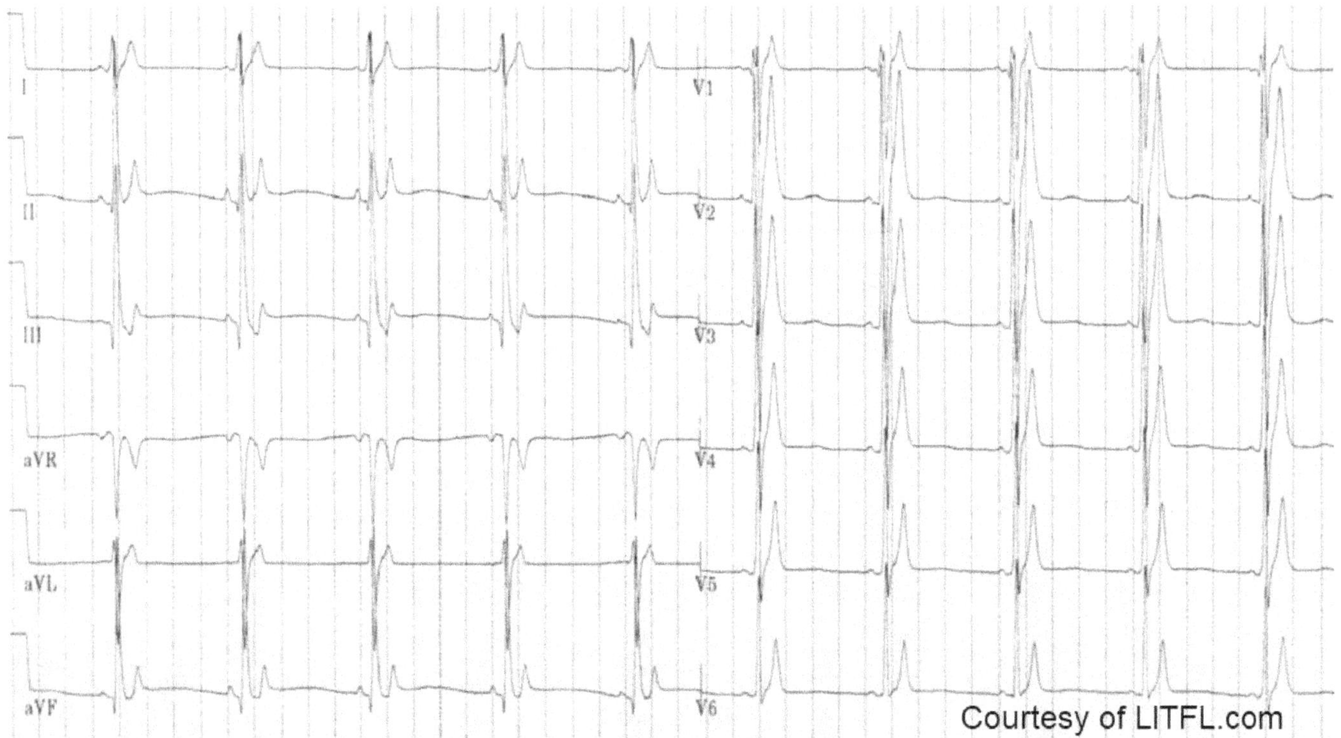

Figure 21-7

It's difficult not to be very impressed with this ECG (Figure 21-7). Note how wide the T-P segment is. There is essentially no ST segment present and the T wave morphology is very distinctive – *tall, sharply peaked*, and *symmetrical*. The T waves are very similar to hyperkalemic T waves, but I have never seen such short ST segments in cases of hyperkalemia. Although hyperkalemia can cause shortening of the ST segment, it won't be to this extent. On the other hand, hypercalcemia can certainly shorten the ST segment like this, but, since the Ca++ channels are not normally operative during Phase 3, the T wave will be normal.

The short QT syndrome is very lethal and affects all ages – infants to the elderly (if there are indeed any elderly still with us who have the short QT syndrome!).

Catecholaminergic Polymorphic Ventricular Tachycardia (CPVT)

CPVT has no pathognomonic characteristic during the normal baseline ECG. Many of those afflicted may have a resting bradycardia, but that is a non-diagnostic finding. This is primarily a tachydysrhythmia of *childhood – from toddlers to teens*, but occasionally in people in their 20s and 30s. If left untreated, up to 50% will die by 30 years of age.

It is a very lethal tachycardia and is initiated by exercise and intense emotion. Diagnosis is confirmed by provocative exercise stress testing. You won't be able to make a definitive diagnosis during acute management unless the patient presents with a very characteristic progression of dysrhythmias, but you can certainly *suspect* it based on the patient's activities surrounding the event.

Catecholaminergic polymorphic VT occurs in a somewhat predictable manner. First, there is an acceleration of the sinus rhythm followed by a ventricular bigeminy. Then follows a narrow complex SVT such as atrial fibrillation. Then a polymorphic VT and/or a bidirectional tachycardia comes next. If ventricular fibrillation does not occur, the tachydysrhythmia just reverses itself, resolving in reverse order.

It also has a predilection to occur during swimming. Always suspect it if a good swimmer experiences a near-drowning episode. It has been reported that up to 25% of patients may also experience CPVT while at rest or during routine daily activities.

> **TIP |** This is a disease of very young people – from toddlers to teens. It may present as a seizure, so be very alert to "seizure" activity following physical or emotional exertion (very active playing, tantrums).

CPVT has three forms of **Electrocardiographic Signature**:

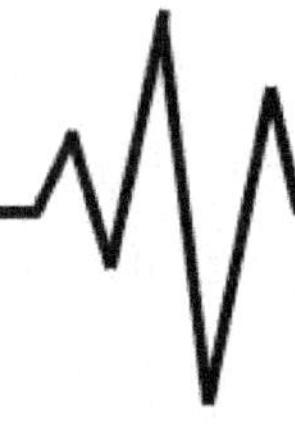

Electrocardiographic Signature

First, the tachycardia may present as just a variation in the QRS complexes, but without the spindle-shaped "torsade" appearance.

Second, it can manifest the same spindle-shaped appearance as torsade de pointes.

Third, it can produce what is called a *bidirectional tachycardia* in which two different polarities or frontal plane axes alternate every second beat. This is not pathognomonic for CPVT since it can also be seen in digoxin or aconitine toxicities.

(Refer back to Chapter 20, Figures 20-2 to 20-4.)

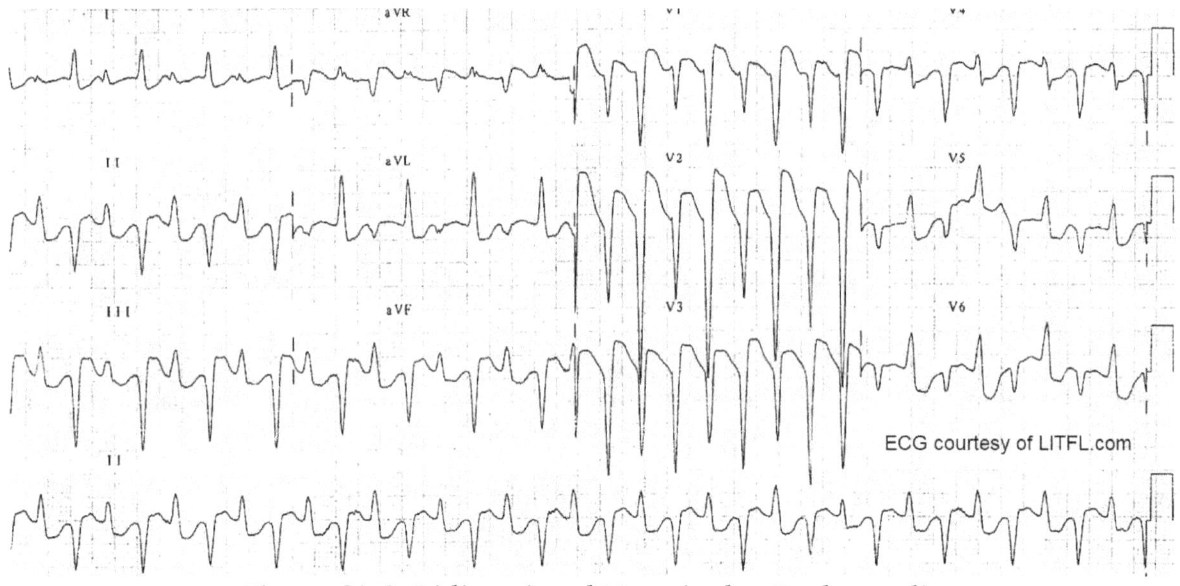

Figure 21-8 Bidirectional Ventricular Tachycardia

If you look at Leads V1 – V3 of Figure 21-8, you will see that not all leads manifest beats with alternating polarities. It's the axis that is changing. In some leads, it will be enough to result in QRS complexes of opposite polarities while in other leads it just results in QRS complexes of differing amplitudes (height or depth).

With progressive exercise or increasing emotional stress, the rhythm progresses from sinus tachycardia to increased ectopy, atrial and junctional dysrhythmias, and eventually polymorphic or bidirectional VT. This rhythm disturbance may result in syncope or degenerate to ventricular fibrillation and sudden death. However, it is frequently self-terminating, following the same dysrhythmia sequence but in reverse.

Bidirectional VT is very characteristic of CPVT – but not *pathognomonic*, since it also occurs in digitalis toxicity and aconitine poisoning. However, given the age range of CPVT victims, it is unlikely that they will be experiencing digitalis toxicity or aconitine poisoning.

CPVT occurs mainly during physical exertion or marked emotional distress. While it was long thought not to occur at rest, recent studies have shown that up to 25% of occurrences can occur while resting. Other tachycardias that may occur during physical exertion or exercise are torsade de pointes due to LQTS 1 and some outflow tract tachycardias – neither of which produce a bidirectional tachycardia.

Like other polymorphic ventricular tachycardias, patient management is more a process of *prevention* rather than *intervention*. Sustained CPVT is lethal, and every effort must be made to intervene by cardioversion. Beta-blockers are a first line of prevention and can be started following cessation and control of the tachydysrhythmia. Termination of the tachycardia can be problematic and multiple attempts may be necessary.

Recommended Reading:

Childers R, MD. Torsades: adjacent and triggering electrocardiographic events. Journal of Electrocardiology. 43 (2010) 515 – 523.

El-Sherif N, MD, Turitto G, MD, Boutjdir M, PhD. Congenital Long QT syndrome and torsade de pointes. Ann Noninvasive Electrocardiol. 2017;22:e12481.

Fitzpatrick JK, MD; Goldschlager N, MD. ECG of the Month. Ann Emerg Med. 2018;71:473-476.

Leenhardt A, MD, Denjoy I, MD, Guicheney G, PhD. Catecholaminergic Polymorphic Ventricular Tachycardia. Circ Arrhythm Electrophysiol. 2012;5:1044-1052.

Pérez-Riera AR, Barbosa-Barros R, deRezende Barbosa MPC, Daminello-Raimundo R, de Lucca AA Jr, de Abreu LC. Catecholaminergic polymorphic ventricular tachycardia, an update. Ann Noninvasive Electrocardiol. 2018;23:e12512. https://doi.org/10.1111/anec.12512.

Roston TM, MD et al. Catecholaminergic Polymorphic Ventricular Tachycardia in Children – Analysis of Therapeutic Strategies and Outcomes From an International Multicenter Registry. Circ Arrhythm Electrophysiol. 2015;8:633-642.

Rudic B, Schimpf R, Borggrefe M. Short QT Syndrome - Review of Diagnosis and Treatment. Arrhythm Electrophysiol Rev. 2014 Aug;3(2):76-9.

Svernhage E, MD, et al. Early Electrocardiographic Signs of Drug-Induced Torsades de Pointes. A.N.E. July 1998;3(3):252-260.

Tiver KD, Dharmaprani D, Quah JX, Lahiri A, Waddell-Smith KE, Ganesan AN. Vomiting, electrolyte disturbance, and medications; the perfect storm for acquired long QT syndrome and cardiac arrest: case report. Journal of Medical Case Reports. 16:9; 2022.

Yap YG, Camm AJ. Drug-Induced QT Prolongation and Torsades de Pointes. Heart. 2003; 89:1363–1372.

Chapter 22

SVT-A's You Should Think About...

What IS an SVT?

Supraventricular tachycardia (SVT) is a general, "catch-all" term for any tachydysrhythmia with its origin above the ventricles. This includes:

- sinus tachycardia

- reentrant sinus tachycardia

- atrial tachycardia

- multifocal atrial tachycardia

- atrial fibrillation

- atrial flutter

- AVNRT (slow-fast, fast-slow, slow-slow)

- AVRT (orthodromic, antidromic)

- focal junctional tachycardia

- permanent junctional reciprocating tachycardia (PJRT)

So you see, telling patients that they have an "SVT" is like telling them they have "fever" or "an infection." "SVT" is not a diagnosis at all. So, is it really important that we try to be more specific about which SVT the patient has?

What if the patient has an AVRT? Sure... you can terminate it with vagal maneuvers or adenosine easily enough – but what if this patient later develops atrial fibrillation? The sudden influx of impulses into the ventricles at a rate between 300 – 600 beats/minute could result in ventricular fibrillation before the patient has a chance to call for help.

PEARL | In all the algorithms and methods discussed in this workbook, the only diagnosis made is *ventricular tachycardia*. **Choosing between VT and SVT is the same as choosing between VT and *not* VT!**

Of course, you may or may not be able to determine which SVT the patient has during the management of an acute episode, but it must be done eventually. The patient will always need a referral to a cardiologist.

PEARL | Ruling out ventricular tachycardia still leaves you with no diagnosis.

Here are some things the heart can do to confuse you a bit. These are all situations involving tachydysrhythmias originating *above* the ventricles.

1. AVNRT with Aberrancy and an Upper Common Pathway Block

You are familiar with AVNRT: a regular, monomorphic NARROW complex tachycardia that develops in or around the AV node. It sometimes manifests pseudo-s waves in the inferior leads and a pseudo-r′ in Lead V1. It frequently responds to vagal maneuvers or, failing that, a rapid injection of adenosine. It also usually converts rather easily with IV calcium channel blockers.

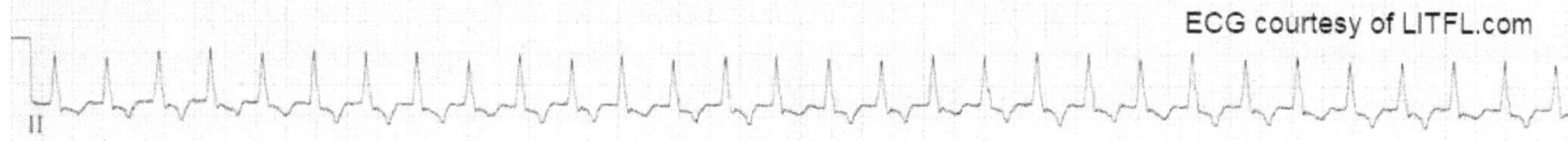

Figure 22-1

But now let's add *aberrant conduction* to this tachycardia, the RBBB type of aberrancy. Now we have the *same tachydysrhythmia* as in Figure 22-1, except that it has a *wide QRS complex* with a classic right bundle branch block morphology (not shown). It still *responds to the same treatment* in the *same way* – very well.

PEARL | If a patient has an accessory pathway and develops a sinus tachycardia or an atrial tachycardia or an atrial flutter... those tachydysrhythmias can only use the accessory pathway as an open door – a bystander pathway. They cannot participate in a reentrant (or reciprocal) rhythm. Why? Because once the reentrant rhythm begins, sinus tachycardia, atrial tachycardia, and atrial flutter are no longer in the picture. ***Once a reentrant rhythm begins, it becomes the de facto dominant pacemaker for the heart until it is terminated.***

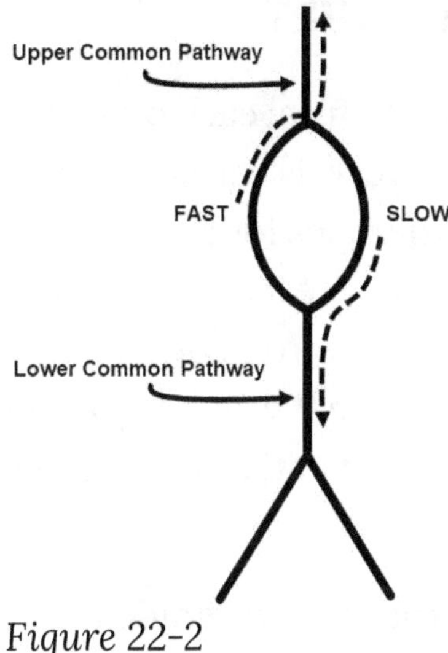

Figure 22-2

(Figure 22-2) At the "top" of the circuit (the *upper common pathway*), the fast pathway sends an impulse to the atria (dashed arrow) which can sometimes be visible at the end of the QRS complex, but it's usually hidden within the QRS. Those P waves are actually P′ (pronounced "P prime") waves since they are not generated by the sinus node (only depolarizations of the sinus node can be called P waves – all others are P′ waves).

But what if there is a block of the atrial exit from that upper common pathway so that no impulse from the AV nodal reentry circuit can enter the atria? The rapid rate of the P′ waves has kept the sinus node suppressed (we call that *overdrive suppression*), but now with a retrograde block into the atria, there are no rapid P′ waves to suppress the sinus node; thus, the sinus node will reactivate and start producing P waves at its intrinsic rate (60-100 beats/minute). So what will the ECG look like now?

There will be a rapid, regular, wide-complex monomorphic tachycardia with AV dissociation – an atrial rate that is slower than the ventricular rate. That fits all the criteria for ventricular tachycardia... except for one thing: the ventricular impulses are originating above the bundle of His! That is NOT ventricular tachycardia.

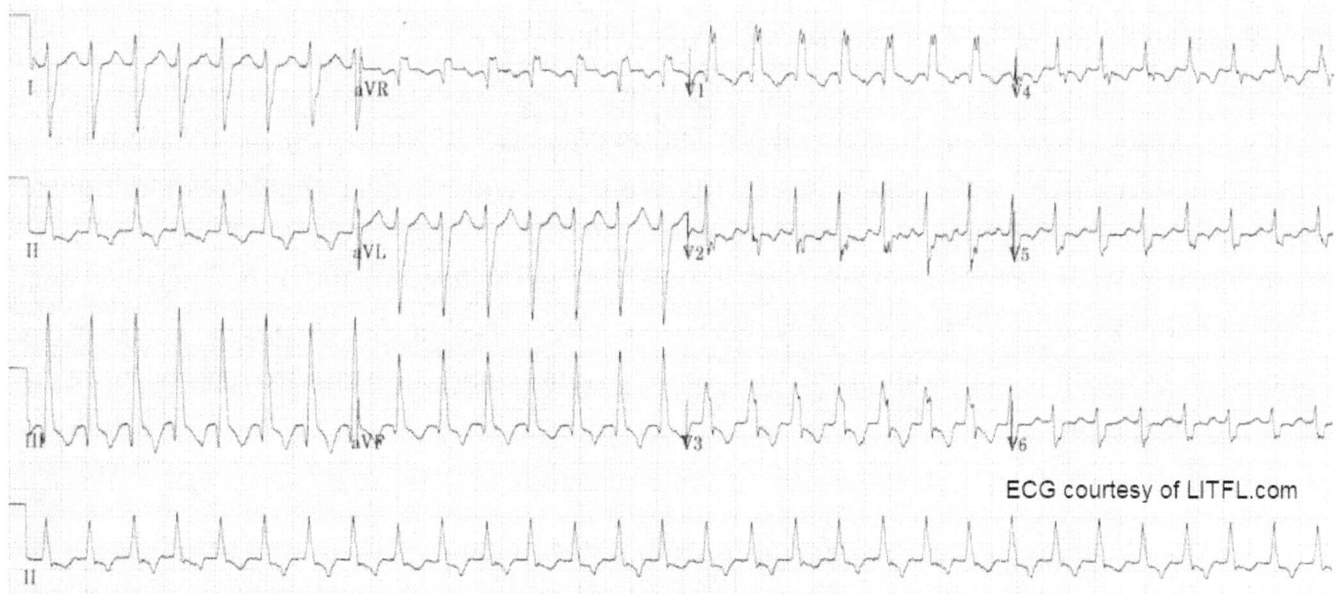

Figure 22-3

Could the ECG above (Figure 22-3) represent an AVNRT with aberrant conduction and a block of the upper common pathway? Yes, it could! Is that likely to be the diagnosis? NO! This is much more *likely* to be an *anterior fascicular tachycardia* or a *left ventricular outflow tract* (*LVOT*) *tachycardia.*

2. Orthodromic AVRT with Aberrancy and Antidromic AVRT

These two tachydysrhythmias should be less of a problem to differentiate from each other, although differentiating an antidromic AVRT from a real ventricular tachycardia can sometimes be very problematic. Orthodromic AVRT with aberrancy will follow the rules for aberrancy since the impulse is entering the ventricles via the His-Purkinje system – Leads V1 and V6 will look more like a classic bundle branch block. You may be able to see retrograde P′ waves following the QRS – usually at least 70 msec from the J point. The retrograde P′ waves following the QRS complex in an AVRT are typically found in the ST segment or the initial slope of the T wave.

Both orthodromic AVRT with aberrancy and antidromic AVRT can produce retrograde P′ waves: orthodromic by traveling up the accessory pathway in a retrograde manner, antidromic by traveling up the bundle of His and on through the AV node. But ventricular tachycardia *can do the same thing*, typically by traveling up the bundle of His and then the AV node. So the production of retrograde P′ waves does not prove either SVT-A or VT. Unless… (to be continued in Chapter 24, "More Practice with AV Dissociation").

3. Atrial Fibrillation with Antegrade Conduction over an Accessory Pathway

An accessory pathway does not always have to participate in a macro-reentry *circuit* – sometimes it can act as an open door between the atria and ventricles. *That is what makes accessory pathways so dangerous!* Atrial fibrillation entering the ventricles via the AV node is controlled by the AV node's "gatekeeper" function. It manifests *decremental conduction*: as the atrial rate *increases*, conduction velocity through the AV node *decreases*. That function protects the ventricles from being overwhelmed by excessively rapid and unmanageable atrial rates. But the presence of an accessory pathway changes all that. Accessory pathways can conduct over a range from somewhat slow to very rapid – and they tend to cluster more towards "very rapid."

> **PEARL |** When you see a ventricular rate this slow (Figure 22-4) during atrial fibrillation, you should always suspect that the patient is taking a rate-controlling medication. The natural ventricular rate for untreated atrial fibrillation is around 120 -130 beats/minute.

Here (Figure 22-4) is atrial fibrillation conducted through the AV node – His-Purkinje system:

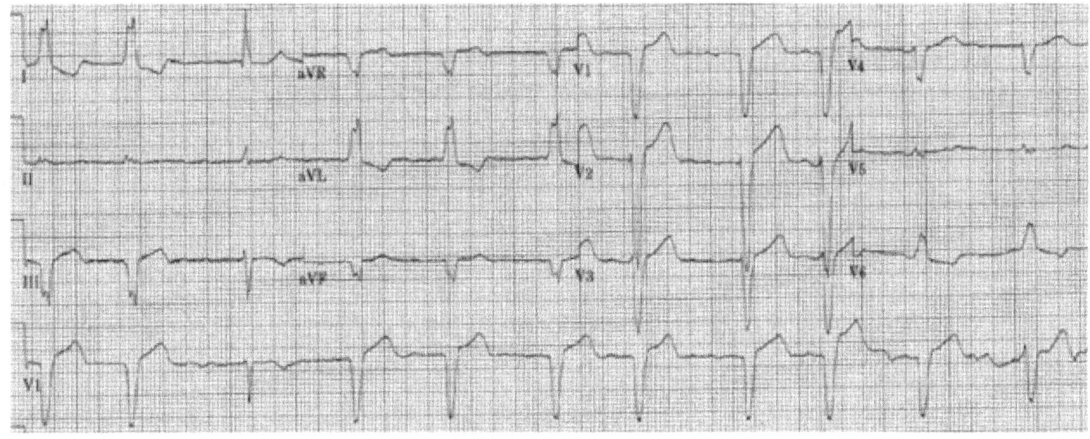

Figure 22-4

Now, here (Figure 22-5) is atrial fibrillation entering the ventricles through an accessory pathway:

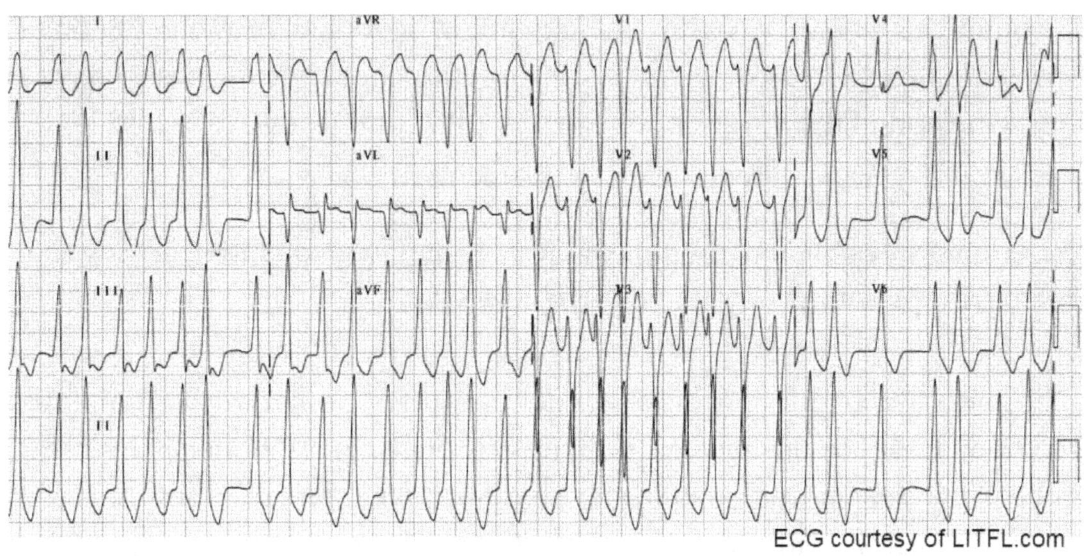

Figure 22-5

This is a rate that will not be tolerated by the ventricles for very long. Eventually, and definitely sooner than later, they will fibrillate. Do you see those pauses scattered throughout the tracing? Those are likely areas where the impulse traveling through the AV node was able to momentarily capture the ventricles. Those pauses may be playing a significant role in keeping this patient alive. That's why one should never give AV nodal blockers to a patient with an irregular, mostly monomorphic*, wide complex tachycardia. This is an atrial problem and not an inherent ventricular problem!

*Because the atrial fibrillatory impulses find the ventricular conduction system in various states of refractoriness, the QRS complexes may exhibit some variable morphologies.

Here (Figure 22-6) is an atrial flutter with a typical 2:1 *conduction* (not 2:1 *block*):

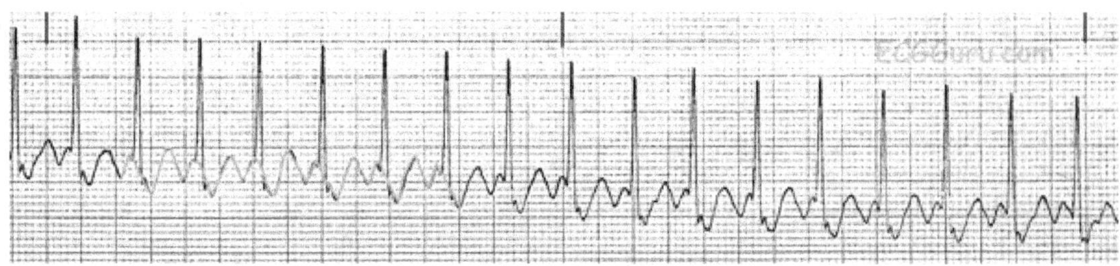

Figure 22-6

Now look at atrial flutter (Figure 22-7) conducting through an accessory pathway:

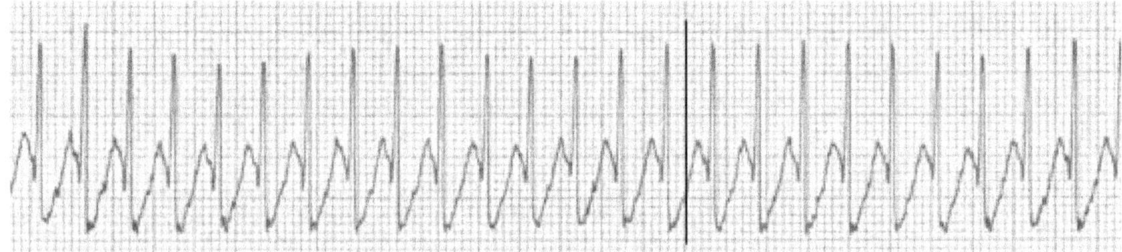

Figure 22-7

These QRS complexes look very narrow and one might be fooled into thinking that it is a very rapid narrow-complex tachycardia – but don't forget to check the S waves! I have drawn a vertical line at the end of the S wave of one of the QRS complexes in Figure 22-7.

> **PEARL |** Sometimes the narrow, peaked R wave can fool you into thinking that the QRS is narrow. But don't forget about the S wave.

This could be aberrant conduction, but I wonder how many people with atrial flutter (usually a more aged population) could transmit impulses through the AV node at this rate? Could the patient possibly have more than one accessory pathway? Or could this be a pathway that connects directly with the Purkinje system (atriofascicular or nodofascicular Mahaim fiber)? What do YOU think? I think it's a case for the electrophysiologist (after the patient has been cardioverted)!

Recommended Reading:

Fisch C, Zipes DP, McHenry PL. Rate Dependent Aberrancy. *Circulation*. 1973;48:714-724.

You can find the online version of this article at: http://circ.ahajournals.org/content/48/4/714.This is one of the *classics* of electrocardiographic literature. Dr. Fisch was a true pioneer in dysrhythmias. He wrote several books – now out of print – that are still available at online booksellers.

Chapter 23

Look-Alike WCTs and How to Distinguish Them...

There are several look-alikes among wide complex tachycardias that can create confusion for healthcare professionals interpreting ECGs. They include:

- RVOT Tachycardia vs. Arrhythmogenic Cardiomyopathy (AC, ARVC/D)

- Ventricular Tachycardia vs. Pre-excited Antidromic Supraventricular Tachycardia

- Posterior Fascicular Tachycardia vs. RBBB with Anterior Fascicular Block

- Torsade de Pointes vs. Non-torsade Polymorphic Ventricular tachycardia

RVOT Tachycardia vs. Arrhythmogenic Cardiomyopathy

It is vitally important that one be able to distinguish these two tachydysrhythmias – one is *benign* and the other is *lethal*. Either one can present as a stable, alert patient with palpitations. RVOTs are usually short and self-limited. In the unlikely event that one should become sustained, the patient will NOT develop cardiovascular collapse! If the patient is unstable – it is arrhythmogenic cardiomyopathy.

There are TWO algorithms to assist you in differentiating between idiopathic ventricular tachycardias and scar-related ventricular tachycardias: the Hoffmayer algorithm and the Wijnmaalen algorithm. There is, however, a difference between the two algorithms in that the Hoffmayer algorithm can be used *during the tachycardia*, and the Wijnmaalen algorithm is used *during sinus rhythm*.

The Hoffmayer Algorithm

A scoring system has been developed to aid in distinguishing between *idiopathic* and *scar-related* ventricular tachycardias. This system is based on the examination of the tachycardia both *during the tachycardia* and *during sinus rhythm*.

- If you have access to a previous ECG – or if the current ECG manifests a non-sustained dysrhythmia with tachycardia interspersed with sinus beats, anterior T wave inversions in Leads V1 – V3, score **3 points**. If you can recognize T wave inversions in Leads V1 – V3 *during* the ventricular tachycardia, score **3 points**. The presence of T wave inversions in *both* sinus rhythm *and* ventricular tachycardia counts only as **3 points** – NOT 6!

- If the QRS duration in Lead I ≥ 120 msec, score **2 points**.

- If QRS notching is present in one or more leads, score **2 points**.

- If the precordial transition is at Lead V5 or later, score **1 point**.

A score of **5 points** or more correctly diagnosed ARVD/C, distinguishing it from idiopathic VT 93% of the time.

SN 84%, SP 100%, PPV 100%, NPV 91%

Using the criteria above, what type of VT do you think this ECG (Figure 23-1) is manifesting?

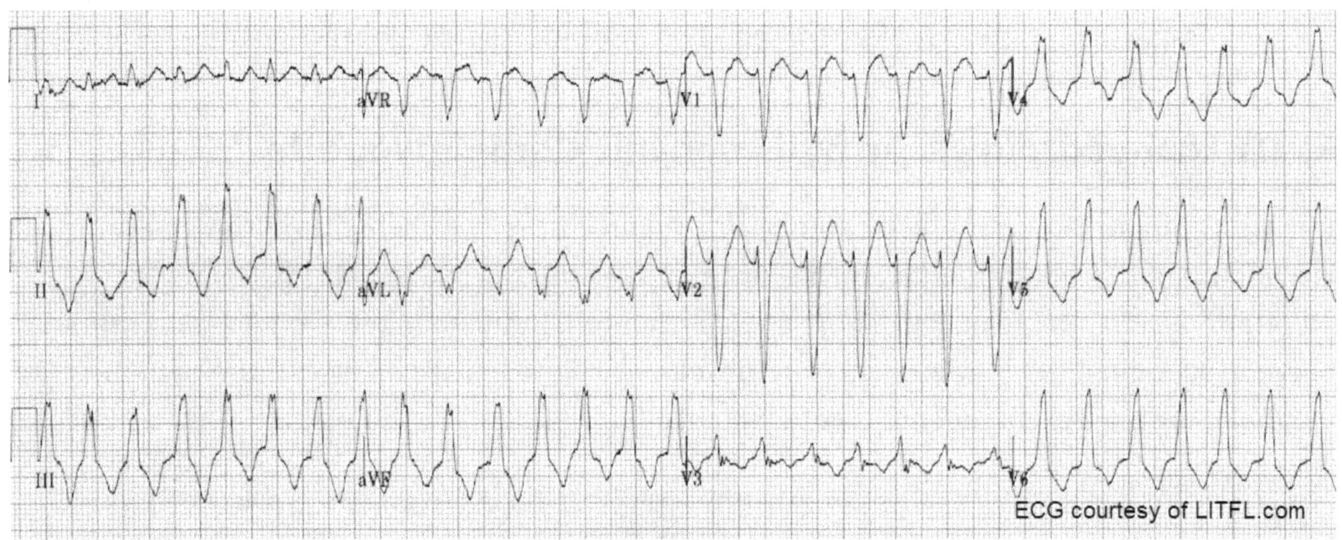

Figure 23-1

PEARL | If the patient has known heart disease, assume any ventricular dysrhythmia to be due to the underlying heart disease until proven otherwise.

Now what type of VT do you think this next ECG (Figure 23-2) manifests?

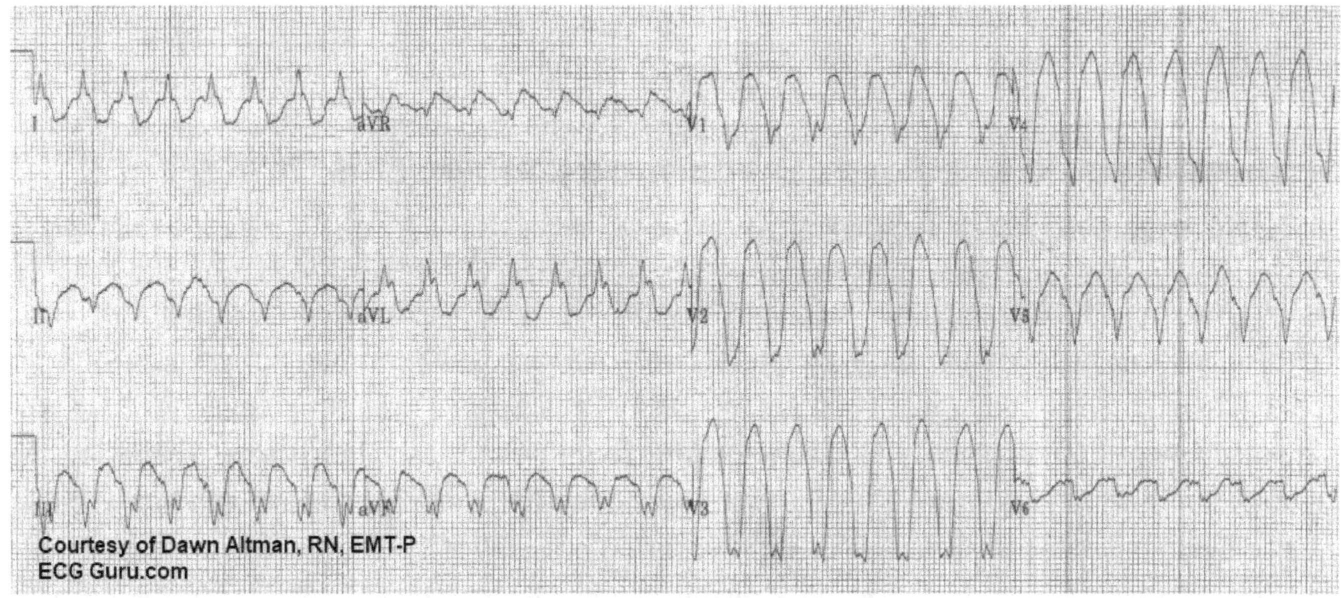

Figure 23-2

The Wijnmaalen Algorithm

In the Wijnmaalen algorithm, we are seeking to diagnose scar-related tachycardia. Three criteria are determined based on a surface ECG (as opposed to an internal electrogram) *during sinus rhythm*:

- Precordial transition beyond Lead V4

- Notching on the downstroke of the S wave in Lead V1 or V2 (aka Josephson's sign)

- QRS to S nadir in Lead V1 > 90 msec

This is not a numbered list because no finding ranks above any of the others. A tachycardia is considered to be *scar-related* if *at least one* of the criteria is present; if *none* of the criteria are present, then the diagnosis is *idiopathic ventricular tachycardia.*

> **TIP** | 1) The diagnosis is made on an ECG *during sinus rhythm – not during the actual tachycardia*; 2) idiopathic ventricular tachycardia remains a *diagnosis of exclusion.*

References:

Hoffmayer KS, et al. An electrocardiographic scoring system for distinguishing right ventricular outflow tract arrhythmias in patients with arrhythmogenic right ventricular cardiomyopathy from idiopathic ventricular tachycardia. Heart Rhythm. 2013 Apr;10(4):477-82.

Wijnmaalen AP. ECG Identification of Scar-Related Ventricular Tachycardia With a Left Bundle-Branch Block Configuration. *Circ Arrhythm Electrophysiol.* 2011;4:486-493.

Scar-Related Ventricular Tachycardia vs. Pre-excited Antidromic Supraventricular Tachycardia

The various algorithms, methods, and criteria typically omit the consideration of antidromic, pre-excited supraventricular tachycardias. Thus, there are "built-in" inaccuracies in these approaches. This allows an "incorrect answer" to be treated as a "correct answer." And, as you may or may not have noticed, the outcome from your use of these algorithms, methods, and criteria is either "VT" or "not VT" – if it isn't ventricular tachycardia, you are still left without a clear diagnosis. (And if you think all supraventricular tachycardias are the same – please enroll in **The Masterclass in Advanced Electrocardiography** or **The Masterclass in Advanced Dysrhythmias**!)

In 1994, Steurer et al. developed a stepwise approach to distinguish *specifically* between *ventricular tachycardia* (mostly scar-related VT) and *pre-excited antidromic supraventricular tachycardia.* Dr. Pedro Brugada was also one of the authors, so this method is also known as the "Brugada method" (with apologies to Dr. Steurer, whose name is listed *first!*). In the group with documented ventricular tachycardia, 89% were related to a previous myocardial infarction, a form of structural or scar-related heart disease. Bear in mind that old myocardial scars are NOT the *only* form of scar-related heart disease. None of the patients with pre-excited antidromic supraventricular tachycardia had any evidence of structural heart disease. Patients with atrial fibrillation were excluded because the diagnosis in those cases was presumed to be obvious.

This is not a scoring system but an *observational* approach. None of the findings ranks higher than any other finding. Findings that are strongly suggestive of a diagnosis of scar-related ventricular tachycardia are:

- The presence of *predominantly negative* QRS complexes in precordial leads V4 – V6

- The presence of a QR complex in one or more of the precordial leads V2 – V6

- AV or VA dissociation

The negative QRS complexes in Leads V4 – V6 need not be monophasic but should have R/S ratios < 1.0 (preferably, much less than 1.0).

In 2023, Vereckei et al. added a fourth criterion to this method – the aVR criterion. This criterion is as follows:

- "...in lead aVR the onset of the QRS complex is positive, and the area above the baseline (R wave area) of the QRS complex is greater than the area below the baseline (S wave area)."

I do not know if Drs. Steurer and Brugada have accepted this addition to their algorithm.

What do the criteria indicate for this ECG (Figure 23-3)?

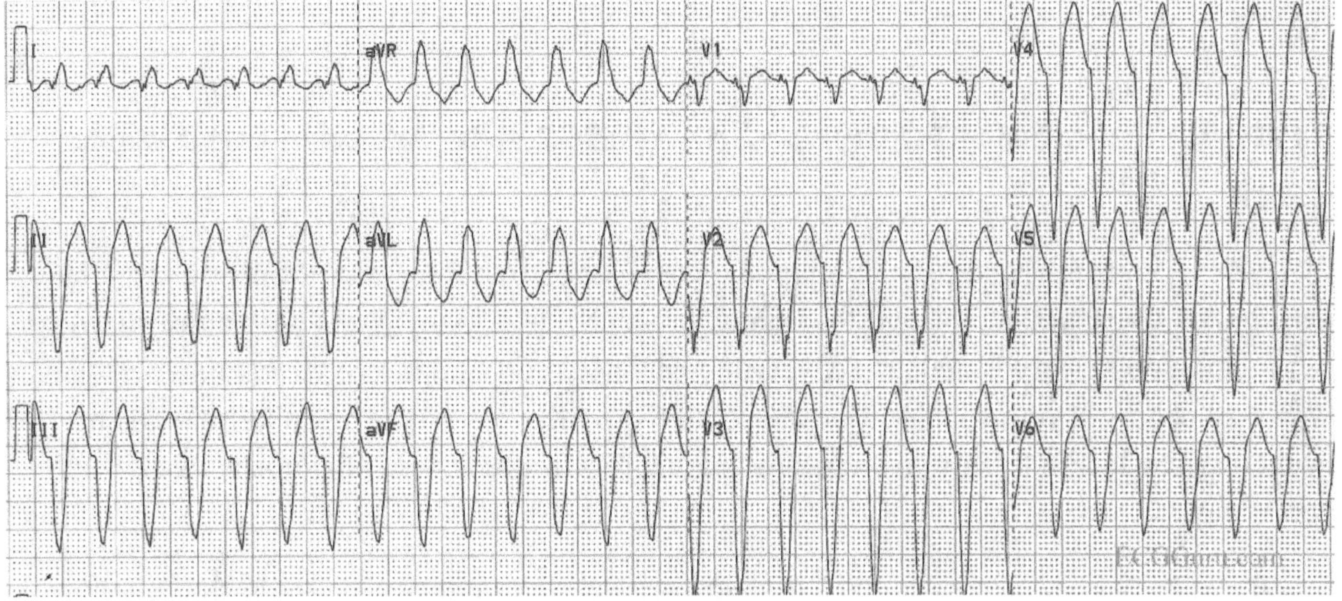

Figure 23-3

And what about this ECG (Figure 23-4)?

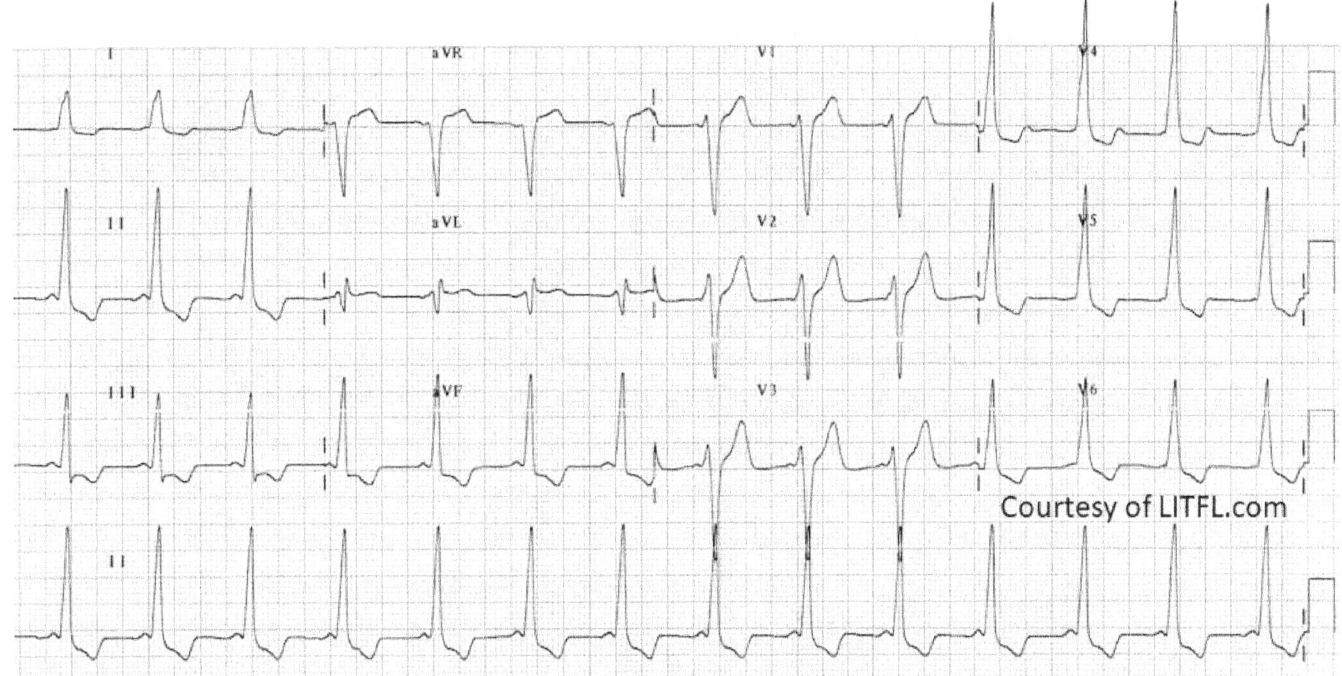

Figure 23-4

References:

Steurer G, Gürsoy S, Frey B, Simonis F, Andries E, Kuck K, Brugada, P. The differential diagnosis on the electrocardiogram between ventricular tachycardia and pre-excited tachycardia. Clin Cardiol. 1994;17:306–8.

Vereckei, A. et al. The Application of a New, Modified Algorithm for the Differentiation of Regular Ventricular and Pre-Excited Tachycardia. Heart, Lung and Circulation (2023) 32: 719-725.

Posterior Fascicular Tachycardia vs. RBBB with Anterior Fascicular Block

Algorithms, methods, and prediction models developed to differentiate ventricular tachycardia with structural abnormalities from supraventricular tachycardia with aberrancy do not include posterior fascicular tachycardia. Because it often has a relatively narrow QRS complex, occurs in young, healthy people, manifests what *appears* to be an RBBB with anterior fascicular block, and is terminated by verapamil, it is frequently misdiagnosed as SVT with aberrancy.

In 2017, Michowitz et al. developed a four-criteria prediction model to aid in the differentiation of posterior fascicular tachycardia from supraventricular tachycardia with RBBB/anterior fascicular block aberrancy.

This is a documented posterior fascicular tachycardia (Figure 23-5):

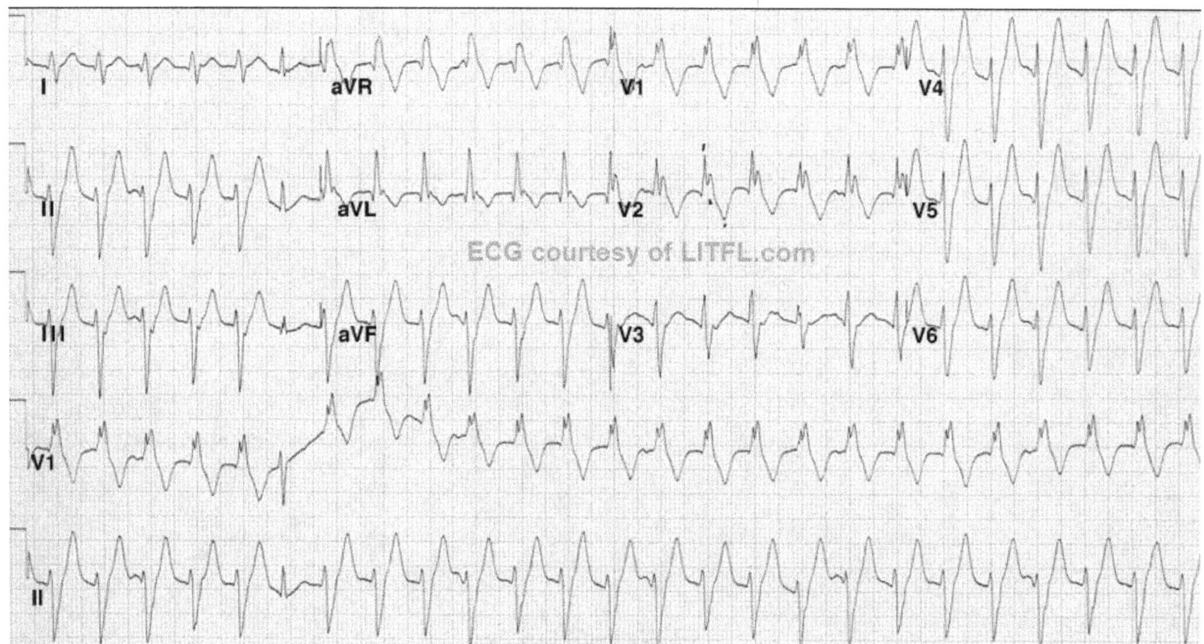

Figure 23-5

QRS morphology in Lead V1

Typical rSR′ morphology → RBBB with LAFB

Atypical Lead V1 morphology → Posterior Fascicular Tachycardia

QRS width

- >140 msec → RBBB with LAFB

- ≤140 msec → Posterior Fascicular Tachycardia (usually ≤130 msec)

Lead V6 R/S ratio

- > 1.0 → RBBB with LAFB

- ≤ 1.0 → Posterior Fascicular Tachycardia

Polarity in Lead aVR

- Negative aVR → RBBB with LAFB

- Positive aVR → Posterior Fascicular Tachycardia

Patients with 3 of 4 positive variables had a high probability of having posterior fascicular tachycardia, while those patients with ≤1 positive variable always had RBBB plus LAFB.

What about this ECG (Figure 23-6)?

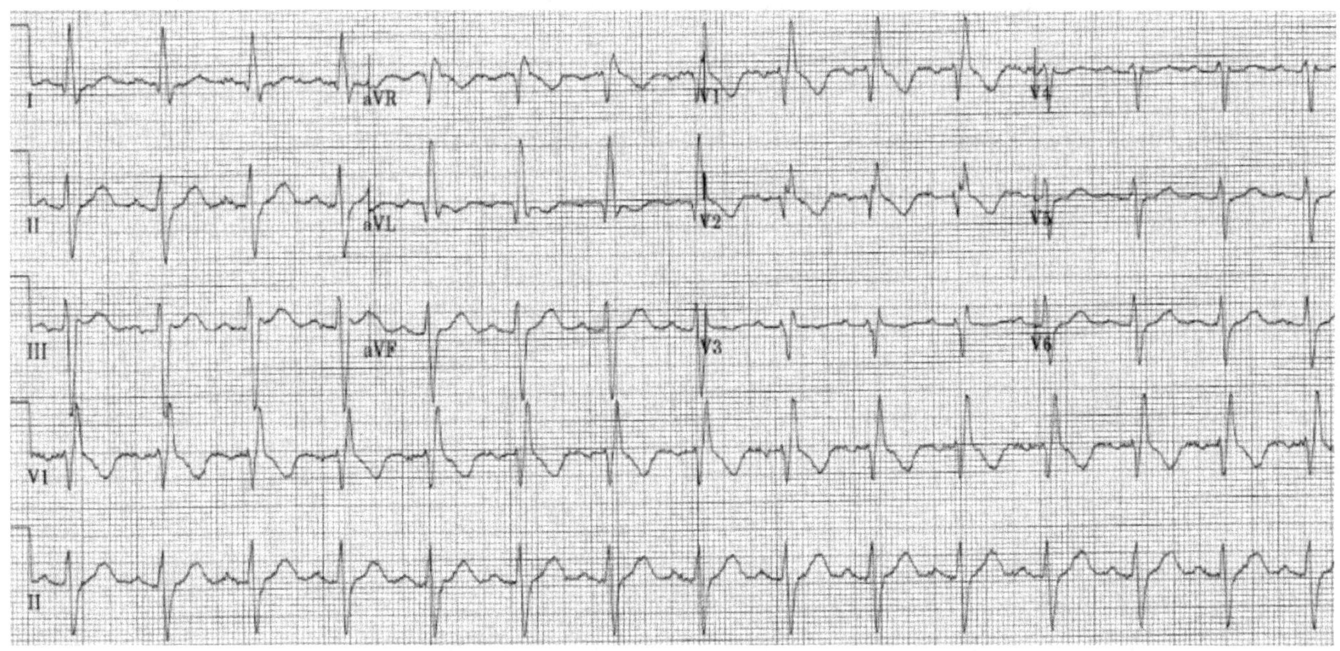

Figure 23-6

References:

Michowitz Y, Tovia-Brodie O, Heusler I, Sabbag A, Rahkovich M, Shmueli H, Glick A, Belhassen B. Differentiating the QRS morphology of posterior fascicular ventricular tachycardia from right bundle branch block and left anterior hemiblock aberrancy. Circ Arrhythm Electrophysiol. 2017

RBBB Tachycardias: Scar-related VT vs. Idiopathic VTs

There are TWO idiopathic ventricular tachycardias in the left ventricle that you should know and be able to distinguish from VT due to structural heart disease, which is by far the most common type of ventricular tachycardia. Now understand, there are several other types of VTs originating in the left ventricle but they are exceedingly rare. Don't worry about them!

Left Ventricular Outflow Tract (LVOT) Tachycardia

The first idiopathic VT is left ventricular outflow tract (LVOT) tachycardia. It is characterized by:

1. an RBBB and an inferior axis (tall R waves in Leads II, III, and aVF) with only moderately wide QRS complexes. There is no specific width to note, but just be aware that if the QRS is very wide (>160 msec, for instance), it is much more likely to be a scar-related tachycardia and not an idiopathic tachycardia.

2. precordial transition *before* Lead V3 (remember: both right and left depolarizations can have a transition at Lead V3, so a transition in V3 is not a great help).

3. responds to adenosine. However, it may also respond to ß-blockers, verapamil, and other antiarrhythmic medications.

This is a left ventricular outflow tract (LVOT) tachycardia (Figure 23-7):

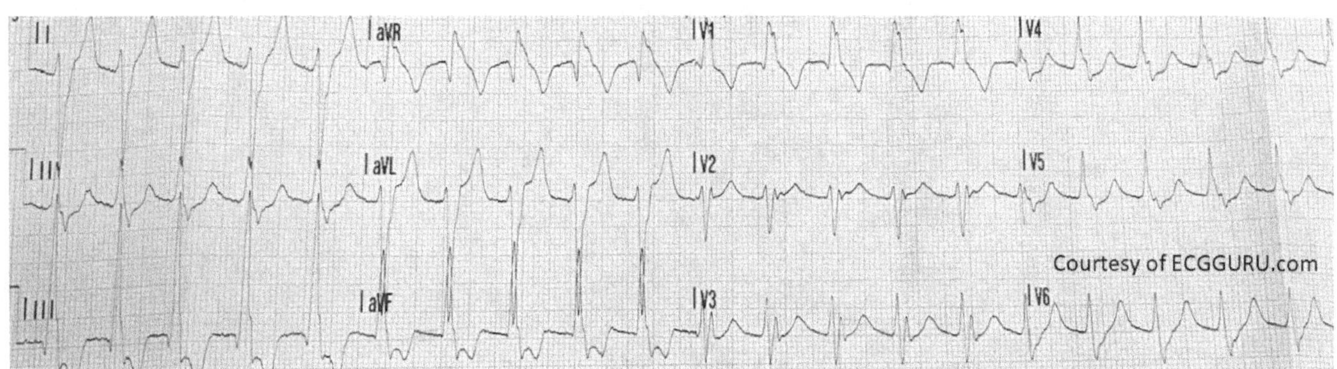

Figure 23-7

Posterior Fascicular Tachycardia

Posterior Fascicular Tachycardia is the other idiopathic VT and the most common *idiopathic* VT of the left ventricle. It is characterized by:

1. RBBB with a superior axis (rS complexes in the inferior leads)

2. relatively narrow QRS complexes, virtually always less than 140 msec and usually less than 130 msec

3. R-to-S -nadir < 80 msec indicating an origin within the conducting system

This is a posterior fascicular tachycardia (Figure 23-8):

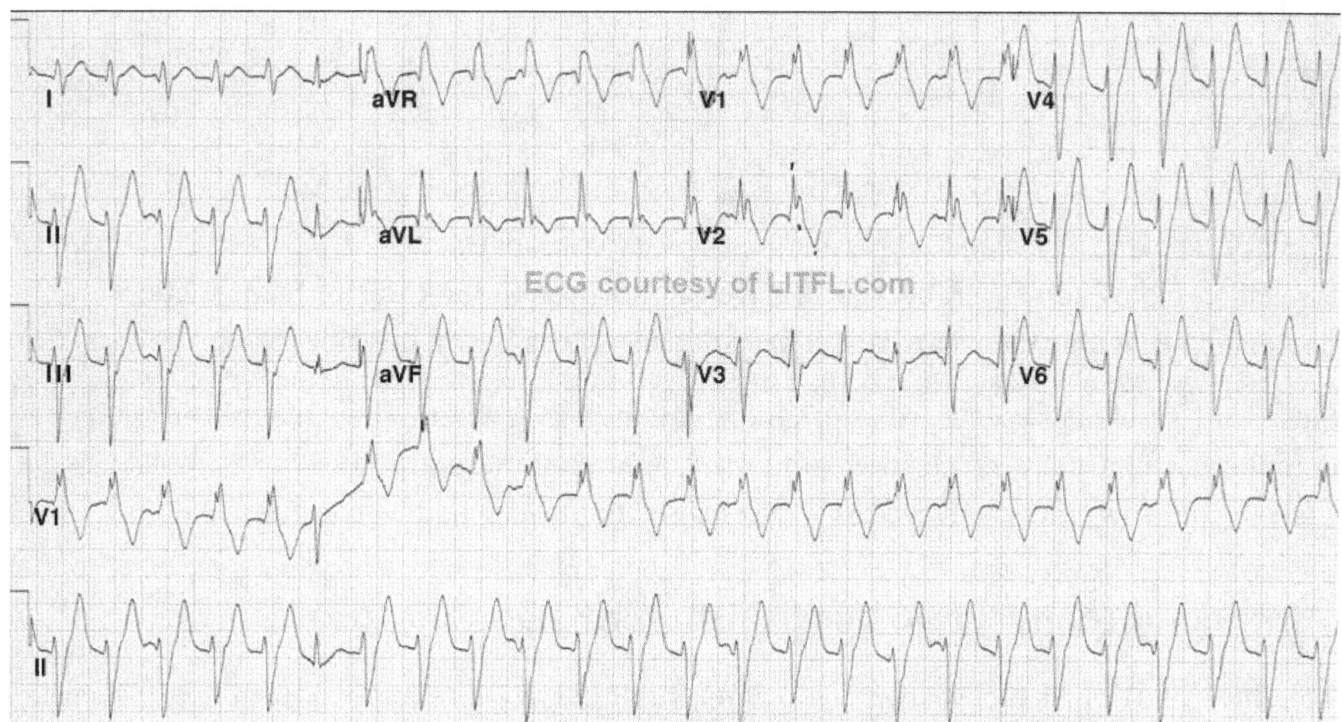

Figure 23-8 (appeared earlier as Figure 23-5)

There is also an **anterior fascicular tachycardia** (Figure 23-9). The only difference is that there is an inferior axis (i.e., all the QRS complexes in the inferior leads consist of tall R waves pointing up) with a tendency to a right axis deviation. Otherwise, treatment and prognosis are the same. Because of the location in the left ventricle, ablation can be a bit more problematic.

PEARL | Posterior fascicular tachycardia looks like an RBBB with anterior fascicular block – but it's not! Anterior fascicular tachycardia looks like an RBBB with a posterior fascicular block – but it's not. Just remember how very *rare* posterior fascicular blocks are compared to anterior fascicular blocks.

Figure 23-9 is an example of *anterior fascicular tachycardia*. Remember: these are *rare*! This may be the only one you'll ever see!

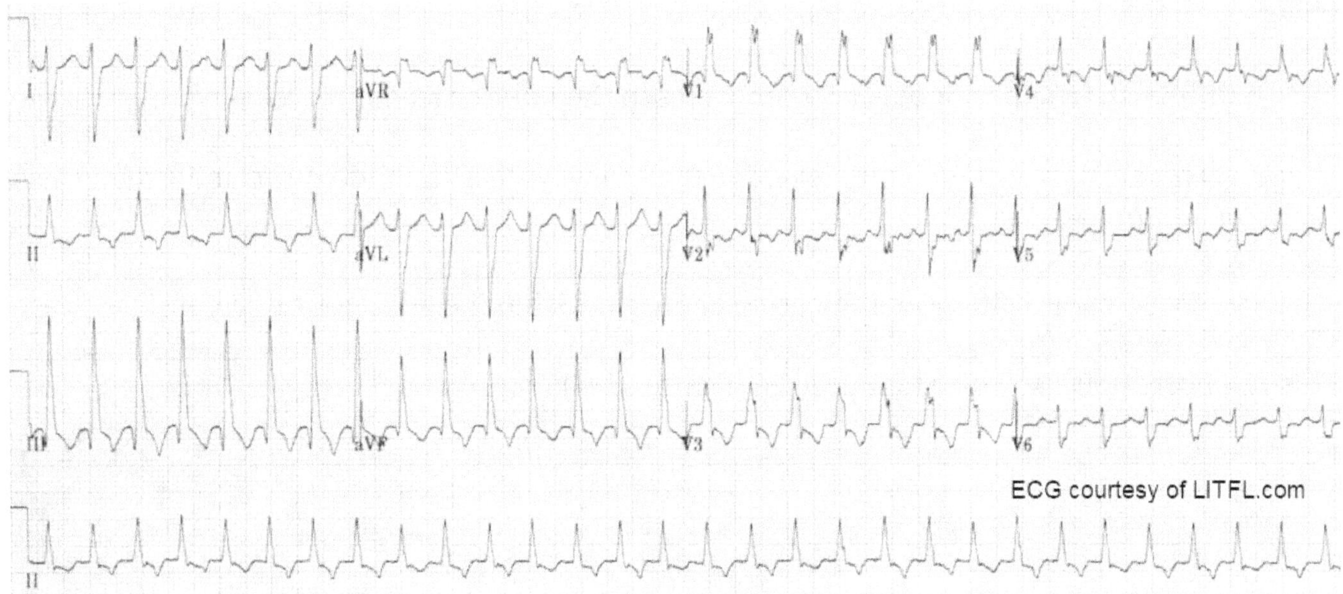

Figure 23-9 Anterior Fascicular Tachycardia - very rare!

The frontal plane axis should differentiate these two idiopathic VTs (LVOT and posterior fascicular) from each other. **LVOT will have tall R waves in the inferior leads while a posterior fascicular tachycardia will have deep S waves in the inferior leads.**

Since both fascicular tachycardias originate in conducting fibers, the onset of the QRS complexes will usually be "cleaner:" smoother, greater slope, and somewhat better formed than the outflow tract tachycardias which originate in working myocardium.

Ventricular Tachycardia Due to Structural Heart Disease

The third ventricular tachycardia to be differentiated is **VT due to structural heart disease**. This is by far **the most common VT of all**, including both the right and left ventricles:

1. widened QRS due to the conduction delay inherent in a structurally damaged myocardium and the re-routing of the depolarization wave through and around the areas of fibrosis

2. notching within the QRS complexes. You may remember "notching" as a characteristic of arrhythmogenic cardiomyopathy, and that is because it represents a structurally damaged myocardium, also.

3. although these VTs can develop just about anywhere in the ventricle, there seems to be a lot that comes from the apical area. While there will be an RBBB with a superior axis – just like a posterior fascicular tachycardia, the QRS complexes will be wider and more

bizarre. Because posterior fascicular tachycardias begin essentially in the posterior fascicle, the onset of the QRS will look a lot more like an aberrantly conducted beat in that the initial deflection onset will be smoother and straighter.

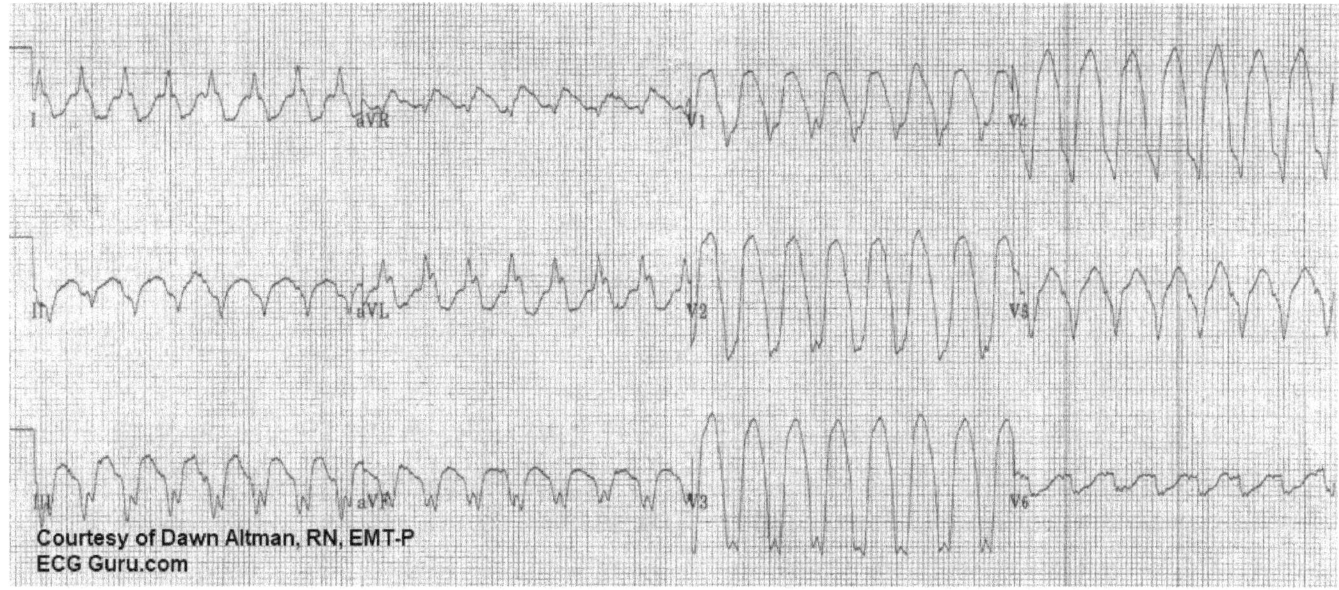

Figure 23-10 (appeared earlier as Figure 23-2)

Torsade de Pointes vs. Non-torsade Polymorphic Ventricular Tachycardia

Torsade de pointes should have a prolonged QT interval while the non-torsade polymorphic ventricular tachycardia should not. However, QT interval prolongation is *not* the best method for differentiating these two very dangerous dysrhythmias, and here is why...

Some patients with one of the long QT syndromes may not consistently manifest a prolonged QT interval on the ECG at all times. Some have an incomplete penetrance of the genetic defect and QT prolongation may be minimal or not apparent at all without some sort of challenge. Some patients with non-torsade polymorphic ventricular tachycardia due to ischemia may have a slightly prolonged QT interval due to conduction delay *caused by the ischemia*. They are not considered to be an acquired long QT syndrome.

The most consistent and reliable differentiating factor is the *coupling interval* created by the last sinus-conducted beat and the ectopic QRS that initiates the tachycardia.

If the *coupling interval is > 400 msec* (two large squares), the rhythm is *torsade de pointes*.

If the *coupling interval is < 400 msec*, the rhythm is *non-torsade polymorphic ventricular tachycardia*.

Is this torsade de pointes or non-torsade polymorphic VT (Figure 23-11)?

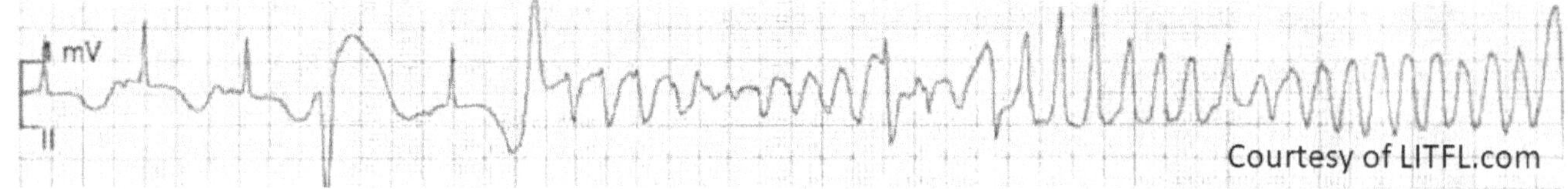

Figure 23-11

How about this rhythm strip – torsade de pointes or non-torsade polymorphic VT (Figure 23-12)?

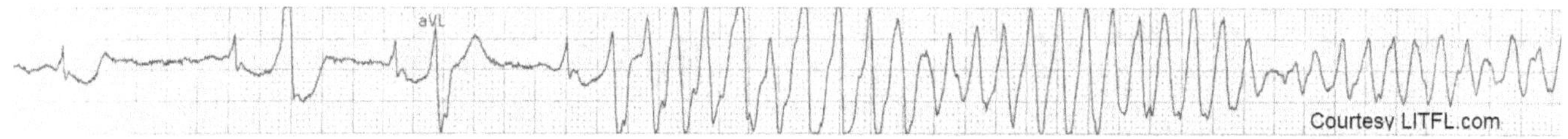

Figure 23-12

CAUTION! | As a reminder, you must see some supraventricular rhythm and preferably the onset of the polymorphic ventricular tachycardia to make the diagnosis and differentiate the two rhythms. If sustained (which is infrequent), the two tachydysrhythmias will look the same. You cannot see a long QT interval *during* the tachycardia.

TIP | Note the wide, bizarre T waves of the PVC and sinus beat just preceding the onset of the tachycardia (Figure 23-11). This occurs frequently in torsade de pointes. Such changes appear to indicate that the onset of torsade de pointes is imminent! Notice that it did *not* occur with the non-torsade tachycardia (Figure 23-12).

ANOTHER TIP | Do not confuse acquired LQTS with non-torsade VT. The non-torsade VT is not associated with a prolonged QTc as a contributory cause of VT and – even when it manifests a spindle shape – it is NOT torsade de pointes!

A Frequent Question...

There is a hierarchy of QRS durations (widths) that sometimes help with the decision-making process. Some QRS complexes are going to be wider than others and some are going to be better formed than others (at least initially).

1. **Widest:** scar-related ventricular tachycardias, antidromic AVRT

2. **Medium:** outflow tract tachycardias

3. **Narrowest:** Fascicular tachycardias, bundle branch tachycardias, interfascicular tachycardias

Scar-related ventricular tachycardias and antidromic AVRTs will generally be wider than 140 msec and very often wider than 160 msec since both begin ventricular activation in working myocardium.

The outflow tachycardias (RVOT, LVOT) will have medium durations of the QRS. They begin in working myocardium, but both are near conducting fibers. They tend to be less than 140 msec in duration.

The third category involves tachycardias that begin in the conduction fibers of the ventricles. Using fascicular tachycardia as our example, the QRS durations of these tachycardias will be less than 140 msec and the majority will be less than 130 msec. What's even more important here is the onset of R-to-S nadir in Lead V1. This will generally be 80 msec or less in tachycardias that originate in conducting fibers.

Here are two questions that I am asked a lot...

1. How do I tell the difference between LVOT tachycardia and fascicular tachycardia?

   a. First, if you are talking about posterior fascicular tachycardia, there should be no problem at all – not even an issue of QRS width! During an LVOT tachycardia, the QRS complexes in the inferior leads will be pointing UP, and during posterior fascicular tachycardia, they will be pointing DOWN.

   b. Now, if the fascicular tachycardia happens to be an *anterior* fascicular tachycardia (a very rare phenomenon!), you will have to assess the width of the QRS complexes and the R-to-S nadir in Lead V1. The fascicular tachycardia will likely be less than 130 msec and the R-to-S nadir will be 80 msec or less.

2. Since scar-related ventricular tachycardias occur most frequently in the left ventricle, how do I differentiate a scar-related VT from an LVOT tachycardia?

   a. The scar-related VT will be wider – usually 160 msec or more – and less well-formed than the QRS complexes of the LVOT tachycardia. The QRS complexes of the LVOT tachycardia should also be 140 msec or less.

Please bear in mind that these values are NOT official, but they are frequently used when assessing wide complex tachycardias.

Recommended Reading:

Hoffmayer KS, et al. An electrocardiographic scoring system for distinguishing right ventricular outflow tract arrhythmias in patients with arrhythmogenic right ventricular cardiomyopathy from idiopathic ventricular tachycardia. *Heart Rhythm.* 2013 Apr;10(4):477-82.

Michowitz et al. Differentiating the QRS Morphology of Posterior Fascicular Ventricular Tachycardia From Right Bundle Branch Block and Left Anterior Hemiblock Aberrancy. *Circ Arrhythm Electrophysiol.* 2017; 1-11.

Moss, JD MD, Scheinman MM MD. Differentiating the QRS Morphology of Posterior Fascicular Ventricular Tachycardia From Right Bundle Branch Block and Left Anterior Hemiblock Aberrancy – Why the Difference (Editorial). *Circ Arrhythm Electrophysiol.* 2017; 1-3.

Steurer G, Gürsoy S, Frey B, Simonis F, Andries E, Kuck K, et al. The differential diagnosis on the electrocardiogram between ventricular tachycardia and pre-excited tachycardia. *Clin Cardiol.* 1994;17:306–8.

Wijnmaalen AP. ECG Identification of Scar-Related Ventricular Tachycardia With a Left Bundle-Branch Block Configuration. *Circ Arrhythm Electrophysiol.* 2011;4:486-493.

Chapter 24

More Practice with AV Dissociation

My philosophy is that you can never get *too* good at recognizing AV dissociation. Although there is no 100% assurance that its presence is pathognomonic of ventricular tachycardia, the other wide complex tachycardias that can produce it are so rare that you need not worry yourself with them.

OK... let's get started!

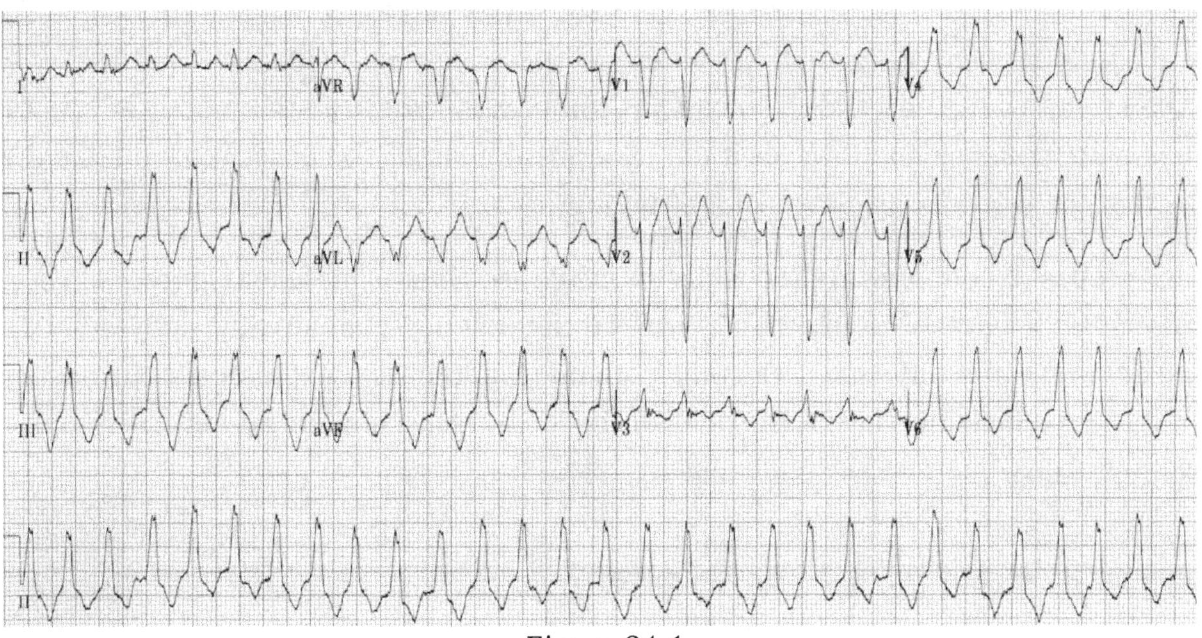

Figure 24-1

(Figure 24-1) There are two ways to go about your search for AV dissociation:

1. Sit back, scan the ECG, and see if anything catches your eye. I call this the *Gestalt approach*; or,

2. Look specifically for changes suggestive of AV dissociation by comparing parts of the baseline from the J point to the onset of the next QRS complex. Don't bother searching *within* the QRS complex – you aren't going to find anything useful. I call this the *Scientific approach*.

Not surprisingly, I have found that many people (if not *most*) use the Gestalt approach and then complain that AV dissociation is too difficult to recognize.

Introducing "The Bank"

Let me help you begin to develop proficiency using the Scientific approach.

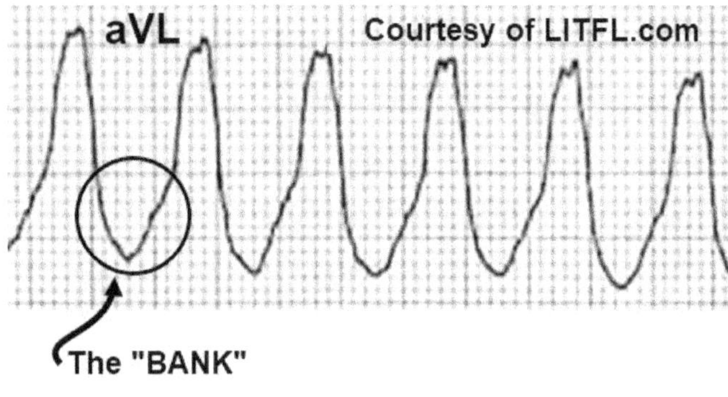

Figure 24-2

First, you want to concentrate on the areas of the lead where you are most likely to see P waves. That, as I said, will be *from the J point of a QRS complex to the onset of the next QRS complex* (Figure 24-2).

I call this area "the Bank" for two reasons. There is a story of an infamous bank robber here in the US many years ago named Willie Sutton. When asked why he robbed banks, Willie *allegedly* replied, "Because that's where all the money is!" Well, that stretch of baseline from the J point to the onset of the next QRS complex is "where all the money is." That is where you are going to find P waves if they are present at all! The other reason I like that term is that the word "bank" saves a lot of typing!

The next step is to compare all the "banks" in the chosen lead. This lead (Figure 24-2) consists of monophasic R waves with inverted T waves (but you knew that already, didn't you). Do you see anything that differs significantly from one bank to the next? I don't, either! This is Lead aVL, so the little notches at the peak of the R waves are characteristic of an LBBB-like morphology.

Is the P or P′ Wave Upright or Inverted?

Let's look at another snippet (Figure 24-3); I've added some lines indicating a bank (a "bank" begins at the J point, *which may be the end of an S wave, as in this snippet*)...

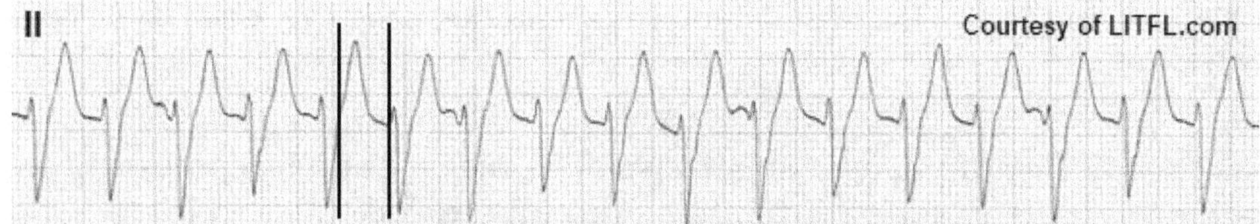

Figure 24-3

You need to use the most "normal" appearing bank as your point of reference. The bank between the first and second QRS complexes appears pretty normal and lacks any suspicious findings. Let's move on to the second bank. We've found something! There is a definite hump (or "blip") in the baseline between the end of the T wave and the small r wave of the rS complex. And it is *upright in Lead II*. That means it is *not* a retrograde P′ wave. There also *appears* to be a small q wave following it; let's take a closer look (Figure 24-4)…

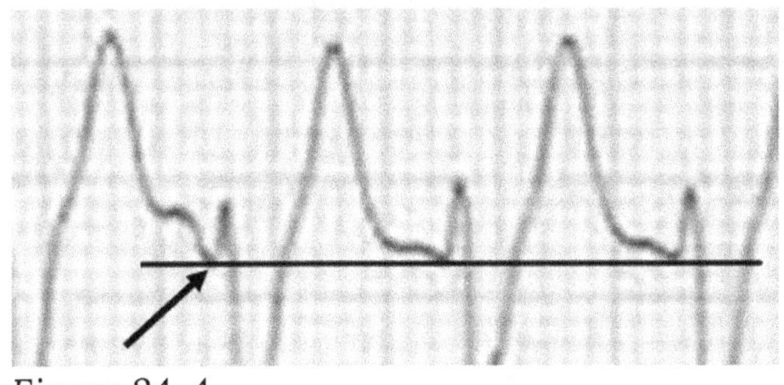

Figure 24-4

The nadir of the suspected "q" wave aligns quite well with the baseline (and onset of all the other r waves). Because there is no negative voltage (any area below the baseline), it cannot be a q wave. This has to be an upright P wave and most likely a *sinus* P wave. The only other upright deflection that could be there would be a U wave, and sizable U waves do NOT appear intermittently in Lead II *during rapid heart rates*. This is a P wave. Now, are there any others?

Yes… there are three more P waves. Now you know how and where to search for sinus P waves and retrograde P′ waves.

AV and VA Dissociation: Which Is Better Proof of Ventricular Tachycardia?

You've seen this rhythm strip (Figure 24-5) before as part of a 12-lead ECG. Using your knowledge about comparing the banks, see if you can discover the finding that is *even more indicative of ventricular tachycardia than AV dissociation.* I've outlined the first bank.

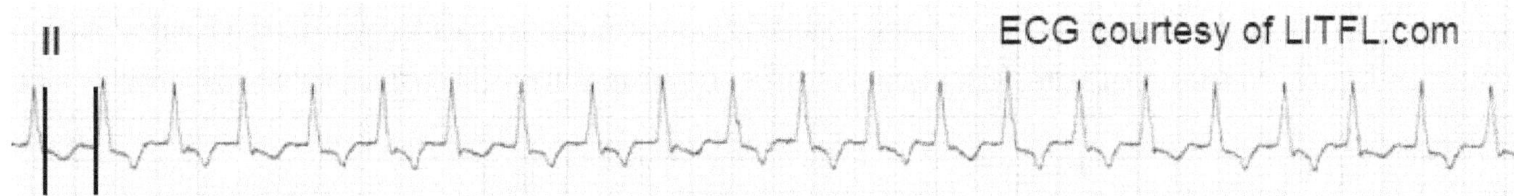

Figure 24-5

You should have noticed that some banks have deeply inverted T waves while others have rather shallow, inverted T waves. There is a pattern here – look very closely. Begin with the very first QRS complex and the first "bank." The T wave is shallow. Now look at the second bank – the T wave is deeply inverted. Now look at the third bank – the T wave is deeply inverted. Now look at the fourth bank – there is just another shallow inversion of the T wave.

Out of three banks, two have deeply inverted T waves. What is the only deflection that can intermittently distort a T wave? A P wave – or more precisely, a P′ wave. "How about U waves during hypokalemia?" you ask. U waves don't appear, then disappear, then reappear again, etc. Only P or P′ waves can do that. What we have here is a 3:2 *ventriculoatrial* (VA) block! The second and third banks manifest retrograde inverted P′ waves occurring around the nadir of the T waves. But the first and fourth banks show no signs of inverted P' waves. Those are the P' waves that were blocked from entering the atria. This is, most likely, a 3:2 Mobitz I VA block. Measuring the R-P' intervals under magnification reveals a subtle lengthening of the second R-P' interval. Now, why is a VA conduction block absolute *proof* of ventricular tachycardia while AV dissociation (though an *excellent* suggestion of VT) is not?

In the case of supraventricular rhythms with wide QRS complexes and retrograde P' waves – which SVT would constitute the only problem in differentiating ventricular tachycardia with retrograde conduction to the atria? It would have to be an SVT that enters the ventricles *and* then exits the ventricles – *antidromic AVRT.*

How does a VA block (Mobitz I or Mobitz II) distinguish between ventricular tachycardia and an antidromic AVRT? Look back at the rhythm strip of this ventricular tachycardia (Figure 24-5): what do you see? You see regular, monomorphic ventricular depolarizations that *continue without stopping or even pausing.* It is a ventricular tachycardia.

Now, what would you see if this were an antidromic AVRT? You would see a *maximum* of two ventricular depolarizations and then the tachycardia would self-terminate. The AVRT would continue until the AV or VA block occurred. VA block = retrograde AV block.

Whether you are going in or out of the room, you are still going through the same door.

The same concept applies to both AV and VA blocks. How do we terminate AVRTs – whether they are orthodromic or antidromic? By blocking the AV node! When we block an orthodromic AVRT we are blocking AV *conduction.* When we block an antidromic AVRT, we are blocking VA *conduction.* But it's still the same AV node! Study this rhythm strip thoroughly. This may not be the last time you see something like this. Let's look at another one...

OK... you are confronted with a wide complex tachycardia (the QRS duration here is 120 msec). I am telling you that this is ventricular tachycardia because I don't have the full 12-lead ECG. Specifically, this is a rather slow *posterior fascicular tachycardia,* which explains the relatively narrow QRS complexes. I don't know why it is so slow, but apparently some part of the tachycardia circuit is causing a delay. I don't have any information about the patient. It could be a medication effect. Remember: you should always diagnose a dysrhythmia from a 12-lead ECG – never just a rhythm strip!

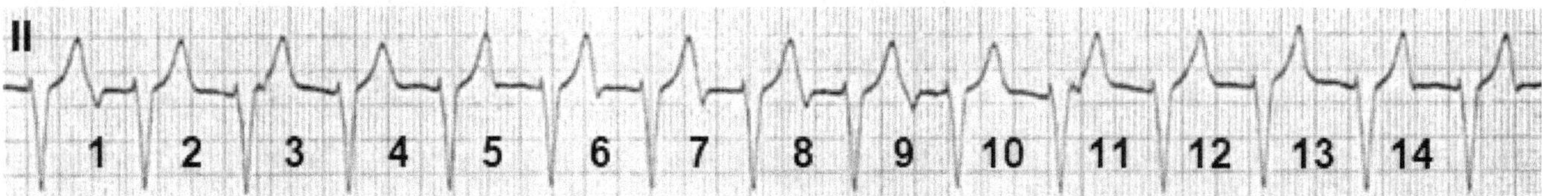

Figure 24-6

(Figure 24-6) To properly approach this dysrhythmia, you should *first know exactly what you are looking for*: you are looking for *retrograde P′ waves* to establish a diagnosis of either AV dissociation or VA dissociation. It is important to note that this is Lead II; if there are any retrograde P′ waves present, they will be *inverted*. Retrograde P′ waves are *always inverted* in Leads II, III, and aVF – the inferior leads. They will be upright (usually) in the *superior* leads – Leads aVR and aVL. Because the vector for retrograde P′ waves travels upward and somewhat perpendicular to Lead I, they are usually very difficult to see in that lead or they are simply not present at all. Retrograde P′ waves are always upright in Lead V1.

> **TIP |** It is not enough to simply find P waves or P′ waves during a wide complex tachycardia. You must know what *type* of P waves you are looking for, *where* you expect to find them, and *how to interpret them* based on their relationship to the QRS complexes.

Now let's find a QRS and its bank (Figure 24-6) that we can use as a "normal" point of reference. There are several: #2, #4 and #10 are good examples. We'll use bank #2. Study it closely. Next, you should carefully compare all the banks – *the area from the J point of one QRS complex to the onset of the next QRS complex*. We see a definite difference between the first and second banks. There is an *inverted deflection* immediately following the first T wave. Could that be a retrograde P′ wave? Yes, it could!

An Eye Exercise

Next, do you see anything in banks 2-5? If not, look more closely! Compare bank #2 with bank #3. Do you see any difference? There appears to be a very small notch in the ST segment of bank #3 at the *base of the ascending limb* of the T wave. Don't assume that it is an artifact. It looks like a very small *negative* deflection. And that's exactly what we are looking for – small, negative deflections. But it isn't present in bank #2 and disappears from banks 4 and 5. Then it appears again in bank #6 – but now it is located at the *base of the descending limb* of the T wave! What is going on here? Follow along with me now very carefully: **I'm about to greatly increase your skill at recognizing AV and VA dissociation!**

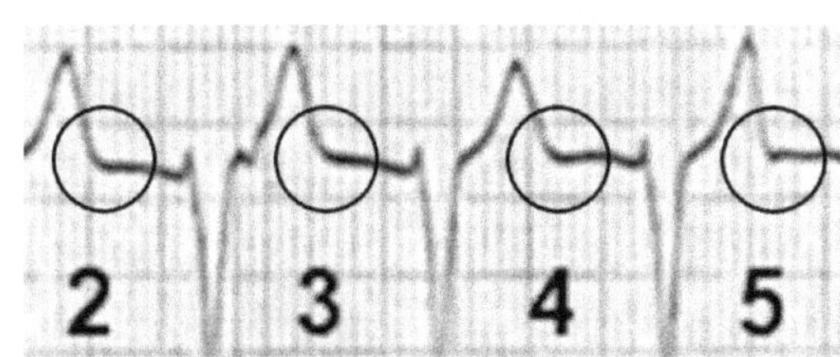

Figure 24-7

We are going to compare banks 2 – 4 with bank #5. But we are going to be even *more specific* because we are focusing on a very localized area. For this, I will enlarge those banks (Figure 24-7):

We are going to focus on the *end of the T wave where it rejoins the baseline*. If you look at banks 2-4, you will see a smooth, gradual curve from the T wave to the baseline. But when you look at bank #5, you will see an abrupt, sharp angle between the end of the T wave and the baseline. Keep studying those banks until you can easily see the difference. It's a very, very subtle difference, but that's why I call this an "Eye Exercise."

Why is the termination of the T wave in bank #5 different from the others? It's because the smooth, gradual termination of the T wave has fused with a more abrupt inverted deflection, creating a sharper angle. And what do you suppose that inverted deflection might be? It's a retrograde P′ wave, of course. But where was it during bank #4? I will answer that by asking you another question: where was it in bank #3 and now where is it in bank #5? In bank #3 it was in *front* of the T wave and in bank #5 it is immediately *following* the T wave. The most plausible answer is that the retrograde P′ wave was hidden within the T wave of bank #4 as it was traveling through it.

What effect does a negative P′ wave (a *negative* voltage area) have on an upright T wave (a *positive* voltage area)? The negative voltage of the retrograde P′ wave will subtract voltage from the positive T wave which should result in a slightly smaller area contained within the T wave; in other words, a slightly smaller T wave. Look at the T wave height in bank #4 and compare it with the T waves on both sides. In bank #5, as the retrograde P′ wave moves out of the T wave, the T wave regains its height (or amplitude). This "subtraction" of negative voltage from positive voltage occurs within the ECG machine during its calculations. It is not something that occurs within the heart itself. Now let's look at the strip once again (Figure 24-8):

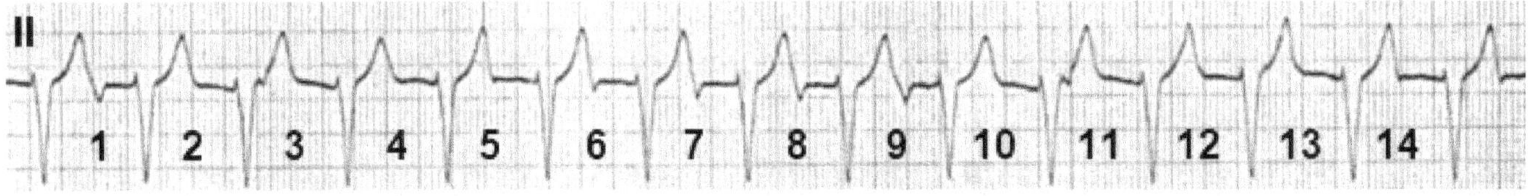

Figure 24-8

What you are seeing is a Mobitz I VA block. Begin with bank #2. There is no evidence of a retrograde P′ wave anywhere in this bank, so this is likely the beat in which the VA impulse was blocked. We are assured that is the case because there is a deep retrograde P′ wave *after* the T wave in the preceding beat. In bank #3, we see a retrograde P′ wave just *before* the onset of the T wave, we see nothing in bank #4 because the retrograde P′ wave is moving through the T wave at this point, in bank #5 the retrograde P′ wave is just beginning to make its appearance after the T wave. In banks #6-#9 the retrograde P′ wave becomes larger and more pronounced as it moves further away from the end of the T wave. Then, the ventricular impulse blocks and fails to appear in bank #10. Following the block, the process starts over again, etc.

PEARL | A typical Mobitz I **AV** block presents with **PR** intervals that get wider and wider until a P *wave fails to conduct.* A typical Mobitz I **VA** block presents with **RP'** intervals that get wider and wider until a P' *fails to appear.*

If these findings seemed difficult to you it's only because you didn't know exactly what you were looking for. And even if you did, you probably didn't realize how closely and carefully you had to assess even the most minute changes. If you are still having difficulty seeing the difference between banks #4 and #5, keep studying them. It will sharpen your skill at recognizing AV and VA dissociation. Even those ECGs that *don't* manifest any dissociation will still help sharpen your eyes and your skill because those ECGs will force you to look as closely and carefully as possible as you try to locate P waves or retrograde P' waves. As a point of reference, it took me about three seconds to detect the difference between the fourth and fifth banks. When you know exactly **WHAT *you are looking for*** and **WHERE *you should be looking*** – the process becomes a lot easier and faster! That takes *practice* and *experience*.

TIP | Although only about 20% of wide complex tachycardias will manifest AV or VA dissociation, just assume that either (or both) are present and try your best to find them. Even when you don't, you will greatly sharpen your eyes and your skills.

PEARL | There are two endpoints from all this that you should strive to achieve. The first, of course, is the ability to recognize the subtle signs of AV or VA dissociation. The second endpoint is that when you *fail* to find any evidence of AV or VA dissociation – you will be both *satisfied* and *confident* that it simply isn't there!

Here is another sign of AV dissociation – a FUSION BEAT!

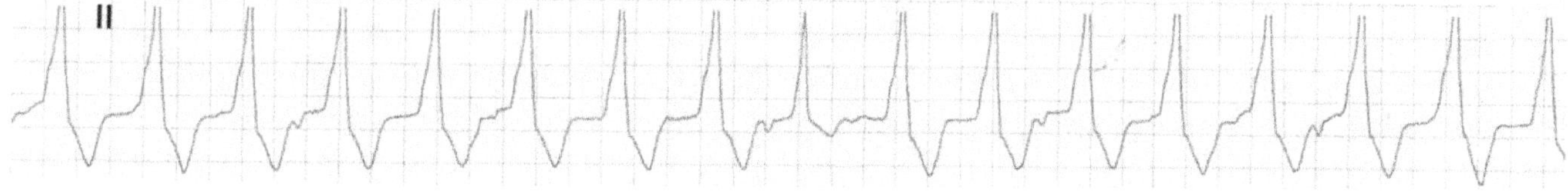

Figure 24-9

(Figure 24-9) The ninth beat is a *fusion beat.* Unfortunately, we don't have a strip of sinus rhythm for perspective, but we know this is a fusion beat because it appears right on time and the QRS appears more normal (i.e., narrower).

PEARL | Do the R-R intervals before and after the fusion beat appear different to you? Does the interval following the fusion beat appear slightly wider than the R-R interval preceding the fusion beat? If it does, then you are viewing the R-R intervals incorrectly! Always measure the intervals between deflections – *any deflections* – from *onset to onset at the baseline!* What you are seeing here is the reason we do that. The R-R interval preceding the fusion beat and the R-R interval following the fusion beat are equal. The decreased width of the fusion QRS makes the R-R interval with the following beat appear wider.

A capture beat would appear early, *before the next expected ectopic beat.* It is preceded by a deflection that is either an upright sinus P wave or an inverted retrograde P′ wave. This is Lead II, so it could be either one.

PEARL | When we look for **AV dissociation** in the inferior leads (II, III, and aVF), we are looking for *upright sinus P waves.* When we look for **VA dissociation** in the inferior leads, we are looking for *inverted retrograde P′ waves.* Don't confuse the fact that retrograde P′ waves are always inverted in the inferior leads with the search for dissociated P waves. The presence of either dissociated upright P waves or dissociated inverted retrograde P′ waves is indicative of an ectopic ventricular rhythm. But remember: inverted retrograde P′ waves that follow *every* QRS complex consistently *at the same RP′ interval* do *not* represent AV or VA dissociation nor should they suggest ventricular tachycardia. I know it *looks* like it should, but trust me – *it doesn't!*

Let's think about this for a moment. What are our options here regarding the rhythm strip in Figure 24-9?

1. A fusion beat caused by a sinus P wave that managed to get through the AV node and activate at least some of the ventricular myocardium, or

2. a retrograde P′ wave that resulted in a reciprocal (echo) beat that returned to the ventricles via the His-Purkinje system and excited part of the ventricular myocardium, fusing with a ventricular ectopic depolarization (yes, that actually happens!).

It all depends on whether the P wave in question is upright or inverted. Let's see how we can find out by taking a closer look...

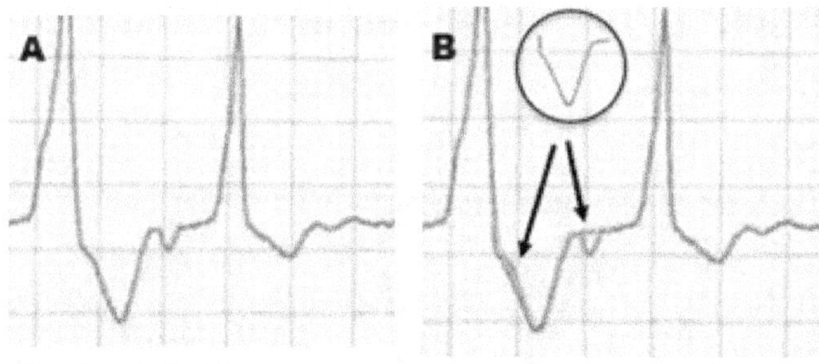

Figure 24-10

(Figure 24-10) I copied a bank (T wave and some baseline) from a preceding repolarization abnormality (circle) and then superimposed it on the bank with the P or P′ wave in question. By doing so, we can see clearly that this deflection is an inverted, retrograde P′ wave.

Not all retrograde P′ waves simply disappear after reaching the atria. (Figure 24-11) After traveling up the fast pathway (Figure 24-11A), the ectopic impulse continued to the slow pathway where it descended to the His bundle (the common final pathway) and reentered the ventricular conduction system. Because this returning impulse is using the His-Purkinje system for conduction, the QRS is much more normal appearing. Whether the reciprocal (echo) beat appears immediately after the QRS complex or further away depends on which pathway in the AV node it used as an ascending pathway.

In this case, it is apparent that since the distance from the onset of the preceding QRS to the P′ wave is greater than the distance from the P′ wave to the fusion beat, the slow pathway transmitted the impulse upward to the atria and the fast pathway was used to return downward to the ventricles and fuse with the next ventricular ectopic beat (Figure 24-11B). Thus, a *reciprocal (echo)* QRS is just the first beat of an AVNRT that immediately self-terminated.

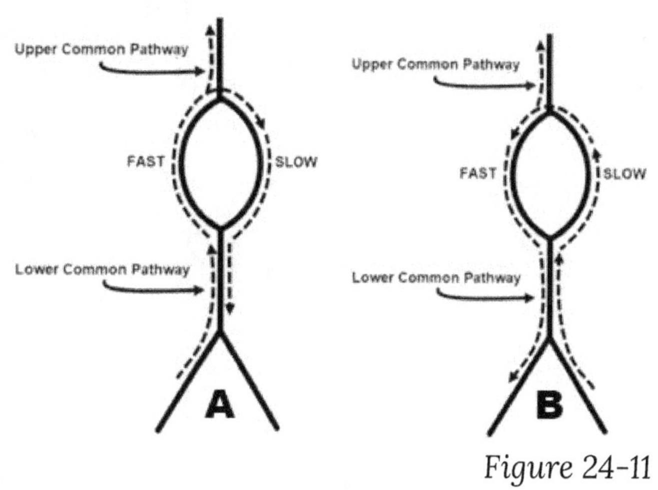

Figure 24-11

There's a lot of information there, but let's not lose our perspective: there is a fusion beat present and that alone *very* strongly suggests that the wide complex tachycardia is ventricular in origin.

I told you about checking the "banks" for evidence of AV or VA dissociation. Now I want to introduce you to the concept of QRS *shoulders*, another area *within the banks* to focus your search for P waves and P′ waves. The shoulders are bits of baseline just preceding the QRS or immediately following the QRS. The shoulders give very important hints that *something other than ventricular depolarization* is happening.

PEARL | When using ECG calipers to check for slight irregularities in a rapid rhythm (such as verifying atrial fibrillation), set the calipers to four or five R-R intervals instead of trying to measure one R-R interval at a time. Any irregularity will become very apparent.

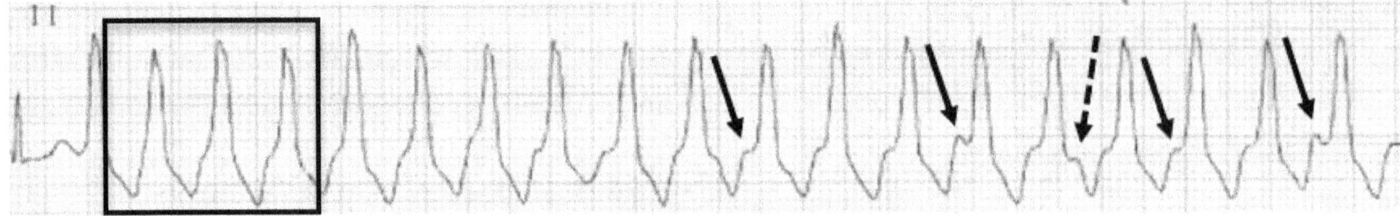

Figure 24-12

In this snippet (Figure 24-12), the black square contains three QRS complexes *without* shoulders. The solid arrows indicate shoulders before the onset of the QRS and the dashed arrow indicates a shoulder following the QRS. These are excellent locations to look for P or P′ waves – as you can already see!

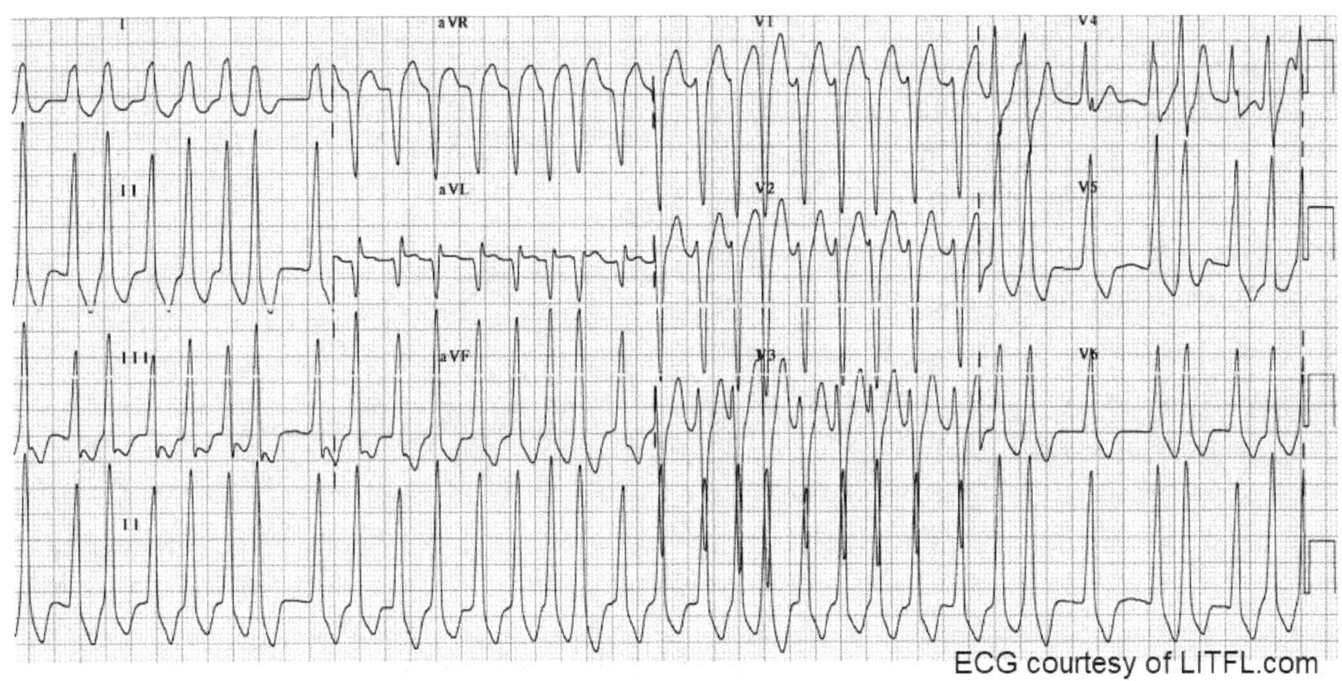

Figure 24-13

Note the shoulders of varying widths in this ECG (Figure 24-13) manifesting atrial fibrillation entering the ventricles through an accessory pathway (WPW).

Chapter 25

Let's Put Your New Skills to the Test!

For each of the following examples of wide complex tachycardias, I want you to see how quickly and accurately you can assess each tachydysrhythmia. Assume the patient is *hemodynamically stable* and *alert*. You should be able to complete your assessment of these six points of information in 30 seconds or less! I want you to do or answer the following:

1. Note the *ventricle* in which the tachycardia originated – *right* or *left*

2. Note the area of the ventricle in which the ectopic focus is located – *outflow tract* or *apex*

3. Is the ectopic focus located *on or near the septum* or did it originate in the *lateral free wall* of the ventricle?

4. Is the tachycardia likely to be a right or left ventricular outflow tract tachycardia?

5. Is the tachycardia likely to be a fascicular tachycardia?

6. Is the patient in any imminent danger?

These questions are placed above each ECG as a memory aid. My assessments for each ECG are on the opposing (left) page.

If you cannot accomplish this in 30 seconds or less – keep practicing these *same* ECGs over and over until you can! *Then* get on the internet and practice with different ECGs.

To paraphrase Thomas A. Edison: "Most people wouldn't recognize success if it were standing right in front of them. That's because it's usually dressed in overalls and disguised as work!"

1. QRS in Lead V1 is primarily negative – RIGHT VENTRICLE!

2. Superior axis in inferior leads; S waves point to the APEX as the origin of the impulse.

3. QRS complexes are relatively wide and the precordial transition is AFTER Lead V6, so likely RIGHT LATERAL WALL.

4. NO! This ectopic focus is in the RIGHT APEX.

5. NO! It's wide and it's located in the right ventricle.

6. YES! This is *not* an outflow tract tachycardia, so the patient is in DANGER. A patient with an outflow tract or fascicular tachycardia who is alert and has a normal blood pressure will likely do just fine as long as you give them food and water. A patient with ventricular tachycardia that is not an outflow tract or fascicular tachycardia may do just fine *for a while* – but they could suffer a cardiovascular collapse at any moment!

An Advanced Thought

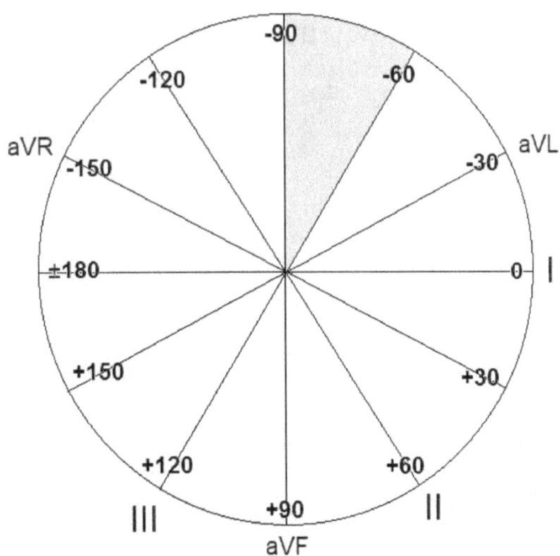

Hexaxial Reference Grid

All the inferior leads have QS complexes, strongly suggesting an epicardial site of origin (SoO), Leads I, aVR and aVL are all upright, meaning that the ectopic impulse is traveling toward ALL of them! How can that be? Lead aVR is on the opposite side of the heart from Leads I and aVL. Look at the Hexaxial Reference Grid:

There is a narrow "window" in which an impulse with a superior axis (i.e., originating in the apical region) can result in positive QRS complexes in Leads I, aVR, and aVL at the same time – between -60° and -90°. If less than -60°, Lead aVR will be negative; if greater than -90°, Lead I will be negative.

1. Note the *ventricle* in which the tachycardia originated – *right* or *left*

2. Note the area of the ventricle in which the ectopic focus is located – *outflow tract* or *apex*

3. Is the ectopic focus located *on or near the septum* or did it originate in the *lateral free wall* of the ventricle?

4. Is the tachycardia likely to be a right or left ventricular outflow tract tachycardia?

5. Is the tachycardia likely to be a fascicular tachycardia?

6. Is the patient in any imminent danger?

ECG 1

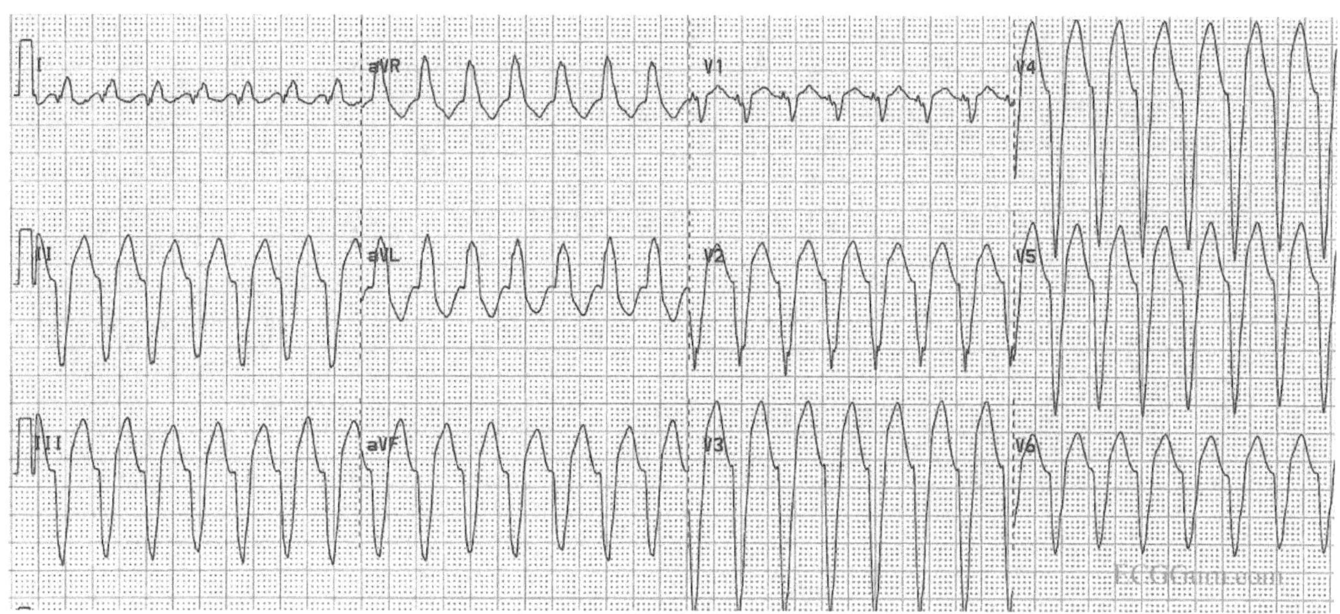

Figure 25-1

1. RIGHT ventricle.

2. APEX

3. The QRS complexes are very wide suggesting an origin in a lateral or free wall, perhaps even in the epicardium (which produces some of the widest QRS complexes). The precordial transition is AFTER Lead V6 (Lead V2 looks out of place), which is compatible with a far-right origin of the impulse, so the ectopic focus is likely in the RIGHT LATERAL APICAL wall.

4. NO!

5. NO!

6. YES!

1. Note the *ventricle* in which the tachycardia originated – *right* or *left*

2. Note the area of the ventricle in which the ectopic focus is located – *outflow tract* or *apex*

3. Is the ectopic focus located *on or near the septum* or did it originate in the *lateral free wall* of the ventricle?

4. Is the tachycardia likely to be a right or left ventricular outflow tract tachycardia?

5. Is the tachycardia likely to be a fascicular tachycardia?

6. Is the patient in any imminent danger?

ECG 2

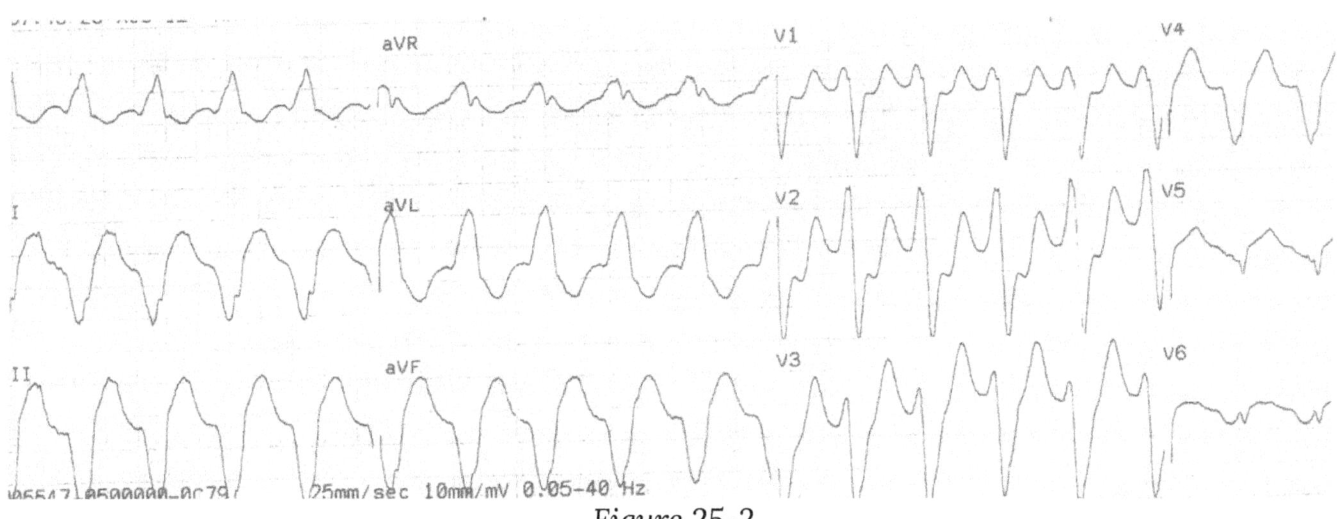

Figure 25-2

1. LEFT ventricle.

2. APEX

3. The QRS complexes are well-formed and relatively narrow, so the ectopic focus is likely on the septum or in or near a Purkinje fiber.

4. NO! An origin in the left ventricular outflow tract (LVOT) would present all tall R waves in the inferior leads.

5. YES! It fits the electrocardiographic signature of a *posterior fascicular tachycardia,* and the QRS is relatively narrow and well-formed (R wave peak time is just 40 msec) indicating an origin in or very near the conducting system of the left ventricle.

6. NO!

1. Note the *ventricle* in which the tachycardia originated – *right* or *left*

2. Note the area of the ventricle in which the ectopic focus is located – *outflow tract* or *apex*

3. Is the ectopic focus located *on or near the septum* or did it originate in the *lateral free wall* of the ventricle?

4. Is the tachycardia likely to be a right or left ventricular outflow tract tachycardia?

5. Is the tachycardia likely to be a fascicular tachycardia?

6. Is the patient in any imminent danger?

ECG 3

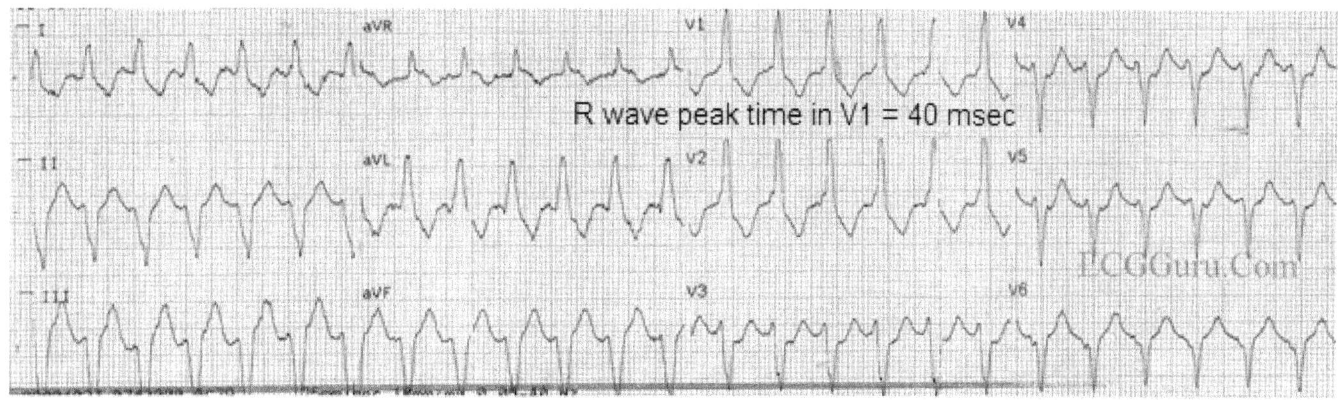

Figure 25-3

1. RIGHT ventricle

2. APEX

3. The QRS is relatively wide and notched, so it is likely not in the septum but rather in the free wall (anterolateral).

4. NO! The QRS complexes in the inferior leads are pointing downward toward the apex.

5. NO! The QRS complexes are wide and notched in some leads, which is very *unlike* fascicular tachycardia.

6. YES! This is not a benign ventricular tachycardia. The patient is stable now, but that could change at any moment. Follow the ACLS protocol.

1. Note the *ventricle* in which the tachycardia originated – *right* or *left*

2. Note the area of the ventricle in which the ectopic focus is located – *outflow tract* or *apex*

3. Is the ectopic focus located *on or near the septum* or did it originate in the *lateral free wall* of the ventricle?

4. Is the tachycardia likely to be a right or left ventricular outflow tract tachycardia?

5. Is the tachycardia likely to be a fascicular tachycardia?

6. Is the patient in any imminent danger?

ECG 4

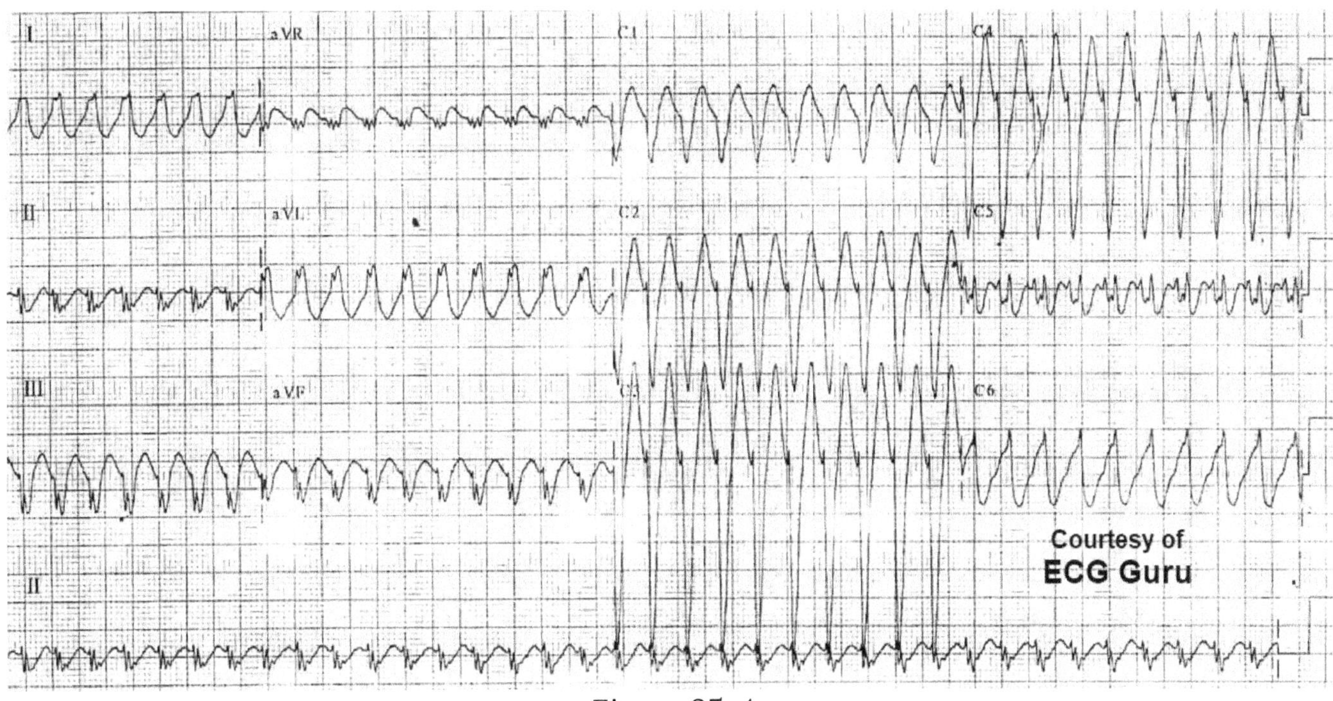

Figure 25-4

1. LEFT ventricle

2. APEX

3. You can see initial slurring on most of the upright QRS complexes. This is *not* WPW; it is likely a sign that the ectopic focus is on the left lateral wall – probably in or very near the *epicardium*. The precordial transition is BEFORE Lead V1, so this focus is *far* to the left laterally (which you should understand by now means *posteriorly*). Note that the QRS changes from a *monophasic* R to a *monophasic* QS between Leads V3 and V4. That is NOT the precordial transition. During the precordial transition, the QRS changes from predominantly NEGATIVE to predominantly POSITIVE – not the reverse! The QRS complexes in Leads I, aVR, and aVL are all positive, so this is a very vertical superior axis that must be located between -60° and -90°.

4. It's coming from the apex (probably the apicolateral area), so it is not an outflow tract tachycardia.

5. NO!

6. YES!

1. Note the *ventricle* in which the tachycardia originated – *right* or *left*

2. Note the area of the ventricle in which the ectopic focus is located – *outflow tract* or *apex*

3. Is the ectopic focus located *on or near the septum* or did it originate in the *lateral free wall* of the ventricle?

4. Is the tachycardia likely to be a right or left ventricular outflow tract tachycardia?

5. Is the tachycardia likely to be a fascicular tachycardia?

6. Is the patient in any imminent danger?

ECG 5

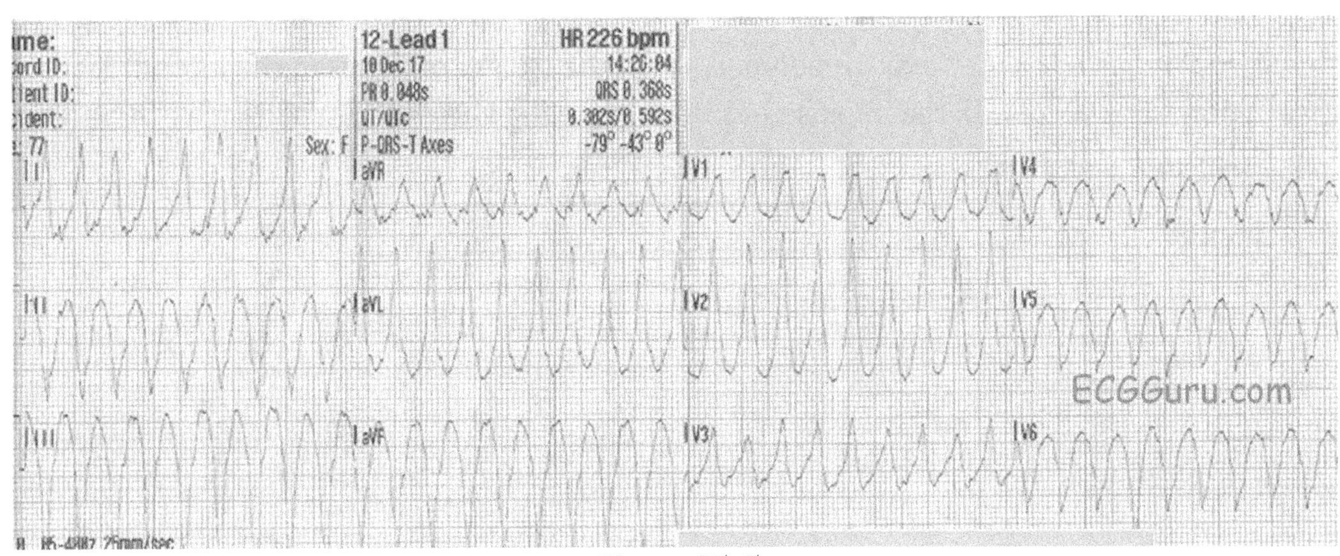

Figure 25-5

1. LEFT ventricle

2. APEX? Not really! In this case – as you will see – we are seeing a fascicular tachycardia. This is a reentrant tachycardia that spends most of its time in the His-Purkinje conduction system. While it is true that the QRS morphology of ectopic tachydysrhythmias that begin in working myocardium reflect the site of origin and not a true block, tachycardias that begin in conducting tissue also do not reflect a block but rather the *order of activation* of the different ventricular areas. That is why there is an exception to my oft-mentioned adage "Nothing good comes out of the apex." This tachycardia is not coming "out of the apex." It's just giving that impression due to the order of activation of the left-sided fascicles.

3. The QRS complexes are relatively narrow and well-formed. The R peak time in Lead V1 is less than 80 msec. This ectopic focus is located in or very near a Purkinje fiber (likely the posterior fascicle).

4. NO! It has a *superior axis* (remember: when the QRS complexes in the inferior leads point DOWNWARD, the impulse has to be traveling UPWARD, making it a SUPERIOR axis.

5. YES!

6. NO!

1. Note the *ventricle* in which the tachycardia originated – *right* or *left*

2. Note the area of the ventricle in which the ectopic focus is located – *outflow tract* or *apex*

3. Is the ectopic focus located *on or near the septum* or did it originate in the *lateral free wall* of the ventricle?

4. Is the tachycardia likely to be a right or left ventricular outflow tract tachycardia?

5. Is the tachycardia likely to be a fascicular tachycardia?

6. Is the patient in any imminent danger?

ECG 6

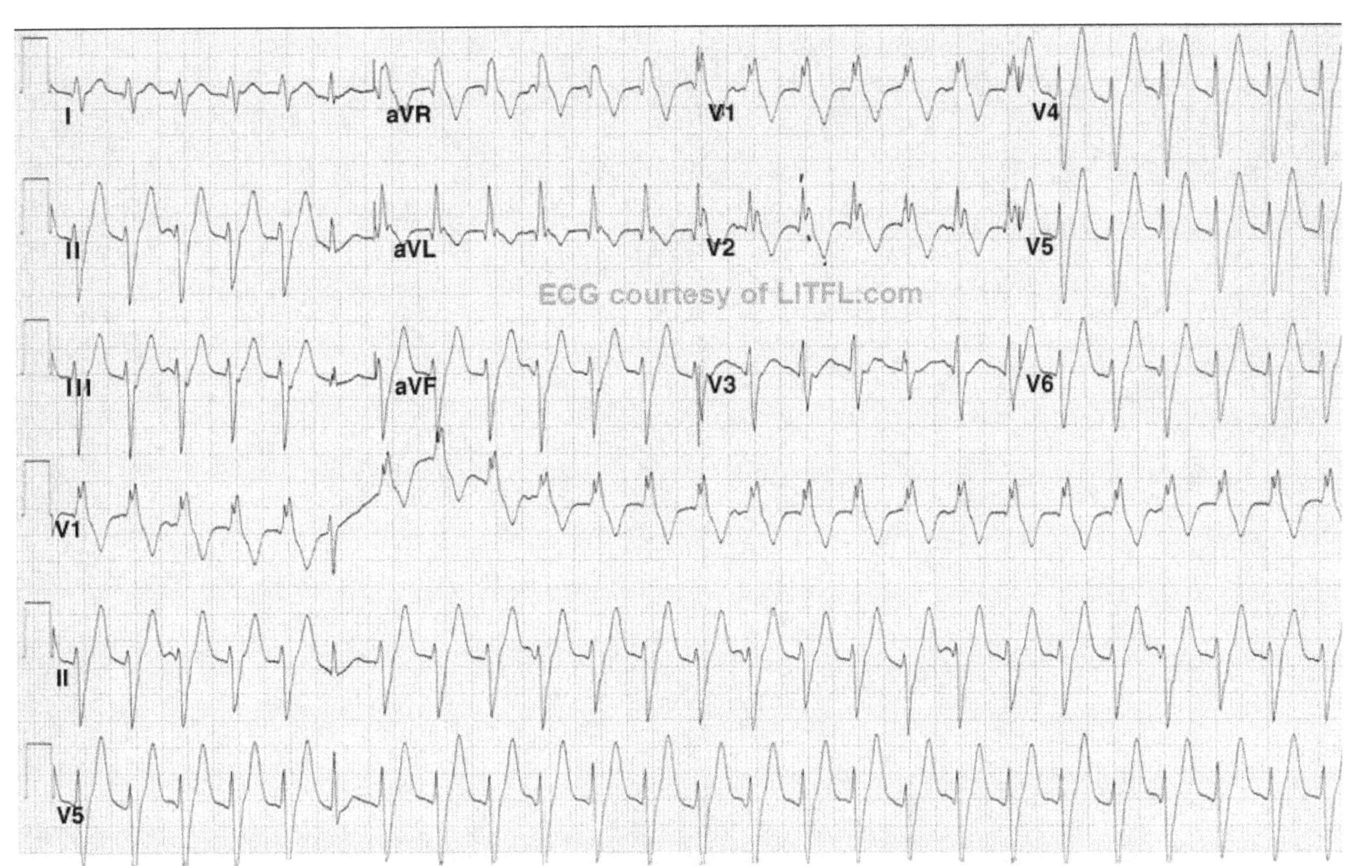

Figure 25-6

1. LEFT ventricle

2. Although Lead II appears to have a somewhat equiphasic QRS, Lead III is positive and Lead aVL is negative, so it appears that this ECG has an inferior axis (an inferior axis always implies a *rightward* axis). That means the origin of the ectopic focus is likely in the outflow tract of the left ventricle.

3. The QRS complexes are very narrow so this ectopic focus is either located in or very near the anterior fascicle – a very rare situation.

4. It is possible but not likely. The thin QRS complexes are more typical of a fascicular tachycardia – in this case, an anterior fascicular tachycardia.

5. YES!

6. NO!

1. Note the *ventricle* in which the tachycardia originated – *right* or *left*

2. Note the area of the ventricle in which the ectopic focus is located – *outflow tract* or *apex*

3. Is the ectopic focus located *on or near the septum* or did it originate in the *lateral free wall* of the ventricle?

4. Is the tachycardia likely to be a right or left ventricular outflow tract tachycardia?

5. Is the tachycardia likely to be a fascicular tachycardia?

6. Is the patient in any imminent danger?

ECG 7

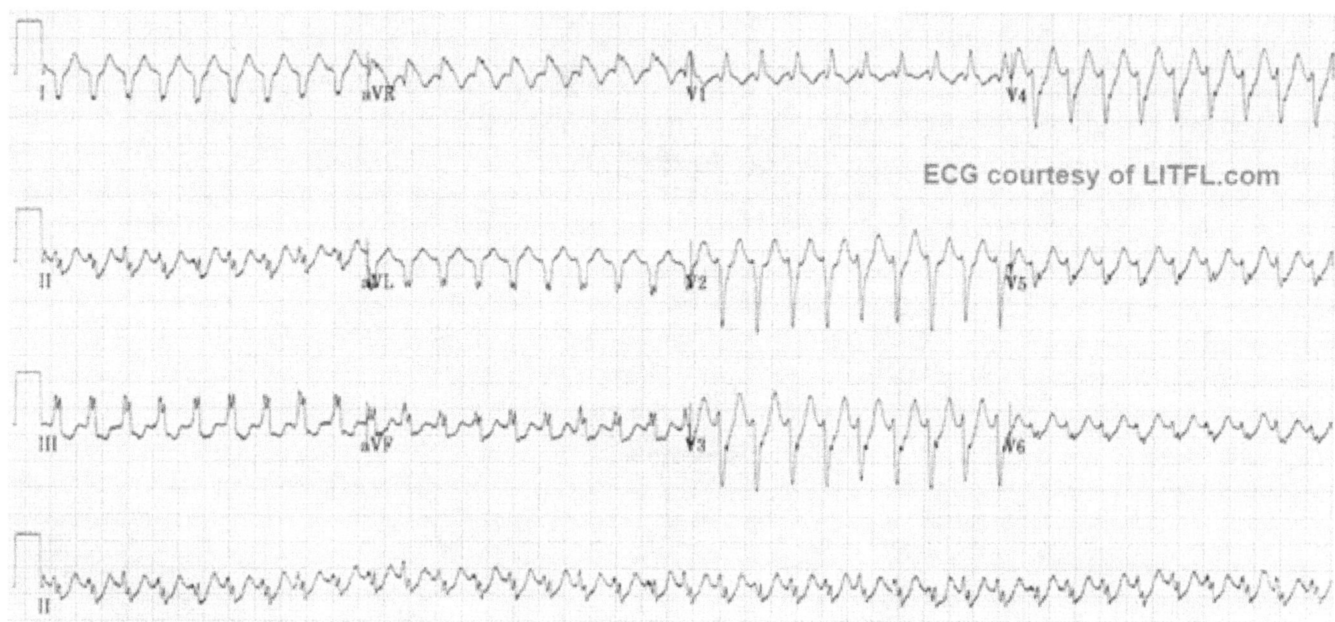

Figure 25-7

1. LEFT ventricle

2. APEX

3. QRS complexes are wide with precordial transition BEFORE Lead V1 indicating an origin in the far left of the left ventricle. Looking at Leads V3 – V6 may give you the impression of narrow QRS complexes – but don't forget about the S waves which give those deflections greater width (actually, *duration* since we are measuring on the horizontal axis).

4. NO!

5. NO!

6. YES!

1. Note the *ventricle* in which the tachycardia originated – *right* or *left*

2. Note the area of the ventricle in which the ectopic focus is located – *outflow tract* or *apex*

3. Is the ectopic focus located *on or near the septum* or did it originate in the *lateral free wall* of the ventricle?

4. Is the tachycardia likely to be a right or left ventricular outflow tract tachycardia?

5. Is the tachycardia likely to be a fascicular tachycardia?

6. Is the patient in any imminent danger?

ECG 8

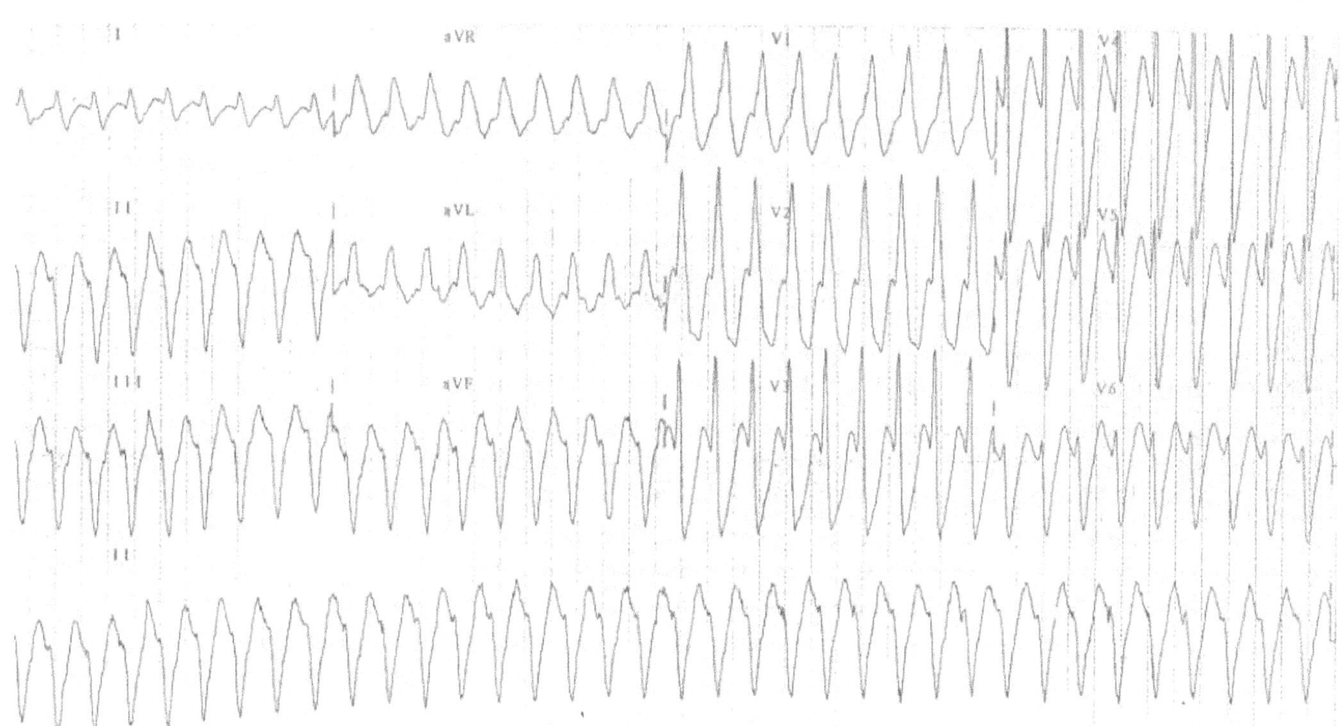

Figure 25-8

1. RIGHT ventricle

2. OUTFLOW TRACT

3. QRS complexes are a bit wide – likely from the endocardial surface of the right ventricular septum since the transition is at Lead V4, which appears equiphasic (R=S). (Review the section on "Precordial Transition" in Chapter 1.)

4. YES!

5. NO!

6. NO!

1. Note the *ventricle* in which the tachycardia originated – *right* or *left*

2. Note the area of the ventricle in which the ectopic focus is located – *outflow tract* or *apex*

3. Is the ectopic focus located *on or near the septum* or did it originate in the *lateral free wall* of the ventricle?

4. Is the tachycardia likely to be a right or left ventricular outflow tract tachycardia?

5. Is the tachycardia likely to be a fascicular tachycardia?

6. Is the patient in any imminent danger?

ECG 9

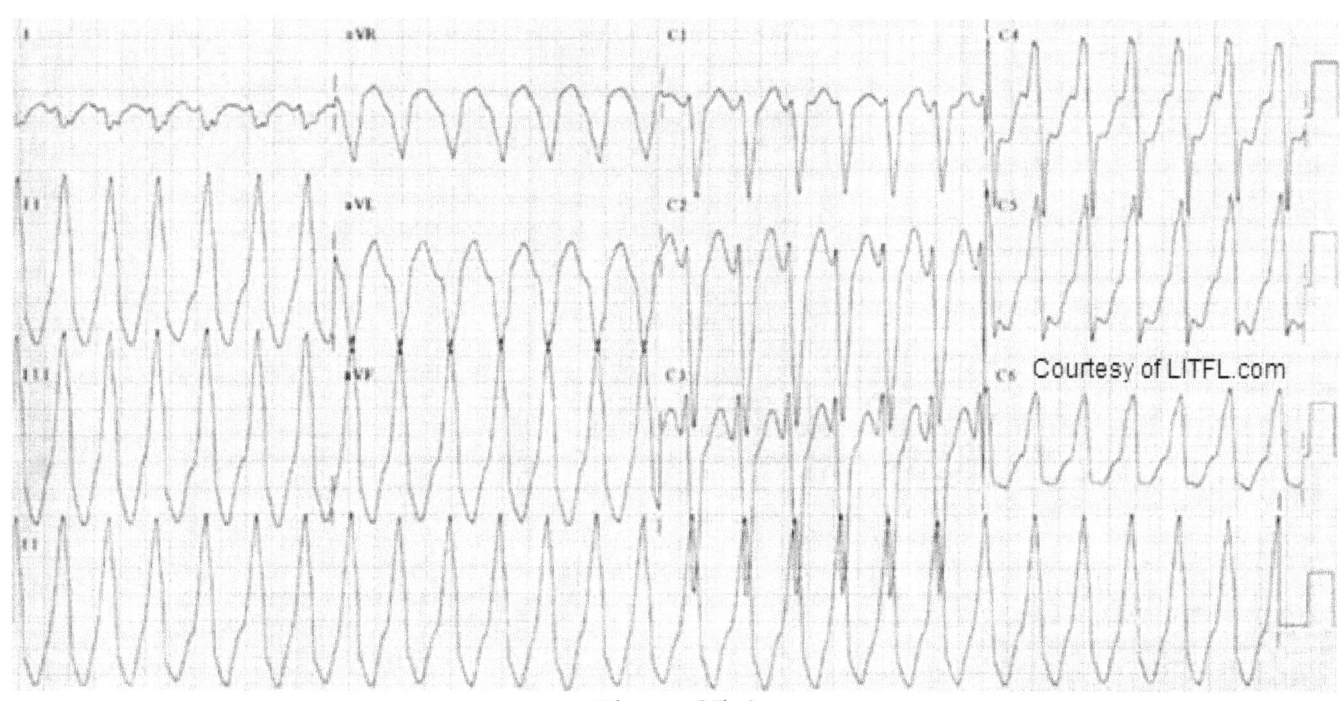

Figure 25-9

1. LEFT ventricle

2. APEX

3. The positive forces in Leads V1 – V4 indicate the ectopic impulse is traveling from posterior to anterior. The origin of this tachycardia is likely in the apicolateral wall of the left ventricle. The precordial transition has already occurred by Lead V1, so the origin of the impulse is far to the left. The mean QRS axis is also in the right upper quadrant of the HRG ("No Man's Land"). This is *not* a benign tachycardia!

4. NO!

5. NO!

6. YES!

1. Note the *ventricle* in which the tachycardia originated – *right* or *left*

2. Note the area of the ventricle in which the ectopic focus is located – *outflow tract* or *apex*

3. Is the ectopic focus located *on or near the septum* or did it originate in the *lateral free wall* of the ventricle?

4. Is the tachycardia likely to be a right or left ventricular outflow tract tachycardia?

5. Is the tachycardia likely to be a fascicular tachycardia?

6. Is the patient in any imminent danger?

ECG 10

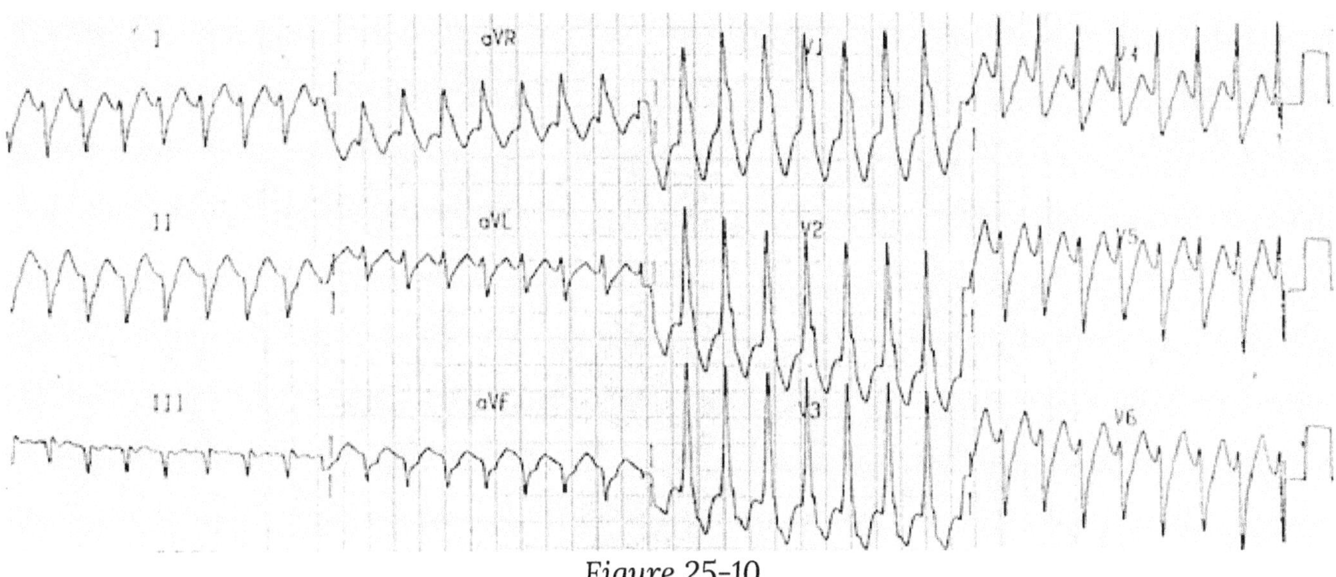

Figure 25-10

Glossary of Terms

Including Abbreviations

I understand that for many of you reading this book, English is a second (or third) language. For that reason, I have included a few "colloquialisms" often used when discussing ECGs.

AKA – also known as

ARVC/D – arrhythmogenic right ventricular cardiomyopathy/dysplasia (AKA arrhythmo-genic cardiomyopathy), sometimes seen as ARVD/C

Axis – the depiction of a vector indicating its direction; a division of a circular grid

Bank – the part of an ECG from the J point to the onset of the following QRS complex. I use the word "bank" to avoid having to write out all those words!

Benign – in the context of a dysrhythmia, neither threatening, debilitating nor dangerous

Blip – a "blip" is a small disruption of the ECG tracing. It can involve the baseline or just one small area of a deflection – *any* deflection. It is very small and the question is always whether it represents some electrocardiographic event or just a small artifact. The term is always used in a very general, non-diagnostic sense.

Bystander pathway – an accessory pathway being used only as a pathway between the atria and the ventricles and not as part of a reentrant circuit

Cherry-picked – carefully selected, selected according to specific criteria, *not* randomly selected, usually implies a selection made specifically to improve an outcome

cLBBB – *complete* left bundle branch block

cRBBB – *complete* right bundle branch block

Delta wave – initial slurring of the onset of depolarization deflection (R or S wave) due to an accessory pathway activating working myocardium before its activation by the His-Purkinje system

Gain-of-function mutation – mutation that increases the activity of an ion channel causing an increase in its usual direction of ion transport

HPS – His-Purkinje system

Incessant – sustained VT present for long lengths of time often requiring intervention, tachycardia may be present more than sinus rhythm

Intrinsicoid deflection – see "R wave peak time"

Isorhythmic – two independent pacemakers firing at exactly the same rate or exact multiples of each other by coincidence; in real life, they are *very rarely exactly the same* and usually lose their synchronization after a short time

Isorhythmic ratio – a coincidental ratio of atrial rate versus ventricular rate, such as an atrial rate of 75/minute and a ventricular rate of 150/minute. The two rhythms may appear related, but in actuality, they are two distinct and independent rhythms.

LAF – left anterior fascicle

LBBB – left bundle branch block

Loss-of-function mutation – mutation that reduces the activity of an ion channel causing a reduction in its usual direction of ion transport

LPF – left posterior fascicle

LVOT – left ventricular outflow tract

Malignant – in the context of a dysrhythmia, dangerous and very possibly lethal; It does not refer to any neoplasms.

Monomorphic – all QRS complexes within a given lead having the same morphology

Monophasic – a completely positive deflection (upright) or completely negative (inverted)

Morphology – shape, appearance

Nadir – the lowest point of a negative (inverted) deflection (*nadir* of S wave vs. *peak* of R wave)

Non-sustained – lasting less than 30 seconds

PAC – premature atrial complex (sometimes seen as APC)

Paroxysmal – intermittent, spontaneous sudden onset and sudden termination

Pathognomonic – describes a finding that occurs in a particular disease or condition and no other, so that its presence is diagnostic of the condition

PJC – premature junctional complex (sometimes seen as JPC)

Pleomorphic – multiple QRS morphologies are present but each type persists for a while before changing to another morphology; they do not change from beat to beat

Polymorphic – a deflection with different morphologies or polarities within a given lead that changes from beat to beat. Spindle-shaped VTs – such as Torsade de Pointes – are polymorphic, but not all polymorphic VTs are spindle-shaped; bidirectional VTs are considered polymorphic. Sometimes seen as *polymorphous*

Pseudo-delta wave – activation of working myocardium by an ectopic ventricular focus before entering the His-Purkinje system. This differs from a delta wave in that the pseudo-delta wave is produced by just one impulse while a true delta wave is a fusion of two separate impulses.

PVC – premature ventricular complex (sometimes seen as VPC)

Repetitive – a tachycardia occurring frequently, usually in short, self-terminating episodes

R wave peak time – formerly known as the intrinsicoid deflection, this interval is measured from the onset of the QRS (whether Q wave or R wave) to the peak of the R wave (if upright) or the nadir of the S wave (if negative)

RBBB – right bundle branch block

RVOT – right ventricular outflow tract

Shoulder – the bit of baseline immediately preceding a QRS complex and/or immediately following a QRS complex

Snippet – a brief portion of an ECG, often just part of one lead

SoO – site of origin

Spindle-shaped – similar to a horizontal oval

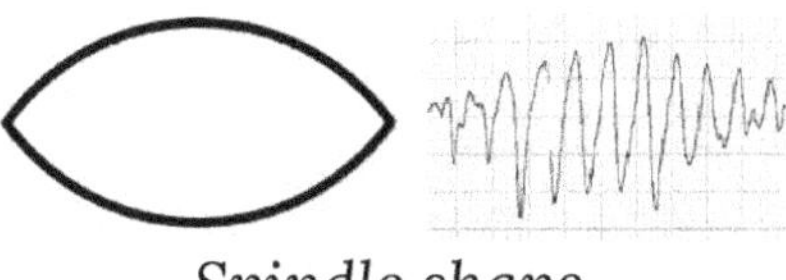

Spindle shape

Straight forward – does not refer to direction or location; a colloquialism meaning "obvious," "very clear;" it can also mean "very direct" and "without circumvention or equivocation"

Sustained – lasting 30 seconds or more or requiring immediate intervention

SVT – supraventricular tachycardia, a general "catch-all" term, not a specific diagnosis

Term of art – a word or expression with a specific meaning relative to a particular discipline, such as law or medicine, which is different from its meaning or connotation in general conversation (e.g., in general conversation, *aberrant* means "different" or "not typical" but in medicine it refers *specifically* to "the activation of one bundle branch before the other due to the residual refractoriness of one of the bundle branches").

VT – ventricular tachycardia

WPW – Wolfe-Parkinson-White

Recommended Reading

1. Abedin Z, MD. Differential diagnosis of wide QRS tachycardia: A review. *Journal of Arrhythmia.* 2021;37:1162–1172.

2. Akhtar M, Shenasa M, Jazayeri M, Caceres J, Tchou PJ. Wide QRS complex tachycardia. Reappraisal of a common clinical problem. *Ann Intern Med.* 1988;109:905–912.

3. Almuzghi F, Kashbour M, Almalti A (November 17, 2022) A Case Report of Fascicular Ventricular Tachycardia in a COVID-19 Patient. *Cureus.* 14(11): e31618. DOI 10.7759/cureus.31618

4. Alzand BS, Crijns HJ. Diagnostic criteria of broad QRS complex tachycardia: decades of evolution. *Europace.* 2011;13:465–472.

5. Anderson RD, MBBS, et al. Differentiating Right- and Left-Sided Outflow Tract Ventricular Arrhythmias – Classical ECG Signatures and Prediction Algorithms. Circ Arrhythm Electrophysiol. June 2019.

6. Antunes E, Brugada J, Steurer G, Andries E, Brugada P. The Differential Diagnosis of a Regular Tachycardia with a Wide QRS Complex on the 12-Lead ECG: Ventricular Tachycardia, Supraventricular Tachycardia with Aberrant Intraventricular Conduction, and Supraventricular Tachycardia with Anterograde Conduction Over an Accessory Pathway. PACE. Vol. 17 September 1994; 1515-1523.

7. Antzelevitch C, PhD, Burashnikov A, PhD. Overview of Basic Mechanisms of Cardiac Arrhythmia. *Card Electrophysiol Clin.* 2011 March 1; 3(1): 23–45.

8. Asirvatham MD, SJ, and Stevenson MD, WG. *Circulation: Arrhythmia and Electrophysiology.* Volume 6, Issue 61, December 2013.

9. Baher AA, MD, et al. Bidirectional Ventricular Tachycardia: Ping Pong in the His-Purkinje System. *Heart Rhythm.* 2011 April; 8(4): 599–605.

10. Baltazar RF, MD, Javillo JS, MD. Ventriculo-Atrial Wenckebach during Wide Complex Tachycardia. *Clin. Cardiol.* 29, 513 (2006).

11. Benito B, and Josephson ME. Ventricular Tachycardia in Coronary Artery Disease. *Rev Esp Cardiol.* 2012;65(10):939–955.

12. Berruezo A, MD, et al. Electrocardiographic Recognition of the Epicardial Origin of Ventricular Tachycardias. *Circulation.* 2004;109:1842-1847.

13. Bhar-Amato J, Davies W, Agarwal S. Ventricular Arrhythmia after Acute Myocardial Infarction: 'The Perfect Storm'. *Arrhythmia & Electrophysiology Review.* 2017;6(3):134–9.

14. Blanck Z, MD, Dhala A, MD, Deshpande S, MD. Sra J, MD, Jazayeri M, MD, Akhtar M. MD. Bundle Branch Reentrant Ventricular Tachycardia: Cumulative Experience in 48 Patients. *Journal of Cardiovascular Electrophysiology.* June, Vol. 4, No. 3; 253-262.

15. Bogaard K, van der Steen MS, Tan HL, Tukkie R. Short-coupled variant of torsade de pointes. *Neth Heart J.* 2008;16:246-9.

16. Brachmann J, MD, Scherlag BJ, PhD, Rosenshtraukh LV, PhD, Lazzara R, M.D. Brady-cardia-dependent triggered activity: relevance to drug-induced multiform ventricular tachycardia. *Circulation.* 68, No. 4, 846-856, 1983; pp. 846-856.

17. Brown DFM, MD, Nadel ES, MD. Wide Complex Tachycardia. *The Journal of Emergency Medicine.* Vol. 21, No. 3, pp. 271–274, 2001.

18. Brugada P, Brugada J, Mont L, Smeets J, Andries EW. A new approach to the differential diagnosis of a regular tachycardia with a wide QRS complex. *Circulation.* 1991;83:1649–1659.

19. Brugada P, MD. Ockham's Razor and Bayes Theorem at Work. JACC : Clinical Electrophysiology. Vol . 8 , No . 7 , 2022 ; 840-842.

20. Bush KNV, MD, Gerasimon GG, MD. Slow, But Dangerous. *Texas Heart Institute Journal.* April 2018, Vol. 45, No. 2.

21. Buxton AE, MD, et al. Prognostic Factors in Nonsustained Ventricular Tachycardia. *Am J Cardiol.* 1984;53:1275-1279.

22. Buxton AE, et al. Right ventricular tachycardia: clinical and electrophysiologic characteristics. *Circulation.* 1983;68:917-927.

23. Callans DJ, MD, et al. Repetitive Monomorphic Tachycardia From the Left Ventricular Outflow Tract: Electrocardiographic Patterns Consistent With a Left Ventricular Site of Origin. JACC. Vol. 29, No. 5 April 1997:1023±7.

24. Chen Q, Xu J, Gianni C, et al. Simple electrocardiographic criteria for rapid identification of wide QRS complex tachycardia: the new limb lead algorithm. *Heart Rhythm.* 2020;17:431–438.

25. Childers R, MD. Torsades: adjacent and triggering electrocardiographic events. *Journal of Electrocardiology.* 43 (2010) 515 – 523.

26. Chiladakis JA, et al. Short-Coupled Variant of Torsade de Pointes as a Cause of Electrical Storm and Aborted Sudden Cardiac Death: Insights into Mechanism and Treatment. *Hellenic J Cardiol.* 2008; 49: 360-364.

27. Cohen SI, MD, Lau SH, MD, Stein E, MD, Young MW, MD, Damato AN, MD. Variations of Aberrant Ventricular Conduction in Man: Evidence of Isolated and Combined Block Within the Specialized Conduction System. *Circulation.* Volume 38, November, 1968; pp. 899-916.

28. Conti GS, MD et al. Right Ventricular Outflow Tract Arrhythmias: Benign Or Early Stage Arrhythmogenic Right Ventricular Cardiomyopathy/Dysplasia? *Journal of Atrial Fibrillation.* Volume 7: Issue 4; Dec 2014-Jan 2015.

29. Corrado D, MD, Link MS, MD, Calkins H, MD. Arrhythmogenic Right Ventricular Cardiomyopathy. *N Engl J Med.* 2017;376:61-72.

30. Corrado D, Basso C, Thiene G. Arrhythmogenic right ventricular cardiomyopathy: diagnosis, prognosis, and treatment. *Heart.* 2000;83:588±595.

31. Corrado D, MD, et al. Right Bundle Branch Block, Right Precordial ST-Segment Elevation, and Sudden Death in Young People. *Circulation.* 2001;103:710-717.

32. Corrado D, MD et al. Spectrum of Clinicopathologic Manifestations of Arrhythmogenic Right Ventricular Cardiomyopathy/Dysplasia: A Multicenter Study. JACC. Vol. 30, No. 6 November 15, 1997:1512±20.

33. De Ferrari GM, MD et al. Clinical Management of Catecholaminergic Polymorphic Ventricular Tachycardia – The Role of Left Cardiac Sympathetic Denervation. *Circulation.* 2015;131:2185-2193.

34. Dendi R, Josephson ME. A new algorithm in the differential diagnosis of wide complex tachycardia – Editorial. *European Heart Journal.* (2007) 28, 525–526.

35. El-Sherif N, MD, Turitto G, MD, Boutjdir M, PhD. Congenital Long QT syndrome and torsade de pointes. *Ann Noninvasive Electrocardiol.* 2017;22:e12481.

36. Elswick BD, MD, Niemann JT, MD. Fascicular Ventricular Tachycardia: An Uncommon but Distinctive Form of Ventricular Tachycardia. *Annals Of Emergency Medicine*. 31(3); March 1998.

37. Ermakov S, Scheinman M. Arrhythmogenic Right Ventricular Cardiomyopathy – Antiarrhythmic Therapy. *Arrhythmia & Electrophysiology Review*. 2015;4(2):86–9.

38. Evans GL, Charles MA, Thornsvard CT. Ventricular tachycardia with retrograde conduction – Simplified diagnostic approach. *British Heart Journal*. 1974, 36, 512-515.

39. Farré J, MD, Wellens HJJ, MD. Unique ECG During Sinus Rhythm in a Patient With a Postmyocardial Infarction–Sustained Ventricular Tachycardia. *Circulation*. 2018;137:527–530.

40. Fitzpatrick JK, MD; Goldschlager N, MD. ECG of the Month. *Ann Emerg Med*. 2018;71:473-476.

41. Francis J, MD, Venugopal K, MD, Sudhayakumar N, Khadar SA, MD, Anoop K. Gupta AK MD FACC. Idiopathic Fascicular Ventricular Tachycardia. *Indian Pacing and Electrophysiology Journal*. 4(3): 98-103 (2004).

42. Gard JJ, MD, Asirvatham SJ, MD. Outflow Tract Ventricular Tachycardia. *Texas Heart Institute Journal*. Volume 39, Number 4, 2012; 526-528.

43. Garmel GM, MD. Wide complex tachycardias: Understanding this complex condition Part 1 – epidemiology and electrophysiology. *WestJEM*. 2008;9:28-39.

44. Garmel GM, MD. Wide complex tachycardias: Understanding this complex condition Part 2 - Management, Miscellaneous Causes, and Pitfalls. *WestJEM*. 2008;9:97-103.

45. Garner JB, Miller JM. Wide complex tachycardia—ventricular tachycardia or not ventricular tachycardia, that remains the question. *Arrhythm Electrophysiol Rev*. 2013;2:23–29.

46. Garratt CJ, et al. Value of physical signs in the diagnosis of ventricular tachycardia. *Circulation*. 1994;90:3103-3107

47. Griffith MJ, Garratt CJ, Mounsey P, Camm AJ. Ventricular tachycardia as default diagnosis in broad complex tachycardia. *Lancet*. Feb 12, 1994;343(8894):386-8.

48. Guo H, Hecker S, Levy S, Olshansky B. Ventricular tachycardia with QRS configuration similar to that in sinus rhythm and a myocardial origin: differential diagnosis with bundle branch reentry. *Europace*. (2001) 3, 115–123.

49. Gupta A, et al. Hyperkalemia Presenting as Wide-Complex Tachycardia in a Dialysis Patient. *Saudi J Kidney Dis Transpl.* 2010;21(2):339-341.

50. Gupta AK, MD, Thakur RK, MD. Wide QRS Complex Tachycardias. *Medical Clinics of North America.* Volume 85, Number 2 March 2001; 245-266.

51. Haqqani HM, MBBS, Marchlinski FE, MD. The Surface Electrocardiograph in Ventricular Arrhythmias: Lessons in Localisation. *Heart, Lung and Circulation.* (2019) 28, 39–48.

52. Hoffmayer KS, et al. An electrocardiographic scoring system for distinguishing right ventricular outflow tract arrhythmias in patients with arrhythmogenic right ventricular cardiomyopathy from idiopathic ventricular tachycardia. *Heart Rhythm.* 2013 Apr;10(4):477-82.

53. Hoffmayer KS, et al. Electrocardiographic Comparison of Ventricular Arrhythmias in Patients With Arrhythmogenic Right Ventricular Cardiomyopathy and Right Ventricular Outflow Tract Tachycardia. JACC. Vol. 58, No. 8, 2011:831– 8.

54. de Holanda-Miranda WR, MD, Furtado FM, MD, Luciano PM, MD, Pazin-Filho A, MD. Lewis Lead Enhances Atrial Activity Detection In Wide QRS Tachycardia. *The Journal of Emergency Medicine.* Article in Press, 2009. doi:10.1016/j.jemermed.2009.08.057.

55. Ilkhanipour K, MD, Berrol R, MD, Yealy DM, MD. Therapeutic and Diagnostic Efficacy of Adenosine in Wide-Complex Tachycardia. *Annals Of Emergency Medicine.* 22:8 August 1993; 152-156.

56. Jastrzebski M, Kukla P, Czarnecka D, and Kawecka-Jaszcz K. Comparison of five electrocardiographic methods for differentiation of wide QRS-complex tachycardias. *Europace.* (2012) 14, 1165–1171 doi:10.1093/europace/eus015.

57. Jastrzębski M,Moskal P, Kukla P, Fijorek K, Kisiel R, Czarnecka D. Specificity of wide QRS complex tachycardia criteria and algorithms in patients with ventricular preexcitation. *Ann Noninvasive Electrocardiol.* 2018;23:e12493.

58. Kallergis E, Goudis C, Simantirakis E, Kochiadakis G, Vardas P. Mechanisms, Risk Factors, and Management of Acquired Long QT Syndrome: A Comprehensive Review. *The Scientific World Journal.* Volume 2012; 1-8.

59. Kannankeril PJ, MD, et al. Efficacy of Flecainide in the Treatment of Catecholaminergic Polymorphic Ventricular Tachycardia – A Randomized Clinical Trial. JAMA *Cardiology.* July 2017; Volume 2, Number 7; 759-766.

60. Kapa S, MD; Gaba P, BS; DeSimone CV, MD PhD, Asirvatham SJ, MD. Fascicular Ventricular Arrhythmias – Pathophysiologic Mechanisms, Anatomical Constructs, and Advances in Approaches to Management. *Circ Arrhythm Electrophysiol.* 2017; 1-14.

61. Kashou AH, Evenson CM, Noseworthy PA et al., Differentiating wide complex tachycardias: A historical perspective. *Indian Heart Journal.* https://doi.org/10.1016/j.ihj.2020.09.006.

62. Kashou AH, MD, et al. Wide Complex Tachycardia Differentiation: A Reappraisal of the State-of-the-Art. *J Am Heart Assoc.* 2020;9:e016598. DOI: 10.1161/JAHA.120.016598.

63. Kindwall KE, MD, Brown J, RN, Josephson ME, MD. Electrocardiographic Criteria for Ventricular Tachycardia in Wide Complex Left Bundle Branch Block Morphology Tachycardias. *Am J Cardiol.* 1988;61:1279-1283.

64. Katritsis DG, and Brugada J. Differential Diagnosis of Wide QRS Tachycardias. *Arrhythmia & Electrophysiology Review.* 2020;9(3):155–60.

65. Kirchhof P, MD, Franz MR, MD, Bardai A, MD, Wilde AM, MD. Giant T–U Waves Precede Torsades de Pointes in Long QT Syndrome – A Systematic Electrocardiographic Analysis in Patients With Acquired and Congenital QT Prolongation. JACC. Vol. 54, No. 2, 2009; 143-149.

66. Kumagai K, MD. Idiopathic ventricular arrhythmias arising from the left ventricular outflow tract: Tips and tricks. *Journal of Arrhythmia.* 30 (2014) 211–221.

67. Kusa S, MD et al. Bundle Branch Reentrant Ventricular Tachycardia With Wide and Narrow QRS Morphology. *Circ Arrhythm Electrophysiol.* 2013;6:e87-e91.

68. Lam P, MD, Saba S, MD. Approach to the Evaluation and Management of Wide Complex Tachycardias. *Indian Pacing and Electrophysiology Journal.* 2(4): 120-126 (2002).

69. Langendorf R, Pick A, Winternitz M. Mechanisms of Intermittent Ventricular Bigeminy : I. Appearance of Ectopic Beats Dependent Upon Length of the Ventricular Cycle, the "Rule of Bigeminy". *Circulation.* 1955;11:422-430.

70. Latif S, MD, Dixit S, MD, Callans DJ, MD. Ventricular Arrhythmias in Normal Hearts. *Cardiol Clin.* 26 (2008) 367–380.

71. Leandro HIC, Lebedev DS, Mikhaylov EN. Discrimination of ventricular tachycardia and localization of its exit site using surface electrocardiography. *J Geriatr Cardiol.* 16: 362-377; 2019.

72. Leenhardt A, MD, Denjoy I, MD, Guicheney G, PhD. Catecholaminergic Polymorphic Ventricular Tachycardia. *Circ Arrhythm Electrophysiol.* 2012;5:1044-1052.

73. Lerman BB, MD. Ventricular Tachycardia – Mechanistic Insights Derived From Adenosine. *Circ Arrhythm Electrophysiol.* 2015;8:483-491.

74. Lo R, MD, Hsia HH, MD. Ventricular Arrhythmias in Heart Failure Patients. *Cardiol Clin.* 26 (2008) 381–403.

75. Long B, MD and Koyfman A, MD. Best Clinical Practice: Emergency Medicine Management of Stable Monomorphic Ventricular Tachycardia. *The Journal of Emergency Medicine.* Vol. 52, No. 4, pp. 484–492, 2017.

76. Marcus FI, MD. Arrhythmogenic Cardiomyopathy Diagnostic Criteria: An Update. *Card Electrophysiol Clin.* 3 (2011) 217–226.

77. Marcus FI, MD. Right Ventricular Dysplasia: A Report of 24 Adult Cases. *Circulation 65,* No. 2, 1982.

78. Marriott HJL, MD. Differential Diagnosis of Supraventricular and Ventricular Tachycardia. *Cardiology.* 1990;77:209-220.

79. Marriott HJL, MD, Rogers HM, MD. Mimics of Ventricular Tachycardia Associated with the W-P-W Syndrome. *J Electrocardiology.* 2 (1), 77-84, 1969.

80. Marriott HJL, Schwartz NL, Bix HH. Ventricular Fusion Beats. *Circulation.* 1962;26:880-884.

81. Mazur, A, MD, Kusniec J, MD, Strasberg B, MD. Bundle Branch Reentrant Tachycardia. *Indian Pacing and Electrophysiology Journal.* 5(2); 86-95; (2005).

82. McCauley M, MD, Vallabhajosyula S, MD, Darbar D, MD. Proarrhythmic and Torsadogenic Effects of Potassium Channel Blockers in Patients. *Card Electrophysiol Clin.* Author manuscript; June 1, 2017.

83. Michowitz et al. Differentiating the QRS Morphology of Posterior Fascicular Ventricular Tachycardia From Right Bundle Branch Block and Left Anterior Hemiblock Aberrancy. *Circ Arrhythm Electrophysiol.* 2017; 1-11.

84. Moccetti F, Yadava M, Latifi Y, et al. Simplified integrated clinical and electrocardiographic algorithm for differentiation of wide QRS-complex tachycardia: the Basel algorithm. *J Am Coll Cardiol EP.* 2022;8(7):831–839.

85. Morita N, MD, Karagueuzian HS, PhD. Cardiac fibrosis as a determinant of ventricular tachyarrhythmias. *Journal of Arrhythmia.* 30 (2014) 389–394.

86. Moss, JD MD, Scheinman MM MD. Differentiating the QRS Morphology of Posterior Fascicular Ventricular Tachycardia From Right Bundle Branch Block and Left Anterior Hemiblock Aberrancy – Why the Difference (Editorial). *Circ Arrhythm Electrophysiol.* 2017; 1-3.

87. Murphy MA, MD, Ferguson JD, CHB MB. The Athlete With Catecholaminergic Polymorphic Ventricular Tachycardia. https://www.acc.org/latest-in-cardiology/articles/2 017/07/27/07

88. Nam G-B, MD, Burashnikov A, PhD, Antzelevitch C, PhD. Cellular Mechanisms Underlying the Development of Catecholaminergic Ventricular Tachycardia. *Circulation.* 2005;111:2727-2733.

89. Napolitano C, Priori SG, Bloise R. Catecholaminergic Polymorphic Ventricular Tachycardia. *GeneReviews®* 2004 Oct 14 [Updated 2016 Oct 13]. In: Adam MP, Ardinger HH, Pagon RA, et al., editors.

90. Neiger JS, Trohman RG. Differential diagnosis of tachycardia with a typical left bundle branch block morphology. *World J Cardiol.* 2011 May 26; 3(5): 127-13.

91. Nishizaki M, MD. Wide QRS complex tachycardia responsive to both ATP and verapamil. *Journal of Arrhythmia.* 28 (2012) 75–77.

92. Novak J, et al. Electrocardiographic differentiation of idiopathic right ventricular outflow tract ectopy from early arrhythmogenic right ventricular cardiomyopathy. *Europace.* (2017) 19, 622–628.

93. Obeyesekere MN, MBBS, Antzelevitch C, PhD, Krahn AD, MD. Management of Ventricular Arrhythmias in Suspected Channelopathies. *Circ Arrhythm Electrophysiol.* 2015;8:221-231.

94. Ohe T, MD, et al. Idiopathic sustained left ventricular tachycardia: clinical and electrophysiologic characteristics. *Circulation.* Vol. 77, No. 3, 560-568, 1988.

95. Ohkubo K, et al. ECG Criteria for Distinguishing Left from Right Ventricular Outflow Tract Tachycardia. *J. Nihon Univ. Med. Ass.* 2015; 74 (3): 95–102.

96. Oksuz F, et al. The classical " R-on-T" phenomenon. *Indian Heart Journal.* 67 (2015) 392e394.

97. Ouyang F, MD, et al. Electroanatomic Substrate of Idiopathic Left Ventricular Tachycardia – Unidirectional Block and Macroreentry Within the Purkinje Network. *Circulation*. 2002;105:462469.

98. Padala SK, et al. Non-sustained wide complex tachycardia: an underappreciated sign to aid in diagnosis. *Europace*. (2016) 18, 1069–1076.

99. Park K-M, MD, Kim Y-H MD, Marchlinski FE, MD. Using the Surface Electrocardiogram to Localize the Origin of Idiopathic Ventricular Tachycardia. *Pace*. Vol.35; December 2012; 1516-1527.

100. Patel RV, et al. Early Repolarization Associated With Ventricular Arrhythmias in Patients With Chronic Coronary Artery Disease. *Circ Arrhythm Electrophysiol*. 2010;3:489-495.

101. Patel VV, MD, PhD, Rho RW, MD, Gerstenfeld EP, MD, Hsia HH, MD, Callans DJ, MD, Marchlinski FE, MD. Right Bundle-Branch Block Ventricular Tachycardias – Septal Versus Lateral Ventricular Origin Based on Activation Time to the Right Ventricular Apex. *Circulation*. 2004;110:2582-2587.

102. Pava LF, Perafan P, Badiel M, et al. R-Wave peak time at DII: a new criterion for differentiating between wide complex QRS tachycardias. *Heart Rhythm*. 2010;7:922–926.

103. Pérez-Riera AR, Barbosa-Barros R, de Rezende Barbosa MPC, Daminello-Raimundo R, de Lucca AA Jr, de Abreu LC. Catecholaminergic polymorphic ventricular tachycardia, an update. *Ann Noninvasive Electrocardiol*. 2018;23:e12512. https://doi.org/10.1111/anec.12512.

104. Perez-Riera AR, MD, et al. Review: R-Peak Time: An Electrocardiographic Parameter with Multiple Clinical Applications. *Ann Noninvasive Electrocardiol*. 2016;21(1):10–19.

105. Pluijmen MJHM, MD, Hersbach FMRJ, MD. Sine-Wave Pattern Arrhythmia and Sudden Paralysis That Result From Severe Hyperkalemia. *Circulation*. 2007;116:e2-e4.

106. Pollack ML, MD, Chan TC, MD, Brady WJ, MD. Electrocardiographic Manifestations: Aberrant Ventricular Conduction. *The Journal of Emergency Medicine*. Vol. 19, No. 4, pp. 363–367, 2000.

107. Prystowsky EN, MD, Padanilam BJ, MD, Joshi S, MD, Fogel RI, MD. Ventricular Arrhythmias in the Absence of Structural Heart Disease. JACC. Vol. 59, No. 20, 2012; 1733-1744.

108. Ramprakash B, Jaishankar S, Hygriv B. Rao, Narasimhan C, Catheter Ablation of Fascic-

ular Ventricular Tachycardia. *Indian Pacing and Electrophysiology Journal.* 8(3): 193-201 (2008).

109. Reviriego SM, Luis Merino JL. Ventricular tachycardia in patients without apparent structural heart disease: Focus on ventricular outflow tract tachycardia. *e-journal of the ESC Council for Cardiology Practice.* Vol. 8, N° 11 - 18 Nov 2009.

110. Riera ARP, et al. Idiopathic intrafascicular reentrant left ventricular tachycardia in an elite cyclist athlete. *Cardiology Journal.* 2009, Vol. 16, No. 4:1-4.

111. Riley MP, MD, Marchlinski FE, MD. ECG Clues for Diagnosing Ventricular Tachycardia Mechanism. *J Cardiovasc Electrophysiol.* Vol. 19, pp. 224-229, February 2008.

112. de Riva M, MD, Watanabe M, MD, Zeppenfeld K, MD. Twelve-Lead ECG of Ventricular Tachycardia in Structural Heart Disease. *Circ Arrhythm Electrophysiol.* 2015;8:951-962.

113. Roberts JD, MD et al. Bundle Branch Re-Entrant Ventricular Tachycardia – Novel Genetic Mechanisms in a Life-Threatening Arrhythmia. JACC: *Clinical Electrophysiology.* Vol. 3, No. 3, 2017; 276-288.

114. Roberts-Thomson KC, Lau DH, Sanders P. The diagnosis and management of ventricular arrhythmias. *Nat. Rev. Cardiol.* advance online publication 22 February 2011; doi:10.1038/nrcardio.2011.15.

115. Rosso, R. et al. Polymorphic ventricular tachycardia, ischaemic ventricular fibrillation, and torsade de pointes: importance of the QT and the coupling interval in the differential diagnosis. *European Heart Journal.* (2021) 42; pp. 3965-3975.

116. Roston TM, MD et al. Catecholaminergic Polymorphic Ventricular Tachycardia in Children – Analysis of Therapeutic Strategies and Outcomes From an International Multicenter Registry. *Circ Arrhythm Electrophysiol.* 2015;8:633-642.

117. Sala MF, MD, et al. Sustained Ventricular Tachycardia as a Marker of Inadequate Myocardial Perfusion during the Acute Phase of Myocardial Infarction. *Clin. Cardiol.* 25, 328–334 (2002).

118. Sandesara CM, MD. Wide Complex Tachycardias: Demystifying the Differential Diagnosis. *EP Lab Digest.* Volume 11 - Issue 1 - February 2011; https://www.printfriendly.com/p/g/cwBXDU.

119. Sandler IA, MD, Marriot HJL, MD. The Differential Morphology of Anomalous Ventricular Complexes of RBBB-Type in Lead V1. *Circulation.* Volume XXXI, April 1965; 551-556.

120. Schiefermueller J. Ventricular Tachycardias in Structurally Normal Hearts - A Case Report and Review of the Literature. *Int J Crit Care Emerg Med.* 4(1); 2018.

121. Shimizu W, MD. Arrhythmias originating from the right ventricular outflow tract: How to distinguish "malignant" from "benign"? *Heart Rhythm.* Vol 6, No 10, pp. 1507-1511; October 2009.

122. Sousa PA, Pereira S, Candeias R, de Jesus I. The value of electrocardiography for differential diagnosis in wide QRS complex tachycardia. *Rev Port Cardiol.* 2014;33(3):165-173.

123. Srivathsan K, MD, et al. Ventricular Tachycardia in the Absence of Structural Heart Disease. *Indian Pacing and Electrophysiology Journal.* 5(2): 106-121 (2005).

124. Steurer G, Gürsoy S, Frey B, Simonis F, Andries E, Kuck K, et al. The differential diagnosis on the electrocardiogram between ventricular tachycardia and pre-excited tachycardia. *Clin Cardiol.* 1994;17:306–8.

125. Subramanian NR, MD, et al. Wide Complex Tachycardia: Diagnosis And Management In The Emergency Department. *Emergency Medicine Practice.* Volume 10, Number 6; June 2008.

126. Sung RK, Boyden PA, Higuchi S, Scheinman M. Diagnosis and Management of Complex Reentrant Arrhythmias Involving the His-Purkinje System. *Arrhythmia & Electrophysiology Review.* 2021;10(3):190–7.

127. Svernhage E, MD, et al. Early Electrocardiographic Signs of Drug-Induced Torsades de Pointes. *A.N.E.* July 1998;3(3):252-260.

128. Szelényi ZDG, Katona G, Fritúz G, et al. Comparison of the "real-life" diagnostic value of two recently published electrocardiogram methods for the differential diagnosis of wide QRS complex tachycardias. *Acad Emerg Med.* 20(11); November 2013; pp. 1121-1130.

129. Thiene G, MD, Bauce B, MD, Corrado D, MD, Basso C, MD. Arrhythmogenic Cardiomyopathy: A [sic] Historical Overview. *Card Electrophysiol Clin.* 3 (2011) 179–191.

130. Tiver KD, Dharmaprani D, Quah JX, Lahiri A, Waddell-Smith KE, Ganesan AN. Vomiting, electrolyte disturbance, and medications; the perfect storm for acquired long QT syndrome and cardiac arrest: case report. *Journal of Medical Case Reports.* 16:9; 2022.

131. Vereckei A, Duray G, Szenasi G, Altemose GT, Miller JM. Application of a new algorithm in the differential diagnosis of wide QRS complex tachycardia. *Eur Heart J.* 2007;28:589–600.

132. Vereckei A. Current algorithms for the diagnosis of wide QRS complex tachycardias. *Curr Cardiol Rev.* 2014 Aug;10(3):262-76.

133. Vereckei A, Duray G, Szenasi G, Altemose GT, Miller JM. New algorithm using only lead aVR for differential diagnosis of wide QRS complex tachycardia. *Heart Rhythm.* 2008;5:89–98.

134. Vereckei A, MD, et al. The Application of a New, Modified Algorithm for the Differentiation of Regular Ventricular and Pre-Excited Tachycardias. *Heart, Lung and Circulation.* (2023) 32, 719–725.

135. Weiss JN, MD et al. Early Afterdepolarizations and Cardiac Arrhythmias. *Heart Rhythm.* 2010 December; 7(12): 1891–1899.

136. Wellens, HJJ, Bär, FW, Lie, KI. The value of the electrocardiogram in the differential diagnosis of a tachycardia with a widened QRS complex. *Am J Med.* 1978;64(1):27–33.

137. Wellens HJJ. Ventricular tachycardia: diagnosis of broad QRS complex tachycardia. *Heart.* 2001;86:579±585.

138. Wichter T, MD, Borggrefe M, MD, Haverkamp W, MD, Chen X, MD, Breithardt G, MD. Efficacy of Antiarrhythmic Drugs in Patients With Arrhythmogenic Right Ventricular Disease Results in Patients With Inducible and Noninducible Ventricular Tachycardia. *Circulation.* Vol 86, No 1 July 1992; pp. 29-37.

139. Wijnmaalen AP. ECG Identification of Scar-Related Ventricular Tachycardia With a Left Bundle-Branch Block Configuration. *Circ Arrhythm Electrophysiol.* 2011;4:486-493.

140. Wilde AAM, Amin AS, Postema PG. Diagnosis, management and therapeutic strategies for congenital long QT syndrome. *Heart.* 2022;108:332–338.

141. Yamada T, MD. Review: Idiopathic ventricular arrhythmias – Relevance to the anatomy, diagnosis and treatment. *Journal of Cardiology.* 68 (2016) 463–471.

142. Yang Z, MD, et al. Azithromycin Causes a Novel Proarrhythmic Syndrome. *Circ Arrhythm Electrophysiol.* 2017;10:e003560.

143. Yap YG, Camm AJ. Drug Induced QT Prolongation and Torsades de Pointes. *Heart.* 2003; 89:1363–1372.

144. Yazdan-Ashoori P, Digby G, Baranchuk A. Failure to Treat Torsades de Pointes. *Cardiol Res.* 2012;3(1):34-36.

145. Ylänen K, Poutanen T, Hiippala A, Swan H, Korppi M. Catecholaminergic polymorphic ventricular tachycardia. *Eur J Pediatr* (2010) 169:535–542.